Neurology

for the Non-Neurologist

SEVENTH EDITION

Steven L. Lewis, MD
Physician in Chief, Lehigh Valley
    Fleming Neuroscience Institute
Farber Institute for Neuroscience
    of Thomas Jefferson University,
    Regional Chief, Lehigh Valley
Timothy M. Breidegam Endowed
    Chair and Chief of Neurology
Lehigh Valley Health Network
Allentown, Pennsylvania

Aaron L. Berkowitz, MD, PhD, FAAN
Professor of Clinical Neurology
Department of Neurology
University of California, San
    Francisco
San Francisco, California

● Wolters Kluwer

Philadelphia • Baltimore • New York • London
Buenos Aires • Hong Kong • Sydney • Tokyo

Acquisitions Editor: Chris Teja, Keith Donnellan
Product Development Editor: Ariel S. Winter
Editorial Coordinator: Thirupura Sundari
Marketing Manager: Kirsten Watrud
Production Project Manager: Matthew West
Design Coordinator: Stephen Druding
Manufacturing Coordinator: Bernard Tomboc
Prepress Vendor: S4Carlisle Publishing Services

Seventh Edition

Library of Congress Cataloging-in-Publication Data

ISBN-13: 978-1-975215-66-8

Cataloging in Publication data available on request from publisher.

shop.lww.com

QUADM1124

Dedication

To Julie, for her continuous support,
and to the lasting memory of my loving parents,
Charles and Phyllis, and my sister Debbie.
Steven L. Lewis

In memory of Dr Martin A. Samuels (1945–2023),
extraordinary neurologist, virtuoso educator, visionary leader, and
generous mentor—a neurology giant on whose shoulders we stand.
Aaron L. Berkowitz

CONTRIBUTORS

Jessica Ailani, MD
Director, Georgetown Headache Center
Department of Neurology
MedStar Georgetown University Hospital
Washington, District of Columbia

Catherine S. W. Albin, MD
Assistant Professor
Department of Neurology and Neurosurgery
Emory University
Atlanta, Georgia

Irena Dujmovic Basuroski, MD
Division Chief, Multiple Sclerosis and Neuroimmunology
Department of Neurology
University of North Carolina at Chapel Hill
Chapel Hill, North Carolina

Aaron L. Berkowitz, MD, PhD, FAAN
Professor of Clinical Neurology
Department of Neurology
University of California, San Francisco
San Francisco, California

Shamik Bhattacharyya, MD, MS, FAAN
Anne Finucane Distinguished Chair in Neurology
Department of Neurology
Brigham and Women's Hospital
Harvard Medical School
Boston, Massachusetts

Joshua A. Budhu, MD, MS, MPH
Assistant Member
Department of Neurology
Memorial Sloan Kettering Cancer Center
Weill Cornell Medical College
New York, New York

Anna Cervantes-Arslanian, MD
Chief, Neurocritical Care and Neuroinfectious Disease
Department of Neurology
Boston Medical Center
Boston University
Boston, Massachusetts

Seemant Chaturvedi, MD
Stewart Greenebaum Endowed Professor of Stroke Neurology
Department of Neurology
University of Maryland School of Medicine
Baltimore, Maryland

Monica M. Diaz, MD, MS
Assistant Professor of Neurology
Department of Neurology
University of North Carolina at Chapel Hill School of Medicine
Chapel Hill, North Carolina

Carrie Dougherty, MD
Associate Professor
Department of Neurology
MedStar Georgetown University Hospital
Washington, District of Columbia

Emily Anne Ferenczi, BM BCh, PhD
Instructor in Neurology
Department of Neurology
Massachusetts General Hospital and Brigham and Women's Hospital
Boston, Massachusetts

Terry D. Fife, MD
Professor of Neurology
Department of Neurology
Barrow Neurological Institute
Phoenix, Arizona

Carrie Katherine Grouse, MD
Associate Professor
Department of Neurology
University of California, San Francisco
San Francisco, California

Amanda C. Guidon, MD, MPH
Assistant Professor of Neurology
Department of Neurology
Massachusetts General Hospital
Harvard Medical School
Boston, Massachusetts

Elan L. Guterman, MD, MAS

Associate Professor of Neurology
Department of Neurology
University of California, San Francisco
San Francisco, California

Kelly Graham Gwathmey, MD

Associate Professor of Neurology
Department of Neurology
Virginia Commonwealth University
Richmond, Virginia

Ethan Hoang, BS, MD

Assistant Professor of Neurology
Department of Neurology
Weill Cornell Medical College
New York, New York

Justin L. Hoskin, MD

Assistant Professor of Neurology
Department of Neurology
Barrow Neurological Institute
Phoenix, Arizona

Lara Jehi, MD, MHCDS

Professor of Neurology
Epilepsy Center
Cleveland Clinic
Cleveland, Ohio

Sara C. LaHue, MD

Assistant Professor of Neurology
Department of Neurology
University of California, San Francisco
San Francisco, California

Steven L. Lewis, MD

Physician in Chief, Lehigh Valley Fleming Neuroscience
    Institute
Farber Institute for Neuroscience of Thomas Jefferson
    University, Regional Chief, Lehigh Valley
Timothy M. Breidegam Endowed Chair and Chief of
    Neurology
Lehigh Valley Health Network
Allentown, Pennsylvania

Nicholas A. Morris, MD

Associate Professor
Department of Neurology
University of Maryland School of Medicine
Baltimore, Maryland

Meabh O'Hare, MB BCh, BAO

Instructor in Neurology
Department of Neurology
Brigham and Women's Hospital
Boston, Massachusetts

Mary A. O'Neal, MD

Chief of General Neurology
Director of the Women's Neurology Program
Department of Neurology
Brigham and Women's Hospital
Boston, Massachusetts

Sashank Prasad, MD

Chief of Neurology, Penn Presbyterian Medical Center
Professor of Clinical Neurology, University of Pennsylvania
    Perelman School of Medicine
Philadephia, Pennsylvania

Vijay K. Ramanan, MD, PhD

Consultant and Assistant Professor
Department of Neurology
Mayo Clinic
Rochester, Minnesota

Megan B. Richie, MD

Associate Professor of Neurology
Department of Neurology
University of California, San Francisco
San Francisco, California

Joseph E. Safdieh, MD

Gertrude Feil Associate Dean of Curricular Affairs
Professor and Vice Chair for Education
Department of Neurology
Weill Cornell Medicine
New York, New York

Erika J. Sigman, MD

Assistant Professor of Neurology and Neurosurgery
Department of Neurosurgery
Emory University School of Medicine
Atlanta, Georgia

Joome Suh, MD

Instructor in Neurology
Department of Neurology
Brigham and Women's Hospital
Harvard Medical School
Boston, Massachusetts

Mark Terrelonge Jr, MD, MPH
Assistant Professor of Neurology
Department of Neuromuscular Medicine
University of California, San Francisco
San Francisco, California

Martina Vendrame, MD, PhD
Associate Professor of Neurology
Lehigh Valley Fleming Neuroscience Institute
Allentown, Pennsylvania

Shadi Yaghi, MD
Associate Professor of Neurology
Department of Neurology
Brown University
Providence, Rhode Island

PREFACE

It has been more than 14 years since the publication of the most recent edition of *Neurology for the Non-Neurologist* and more than 43 years since the first edition of this pioneering textbook, which was the brainchild of Christopher G. Goetz and the late William J. Weiner. Throughout the long history of this book, *Neurology for the Non-Neurologist* has sought to clarify neurologic concepts for non-neurologist clinicians, providing a practical and up-to-date approach to the diagnosis and treatment of the countless patients who initially present to them with neurologic symptoms and conditions.

The impetus for this seventh edition came from Chris Teja, senior acquisitions editor for Wolters Kluwer Health. Chris approached one of us (Steven L. Lewis, who was one of the editors of the previous two editions) about the creation of a long-overdue new edition of this now classic textbook. Steven immediately invited Aaron L. Berkowitz, a like-minded academic general neurologist with similar extensive clinical and educational experience locally and globally, to partner in this important endeavor. Together we decided to start fresh with an entirely new structure and new authors throughout, given the long period since the last edition and the remarkable advances in neurologic diagnosis and treatment over the last decades. Although completely new in content and structure, we have kept the original philosophy and goals of the book intact, ensuring that basic concepts in neurologic diagnosis and treatment are presented clearly for the non-neurologist. Given the global shortage of neurologists, we hope that this book will serve as a helpful companion in the initial diagnosis and treatment of neurologic conditions for front-line providers around the world.

The new edition of this book is divided into three sections. Section 1 provides a general overview of neurologic diagnosis, Section 2 presents the clinical approach to common neurologic symptoms, and Section 3 discusses the diagnosis and treatment of neurologic disorders. Since precise treatment protocols and available drug formulations change frequently, we have opted to discuss the principles of which treatments to use in which circumstances rather than including precise dosing regimens (which can be sought in other continually updated sources).

In Section 1, we have authored several introductory chapters that discuss neurologic diagnosis (Chapter 1), the neurologic history (Chapter 2), the neurologic examination (Chapter 3), and neurodiagnostic testing such as neuroimaging, cerebrospinal fluid analysis, electroencephalography, and nerve conduction studies/electromyography (Chapter 4). These chapters provide a foundation for the subsequent sections by discussing unique aspects of clinical reasoning in neurology such as localization, how to perform and interpret the neurologic examination, and basic principles of understanding when to order neurodiagnostic tests and how to interpret them.

In Section 2, the principles from Section 1 are applied in the context of specific neurologic symptoms commonly encountered in clinical practice. Each chapter provides a concise, expert, and practical discussion of the history, examination, and diagnostic evaluation of patients presenting with a particular neurologic symptom or syndrome including cognitive changes (Chapter 5); disorders of consciousness such as delirium and coma (Chapter 6); transient neurologic symptoms (Chapter 7); headache (Chapter 8); dizziness and vertigo (Chapter 9); sensory symptoms such as numbness and paresthesia (Chapter 10); weakness (Chapter 11); visual symptoms such as visual loss, double vision, pupillary abnormalities, and ptosis (Chapter 12); abnormal movements such as parkinsonism, tremor, dystonia, myoclonus, chorea, tics, and ataxia (Chapter 13); and abnormal gait (Chapter 14). Neurologic conditions mentioned in the chapters of Section 2 are discussed in detail in Section 3.

In Section 3, neurologic disorders are discussed with a focus on presenting symptoms and signs, diagnostic evaluation, and treatment considerations. Headache disorders such as migraine, tension headache, and others are discussed in Chapter 15. Ischemic stroke, intracerebral hemorrhage, and subarachnoid hemorrhage are discussed in Chapter 16. Seizures and epilepsy are discussed in Chapter 17. Causes of dementia such as Alzheimer disease, vascular dementia, dementia with Lewy bodies, frontotemporal dementia, normal pressure hydrocephalus, and Creutzfeldt-Jakob disease are discussed in Chapter 18. Movement disorders such as Parkinson disease, atypical parkinsonian disorders (multiple system atrophy, corticobasal syndrome, and progressive supranuclear palsy), essential tremor, and Huntington disease are discussed in Chapter 19. Multiple sclerosis and other neuroimmunologic disorders such as neuromyelitis optica spectrum disorder, acute disseminated encephalomyelitis (ADEM), and the recently described myelin oligodendrocyte glycoprotein antibody-associated disease (MOGAD) are discussed in Chapter 20. Neurologic infections including meningitis, encephalitis, central nervous system abscess, and neurologic complications of HIV are discussed in Chapter 21. Vestibular disorders such as benign paroxysmal positional vertigo (BPPV), Ménière disease, vestibular neuritis, and vestibular migraine are discussed in Chapter 22. Common conditions affecting the spinal cord and nerve roots and considerations of when to perform neuroimaging and consider surgical referral for these conditions are discussed in Chapter 23. Peripheral neuropathies (including diabetic neuropathy, Guillain-Barré syndrome, and common entrapment neuropathies such as carpal tunnel syndrome) and amyotrophic lateral sclerosis (ALS) are discussed in Chapter 24. Neuromuscular junction disorders (myasthenia gravis and Lambert-Eaton syndrome) and muscle diseases (including dermatomyositis, polymyositis, inclusion body myositis, and statin-associated myopathy) are discussed in Chapter 25. Primary nervous system tumors, nervous system metastases, paraneoplastic syndromes, and complications of cancer therapies are discussed in Chapter 26. Neurologic complications of systemic conditions are discussed in Chapter 27. Diagnosis and treatment of neurologic disorders in pregnancy are discussed in Chapter 28. Sleep disorders including sleep apnea, narcolepsy and idiopathic hypersomnia, insomnia, restless legs syndrome, and rapid eye movement (REM) sleep behavior disorder are discussed in Chapter 29. The diagnosis and treatment of acute head trauma and the sequelae of concussion are discussed in Chapter 30.

We are grateful to the 31 authors who contributed to this textbook. These neurologists are not only masters of their clinical craft but incredibly dedicated to teaching it to others. We thank each one of them for working so closely with us to provide clear, detailed, up-to-date, and practical discussions of the conditions they expertly care for in the clinic and hospital. We would also like to thank Ariel S. Winter, senior development editor at Wolters Kluwer, for skillfully moving this book from concept to publication.

It is our sincere hope that this textbook will help our non-neurologist colleagues provide the best possible neurologic care to their patients.

Steven L. Lewis, MD
Aaron L. Berkowitz, MD, PhD, FAAN

CONTENTS

CHAPTER

1

Approach to Neurologic Diagnosis

Steven L. Lewis and Aaron L. Berkowitz

INTRODUCTION

The diagnostic process in neurology is distinct from the diagnostic process in other medical specialties because the cause of a neurologic symptom may be anatomically remote from the location of the symptom itself. For example, a patient's report of numbness in the hand could be caused by a lesion on one or more peripheral nerves, the brachial plexus, one or more nerve roots, the spinal cord, or the brain.

This chapter provides a basic overview of the neurologic diagnostic process to provide the clinician with a framework for the assessment of a patient with neurologic symptoms. Chapters 2, 3, and 4 provide more specific details about the neurologic history, examination, and neurodiagnostic testing, which are key components of the stepwise diagnostic approach to patients with neurologic symptoms. Chapters 5 to 14 discuss an approach to the history, examination, and

neurodiagnostic testing in patients with specific neurologic symptoms, such as cognitive changes (Chapter 5), alterations in consciousness (Chapter 6), spells (Chapter 7), headache (Chapter 8), dizziness (Chapter 9), numbness (Chapter 10), weakness (Chapter 11), visual changes (Chapter 12), abnormal movements (Chapter 13), and difficulty walking (Chapter 14).

THE NEUROLOGIC DIAGNOSTIC METHOD

Neurologic diagnosis begins with a detailed neurologic history (Chapter 2) followed by a neurologic examination (Chapter 3) informed by the diagnostic considerations based on the history. Using the information gathered during the neurologic history and examination, the clinician's goal is, first, to determine the most likely localization of the process within the nervous system (ie, "Where is the lesion?"), and, second, to determine the most likely mechanism of dysfunction at that lesion site (ie, "What is the lesion?"). Diagnostic testing (eg, laboratory testing, neuroimaging) can then be performed to evaluate the implicated level of the nervous system to arrive at a diagnosis (Chapter 4).

Determining the localization within the nervous system (eg, brain vs spinal cord vs peripheral nervous system) is critical to accurate neurologic diagnosis. Neuroimaging and electrophysiologic testing such as nerve conduction studies/electromyography may detect incidental and/or subclinical abnormalities with no relation to the patient's presenting symptoms. Therefore, ordering only the appropriate testing to evaluate the implicated level of the nervous system and interpreting findings in the context of the history and examination is critical to avoid incorrectly attributing a patient's symptoms to incidental unrelated findings.

LOCALIZATION OF NEUROLOGIC DISEASE

Although neuroanatomy is complex and its study can be daunting, recognition of a few common patterns will usually suffice to provide the general localization that is typically needed in clinical practice, specifically whether the lesion is in the central nervous system (ie, brain, brainstem, cerebellum, spinal cord) or the peripheral nervous system (ie, nerve roots, peripheral nerves, neuromuscular junction, or muscle). Table 1.1 summarizes the basic concept of neurologic localization, correlating common patterns of

neurologic symptoms and signs with the most likely localization within the nervous system.

MECHANISM OF NEUROLOGIC DISEASE

Once the most likely localization(s) of the patient's condition is deduced from the patient's presenting symptoms and examination findings, the next step is for the clinician to determine the most likely mechanism(s) of dysfunction affecting that region of the nervous system. The major mechanisms of neurologic disease are summarized and described in Table 1.2. Categorization into one or several of the most likely mechanism(s) underlying the patient's symptoms takes into account the additional factors elicited from the history, such as the patient's age, the time course of symptom development, the patient's past medical history (including delineation of risk factors for various neurologic disorders), medications, social history, family history, review of systems, and regional epidemiology (see Chapter 2).

Thinking in terms of the likely general mechanism(s) of disease helps ensure diagnostic breadth and avoids prematurely excluding potentially causative specific diseases early in the diagnostic process.

TABLE 1.1	Characteristic Symptoms and Signs of Neurologic Disease at Different Locations	
General location	**Characteristic symptoms and signs suggestive of localization to this region[a]**	**Examples[b]**
Brain	Cognitive dysfunction Speech and language dysfunction Hemiparesis Hemisensory loss Visual field deficits Headache Upper motor neuron signs[c]	Stroke (ischemic stroke or hemorrhage) Neoplasm Cerebral abscess Demyelinating plaque
Brainstem	Diplopia, dysarthria, nausea, vomiting, vertigo Alterations in level of consciousness Ataxia of gait or extremities Unilateral or bilateral weakness or sensory loss Crossed hemiparesis (eg, weakness of one side of the face and the opposite side of the body) Crossed hemisensory loss (eg, numbness of one side of the face and the opposite side of the body) Upper motor neuron signs[c]	Stroke (ischemic stroke or hemorrhage) Neoplasm Demyelinating plaque
Cerebellum	Ataxia of gait or extremities Diplopia, dysarthria, nausea, vomiting, vertigo	Stroke (ischemic stroke or hemorrhage) Demyelinating plaque

TABLE 1.1	Characteristic Symptoms and Signs of Neurologic Disease at Different Locations (*continued*)

General location	Characteristic symptoms and signs suggestive of localization to this region[a]	Examples[b]
Spinal cord (myelopathy)	Unilateral or bilateral weakness and sensory loss Bowel and/or bladder dysfunction Upper motor neuron signs[c]	Degenerative arthritis of the spine Myelitis (inflammation and/or demyelination of the spinal cord) Spinal cord compression (eg, from tumor, abscess, disk) Spinal cord infarct
Nerve root (radiculopathy)	Radiating pain corresponding to a nerve root distribution Numbness or weakness in a nerve root distribution Diminished reflex (lower motor neuron signs) in territory of nerve root	Degenerative arthritis of the spine
Peripheral nerve (neuropathy)	Paresthesia, sensory loss, or weakness in the territory of an individual peripheral nerve Distal paresthesia, sensory loss, or weakness in lower extremities ("stocking distribution") or both lower and upper extremities ("stocking-glove distribution") Lower motor neuron signs[c]	Compressive mononeuropathy (eg, ulnar, radial, or median neuropathy) Distal symmetric polyneuropathy (eg, from diabetes)
Neuromuscular junction	Waxing and waning weakness (dysarthria, dysphagia, ptosis, diplopia) No sensory signs or symptoms	Myasthenia gravis Lambert-Eaton myasthenic syndrome
Muscle (myopathy)	Weakness (especially proximal) No sensory signs or symptoms	Inflammatory myopathy Muscular dystrophy

[a] Not all symptoms/signs will be present in a patient with a lesion in each region.
[b] Just a few of many examples of causative lesions/disorders in these locations.
[c] Upper motor neuron signs on examination include hyperreflexia, clonus, increased tone (spasticity), and the Babinski sign. Lower motor neuron signs on examination include hyporeflexia or areflexia, decreased (flaccid) tone, muscle atrophy, and fasciculations (see Chapter 11).
Modified from Lewis SL. *Field Guide to the Neurologic Examination* (Table 2.2). Lippincott Williams & Wilkins; 2005.

TABLE 1.2	Mechanisms of Neurologic Disease

Mechanism[a]	Comments	Examples[b]	Typical time course
Compressive	Includes any process that produces dysfunction by compression of nervous system structures	Tumors (benign or malignant); intervertebral discs compressing nerve roots or spinal cord; aneurysm compressing a cranial nerve; subdural hematoma exerting mass effect on the brain	Depends on etiology (acute, subacute, or chronic)
Degenerative	Includes any process that causes progressive dysfunction due to nervous system degeneration	Many dementing illnesses (eg, Alzheimer disease, frontotemporal dementia); many movement disorders (eg, Parkinson disease, Huntington disease); some neuromuscular disorders (eg, amyotrophic lateral sclerosis)	Chronic
Epileptic	Produces intermittent dysfunction by abnormal brain electrical activity	Focal or generalized seizure disorders	Acute
Hemorrhagic	Produces dysfunction by bleeding into (or surrounding) the brain or other tissues	Intraparenchymal (intracerebral) brain hemorrhage; intraventricular hemorrhage; subarachnoid hemorrhage (note that subdural hematoma is placed in the compressive category as it causes dysfunction primarily due to mass effect)	Acute

(*continued*)

TABLE 1.2 **Mechanisms of Neurologic Disease (*continued*)**

Mechanism[a]	Comments	Examples[b]	Typical time course
Infectious	Dysfunction occurring due to a micro-organism invading nervous system structures	Bacterial, viral, or parasitic processes	Depends on microbe (acute, subacute, or chronic)
Inflammatory/demyelinating	Includes disorders that cause demy-elination or inflammation in the CNS or PNS	CNS: multiple sclerosis, neuromyelitis optica; neurosarcoidosis; autoimmune encephalitis; spinal cord inflammation (myelitis) of any cause PNS: acute or chronic inflammatory polyradiculoneuropathies	Subacute
Ischemic	Dysfunction due to insufficient blood supply to a nervous system struc-ture or region	Cerebral infarction due to thrombosis or em-bolus; spinal cord infarction; mononeuropathy due to occlusion of vasa nervorum from peripheral nerve vasculitis	Acute or transient
Metabolic/toxic	Mechanism of (typically diffuse) brain or brainstem dysfunction due to endogenous metabolic dysfunction or exogenous substances (eg, tox-ins). Also a common cause of PNS dysfunction	Endogenous metabolic dysfunction: hypona-tremia; hepatic or uremic encephalopathy; thiamine deficiency; peripheral neuropathy related to diabetes Exogenous toxins: carbon monoxide; medication adverse effects on CNS or PNS	Depends on etiology (acute, subacute, or chronic)
Migrainous	A mechanism of (typically transient) brain dysfunction thought to be due to spreading waves of depression of cortical activity	Headache due to migraine; migrainous visual (or other) aura	Acute
Traumatic	CNS or PNS dysfunction due to any kind of direct injury to these struc-tures from an outside force (often immediately evident by history)	Concussion; contusion; laceration; gunshot wound; transection of peripheral nerve (note: most spinal cord injury due to trauma is com-pressive from spinal structures)	Acute

CNS, cerebral nervous system; PNS, peripheral nervous system.

[a] In addition to the disease mechanisms in this list, some *congenital* processes (some of which are genetic) may produce dysfunction due to absence, malformation, or other developmental abnormality of nervous system structure or function since birth; this mechanism is more commonly relevant in pediatric neurologic diagnoses, but may present in adulthood.

[b] Just a few of many examples of each category.

Modified from, Lewis SL. *Field Guide to the Neurologic Examination* (Table 3.1). Lippincott Williams & Wilkins; 2005.

SUMMARY

In summary, the process of neurologic diagnosis in-volves a detailed history and neurologic examination (in that order) to determine the most likely localization(s) of disease and the most likely mechanism(s) of disease affecting the implicated level(s) of the nervous system. Diagnostic testing based on the most likely "where" of localization, and the most likely "what" of mechanism then follows to determine which one of the many pos-sible more specific diagnoses (ie, the differential diag-nosis) within the broad mechanistic category is the cause of the patient's presentation.

Diagnostic test results must always be interpreted in the context of the clinical hypothesis of the most likely localization and mechanism, since neuroimaging, neurophysiologic testing, and other diagnostic test results may reveal incidental and/or subclinical findings unrelated to the patient's symptoms and signs.

Chapters 2, 3, and 4 provide further details on taking a detailed neurologic history, performing a comprehensive neurologic examination, and ordering and interpreting neurodiagnostic tests.

CHAPTER 2

The Neurologic History

Aaron L. Berkowitz and Steven L. Lewis

INTRODUCTION

As is the case when obtaining the general medical history, the goal of the neurologic history is to characterize the patient's symptom(s) with respect to time course of onset and evolution, quality and severity, alleviating and exacerbating factors, and associated symptoms, and to contextualize the symptom(s) in relation to the patient's past medical history, medications, and social and family history.

As discussed in Chapter 1, a fundamental element of neurologic diagnosis is localization: determining the site of pathology within the nervous system. The process of localization begins with the history. For example, cognitive symptoms localize to the brain (see Chapter 5), visual loss localizes along the visual pathway (from the eye to the brain; see Chapter 12), and so on. By the end of the history, the clinician should have an initial hypothesis about possible localizations, which can then be tested on the neurologic examination (see Chapter 3).

HISTORY OF PRESENT ILLNESS

Neurologic symptoms can be difficult for patients to describe. For example, a patient may use the word "dizziness" to refer to vertigo, lightheadedness, or imbalance; "numbness" to refer to sensory loss, paresthesia, weakness, or clumsiness; "weakness" to refer to loss of strength (ie, weakness), loss of coordination (ie, ataxia), or slowing of movement (ie, bradykinesia); or "blurry vision," to refer to visual loss, double vision, or higher order visuospatial dysfunction.

After listening to the patient provide an uninterrupted description of their symptoms, questions should be posed to clarify the domain(s) of neurologic involvement and begin the process of localization (eg, vertigo suggests a lesion of the vestibular pathway [see Chapter 9], weakness suggests a lesion along the motor pathway [see Chapter 11], sensory loss suggests a lesion along the somatosensory pathways [see Chapter 10]). Some neurologic symptoms do not fit a pattern that localizes to the nervous system and may instead be due to systemic conditions rather than primary neurologic disease. For example, a patient may feel weak from cancer, anemia, or systemic infection without focal loss of muscular force (referred to as *asthenia*); a patient may be dizzy due to a cardiovascular condition or a medication without involvement of the vestibular system; or a patient may report stiffness of movement due to arthritis rather than rigidity or spasticity.

For symptoms such as weakness, numbness, incoordination, and visual loss, the distribution of symptoms should be ascertained. For example, does the weakness, numbness, or incoordination affect one limb, the upper and lower extremity on one side of the body, both upper extremities, both lower extremities, or all four limbs? Is there weakness or numbness in the face in addition to the limb(s)? Does visual loss affect one eye or both eyes? The regional pattern of involvement is a key element in determining the localization that is discussed in the chapters of Section 2.

Once the type and regional distribution of symptoms is understood, the time course should be established. Did the symptoms come on suddenly or gradually? Are the symptoms constant or episodic? Time course is a key element in determining the etiology of neurologic symptoms. Sudden-onset neurologic symptoms (eg, over seconds to minutes) can occur in stroke (see Chapter 16) and seizure (see Chapter 17). Acute onset and evolution of symptoms (over hours to days) can be caused by infectious (eg, meningitis, encephalitis; see Chapter 21) and immune-mediated conditions (eg, Guillain-Barré syndrome [see Chapter 24] and flares of multiple sclerosis and neuromyelitis optica [see Chapter 20]). Subacute onset and evolution of symptoms (over weeks to months) can be seen in neoplastic (see Chapter 27), immune-mediated (see Chapter 20), and some infectious (eg, fungal, tubercular, parasitic; see Chapter 21) conditions. Chronic onset of neurologic symptoms (over years) can be seen in degenerative conditions such as Alzheimer disease (see Chapter 18) and Parkinson disease (see Chapter 19). Episodic symptoms can occur with migraine (see Chapter 15), seizure (see Chapter 17), and rarer conditions such as periodic paralysis and paroxysmal movement disorders. Over any of these time courses, medical conditions and medication or drug toxicity can also cause neurologic symptoms and should be considered in the differential diagnosis (see Chapter 27).

Although patients often present with a chief concern, they may also have other symptoms that are less prominent to them and therefore not reported spontaneously. Such symptoms should be inquired about since they can aid in localization and differential diagnosis. For example, is weakness also accompanied by sensory changes? Are bilateral leg symptoms accompanied by bladder or bowel dysfunction? Is tremor accompanied by other features of Parkinson disease such

as slowing of movements, stiffness, and nonmotor features such as anosmia (loss of smell), rapid eye movement (REM) sleep behavior disorder (physically acting out dreams), and/or constipation (see Chapters 13 and 19)? Do a patient's headaches have any associated "red flag" features (eg, awakening them at night, worse in the morning, or new and progressive) that suggest a secondary cause of headache (eg, intracranial lesion) rather than a primary headache disorder (eg, tension headache, migraine; see Chapter 8)? Such questions serve as a review of systems relevant to the patient's chief concern that aid in further characterizing it and localizing the most likely site of pathology in the nervous system.

PAST MEDICAL HISTORY

The patient's past medical history should be evaluated for systemic conditions that may be associated with the patient's neurologic condition. For example, cardiovascular conditions such as hypertension, diabetes, hyperlipidemia, and atrial fibrillation increase the risk of stroke (see Chapter 16); diabetes is a common cause of peripheral neuropathy (see Chapter 24); bariatric surgery may lead to vitamin and mineral deficiencies that can cause neurologic complications (see Chapter 27); systemic cancer can be associated with nervous system metastases, paraneoplastic syndromes, or complications of chemotherapy or radiation therapy (see Chapter 26); immunocompromise predisposes to opportunistic infections (see Chapter 21); and many rheumatologic diseases can have neurologic manifestations (see Chapter 27). However, many neurologic conditions can occur that are unrelated to the patient's past medical history or in patients with no significant past medical history. For example, if stroke occurs in a patient with no cardiovascular risk factors, the evaluation for etiology is extended to rarer potential causes beyond cardiovascular risk factors (see Chapter 16).

MEDICATIONS

The patient's medications should be reviewed for any with potential neurologic toxicities. For example, neuroleptics and dopamine-blocking antiemetics can cause drug-induced parkinsonism (see Chapter 19), statins can cause myopathy (see Chapter 25), bupropion and tramadol can lower the seizure threshold (see Chapter 17), and antibiotics such as cefepime can rarely cause encephalopathy.

FAMILY HISTORY

Patients should be asked about other members of the family with neurologic conditions to evaluate for potential hereditary neurologic conditions such as Charcot-Marie-Tooth (which causes neuropathy), muscular dystrophy (which causes myopathy), spinocerebellar ataxia (which causes ataxia), or Huntington disease (which causes chorea and neuropsychiatric symptoms).

SOCIAL HISTORY

Patients should be asked about alcohol and drug use (eg, chronic alcohol use can cause neuropathy and/or cerebellar degeneration, nitrous oxide use can lead to myelopathy [spinal cord dysfunction], intravenous drug use may result in endocarditis [which can be complicated by stroke] or wound botulism); occupation and occupational exposures (eg, repetitive movements may cause compressive neuropathy; heavy metal exposure can cause neuropathy; manganese toxicity can cause parkinsonism); diet (eg, a vegan or vegetarian diet may lead to vitamin B_{12} deficiency, which can cause a neuropathy, myelopathy, or both); and malnutrition may lead to thiamine deficiency, which can cause neuropathy and/or Wernicke encephalopathy (see Chapter 27). Inquiring about the patient's educational history can be helpful in interpreting the results of cognitive testing in patients with symptoms related to cognition (see Chapter 5).

SUMMARY

A neurologic history should establish the nature of the patient's chief concern with respect to the neurologic system involved (eg, cognition, motor, somatosensory, visual, vestibular) to generate an initial hypothesis regarding the most likely localization. The time course of symptom onset and evolution, associated symptoms, and context of the past medical, family, and social histories alongside the localization should allow for an initial hypothesis regarding the differential diagnosis. The neurologic examination (see Chapter 3) can then be approached as a way to test and refine the localization and differential diagnosis generated by the history.

3

The Neurologic Examination

Steven L. Lewis and Aaron L. Berkowitz

INTRODUCTION

As described in Chapter 2, the neurologic history allows for the development of an initial impression about the potential cause(s) of a patient's symptoms. The neurologic examination is then used to evaluate for signs that help further determine the most likely localization and diagnosis. The basic components of the neurologic examination presented in this chapter assess the functions of the nervous system. The examination maneuvers performed on each patient should be selected and interpreted in light of the diagnostic hypotheses generated by the neurologic history.

The neurologic examination is generally performed and reported in the following order: mental status, cranial nerves, motor, sensory, reflexes, cerebellar, and gait. Although the exact order of the examination is not critical, it is helpful for each clinician to have a consistent approach to avoid inadvertently leaving out critical components.

THE MENTAL STATUS EXAMINATION

The examination of mental status includes assessing both the level of consciousness (ie, whether the patient is awake and alert, comatose, or somewhere in between) and the content of consciousness (ie, the patient's cognition, such as their attention, memory, and language). Often, the history obviates the need for a formal mental status examination since the ability to provide a history requires intact attention, memory, and language function. When the patient presents for evaluation of cognitive concerns—or the examiner has concerns about impaired cognition based on the history—a complete mental status examination should be performed. The domains of cognitive function to assess and how to assess them are listed in Table 3.1.

TABLE 3.1	Assessment of Cognition
Cognitive domain	**Typical tests to assess that domain**
Orientation	Place, date, day of the week, season, month, year
Attention (working memory)	Immediate recall of three words; serial 7s (asking the patient to start from 100 and subtract by 7s); spelling a five-letter word backward; stating days of the week backward
Memory (long-term memory)	Recalling three or more presented words after a delay of several minutes
Language	Spontaneous speech, language comprehension, repetition, object naming, reading
Visuospatial	Copying a picture such as two intersecting pentagons; drawing a clock
Executive function	Often assessed using the trail-making test on the Montreal Cognitive Assessment

Many clinicians find it useful to use scored, standardized tests (eg, the Mini-Mental State Examination [MMSE][1] or the Montreal Cognitive Assessment [MoCA][2]) to assess the major domains of cognition and allow for comparison of performance over time through serial assessment. See Chapter 5 for further discussion of the approach to evaluating patients with cognitive symptoms.

THE CRANIAL NERVE EXAMINATION

The cranial nerves are 12 paired nerves that innervate the structures of the head and neck (and, in the case of the vagus nerve, provide visceral innervation to structures in the thorax and abdomen). The cranial nerve examination tests the function of these nerves as well as their connections in the brainstem and cerebrum. The cranial nerve examination is summarized in Table 3.2.

Examination of Smell (Assesses Cranial Nerve 1)

Although not typically tested in routine neurologic assessment, smell should be evaluated in any patient with a concern related to this sense. To test smell, an easily recognized nonnoxious scent (such as coffee grounds from a clinic kitchen) can be placed under the patient's nostrils with their eyes closed, testing each nostril separately with the patient holding the other nostril closed while asked to identify the smell.

Funduscopic Examination (Assess Cranial Nerve 2 and Intracranial Pressure)

Assessment of the ocular fundus in patients with neurologic disease evaluates for increased intracranial pressure (visible as swelling of the optic disc, known as *papilledema*) or inflammation of the optic nerve head (visible as *papillitis*). In addition, some patients with subarachnoid hemorrhage may have subhyaloid hemorrhages visible on funduscopic examination.

When examining the fundus with an ophthalmoscope, it is helpful to ask the patient to fixate on a distant point at the end of the room and for the examiner to approach the patient from the side (since the optic disc sits slightly medially). Once the ophthalmoscope is close to the patient's eye and

TABLE 3.2	Assessment of Cranial Nerves	
Examination maneuver	**Cranial nerve(s) assessed by examination maneuver**	**Additional notes**
Smell	1 (Olfactory)	Not typically tested in routine neurologic assessment
Funduscopic examination	2 (Optic)	To evaluate the optic disc
Visual acuity	2 (Optic)	May be affected by ocular or optic nerve disease
Visual fields	2 (Optic)	Assesses for abnormalities anywhere along the visual pathways (see Chapter 12)
Pupillary reaction to light	2 (Optic), 3 (Oculomotor)	Pupillary size and reaction may also be affected by cataract surgery or medications/drugs
Eye movements	3 (Oculomotor), 4 (Trochlear), 6 (Abducens)	Beyond weakness, also assesses for the presence of other eye movement abnormalities, for example, nystagmus (suggestive of brainstem, cerebellum, or vestibular dysfunction)
Facial sensation	5 (Trigeminal)	Also assesses for facial sensory changes due to central lesions
Facial strength	7 (Facial)	Also assesses for facial weakness due to central lesions
Hearing	8 (Vestibulocochlear)	Hearing loss may be due to a problem with the ear or cranial nerve 8
Palate position and rise	9 (Glossopharyngeal), 10 (Vagus)	Can be assessed by gag reflex in comatose patients
Shoulder shrug and head turn	11 (Spinal accessory)	Rarely affected
Tongue position and movement	12 (Hypoglossal)	Also assesses for tongue weakness due to central lesions

the optic disc comes into view, the ophthalmoscope lens can be adjusted positively or negatively (starting at zero diopters) until the optic disc and blood vessels are in focus.

Although the assessment of the ocular fundus is challenging when the pupil is not dilated, the increasing use of portable fundus photographic technology will hopefully make this assessment more widely available.

Visual Acuity (Assesses Cranial Nerve 2)

Visual acuity should be assessed if the patient reports impaired vision or has a potential diagnosis that can impair vision (eg, multiple sclerosis or idiopathic intracranial hypertension). Visual acuity can be tested at the bedside using a pocket-sized visual chart, known as a *near card*. The patient holds the card about 12 inches from the eyes and is asked to read the smallest line of letters visible with one eye while covering the opposite eye. The findings from this assessment are recorded as the smallest line the patient can read most of the letters from, with any errors on that line reported as a "minus." For example, if the patient can read all of the letters on the 20/25 line with the right eye and most of the letters on the 20/25 line with the left eye (but two of the letters are incorrect), this is reported as "20/25" for the right eye and "20/25 minus 2" for the left eye. If the patient uses reading glasses, these should be used during the examination since the neurologic assessment of vision is to assess best corrected acuity, which should be 20/20 with normal visual function.

Visual Fields (Assesses Cranial Nerve 2 and Visual Pathways Through the Brain)

In confrontation visual field testing, the examiner stands in front of the patient at eye level and asks the patient to look at the examiner's nose. The examiner then holds either one, two, or all five fingers up in each of the four quadrants (left upper quadrant, left lower quadrant, right upper quadrant, or right lower quadrant), and asks the patient how many fingers are being held up. The visual fields should be tested in each eye separately by having the patient close or

cover one eye while the examiner tests the open eye; the examiner generally also closes the corresponding eye to have a similar sense of the extent of the visual fields being tested. The examiner evaluates for the presence of monocular or binocular dysfunction in counting fingers. Common bilateral deficits are homonymous hemianopia, quadrantanopia, and bitemporal hemianopia, which have precise localizing values (see Chapter 12).

Patients can be tested for neglect by asking the patient to count the fingers presented individually on the left and right, and then together on the left and right. If the patient has neglect (which usually occurs on the left side due to a right parietal lesion), they will be able to count fingers on each side individually but will only notice the fingers on the right when fingers are presented on both the left and right simultaneously (a phenomenon known as *extinction to double simultaneous stimulation*).

Examination of Pupillary Function (Assesses Cranial Nerves 2 and 3 and Their Interconnection in the Brainstem)

The pupils should be examined with respect to their size, symmetry, and response to light.

An abnormally large (mydriatic) pupil can be caused by a cranial nerve 3 palsy (often associated with ptosis and extraocular muscle weakness, yielding a "down and out" eye); an abnormally small (miotic) pupil can be seen in Horner syndrome caused by a lesion of the oculosympathetic pathway (accompanied by mild ptosis). See Chapter 12 for further discussion.

To assess pupillary responses to light, the patient should be in a dimly lit room and asked to look at a distant site at the end of the room. The examiner then shines a bright light into each eye, looking for constriction in response. This is repeated for the other eye, and the ability of each pupil to constrict is noted.

If either pupil fails to constrict to light, the ability of the pupil to constrict to accommodation should be tested by asking the patient to look at their nose or follow the examiner's finger as it moves toward their nose. If the pupil constricts to a near stimulus but not to a bright light, this is known as *light-near dissociation* and can be seen in syphilis (called *Argyll Robertson pupils*) or with a tonic (Adie) pupil. Accommodation does not need to be tested if both pupils react to light.

The "swinging flashlight test" to assess for a relative afferent pupillary defect from an optic nerve lesion (eg, optic neuritis) in a patient with unilateral visual loss is discussed in Chapter 12.

Examination of Eye Movements (Assesses Cranial Nerves 3, 4, and 6 and Their Interconnection in the Brainstem)

The examination of eye movements assesses the cranial nerves and muscles that move the eyes and also evaluates for findings such as nystagmus, which can be seen in vestibular disorders (which may be peripheral or central; see Chapter 9).

To examine a patient's eye movements, the examiner should ask the patient to follow the examiner's index finger slowly moving horizontally (typically from the examiner's left side to the right and then back) and then slowly moving vertically. This examination can help elucidate the cause of a patient's double vision (diplopia), which may be due to a problem with the extraocular muscles (eg, thyroid eye disease), the neuromuscular junction (eg, myasthenia gravis), cranial nerves 3, 4, and/or 6 (eg, microvascular ocular motor palsy), or a brainstem lesion (eg, internuclear ophthalmoplegia). For additional discussion, see Chapter 12.

Facial Sensation (Assesses Cranial Nerve 5 and Its Central Nervous System Pathway)

Facial sensation is evaluated by lightly touching each side of the face (or touching it with a pin if more detailed testing is needed) making sure to assess the distribution of each of the three divisions of the trigeminal nerve (V1: forehead; V2: cheek; and V3: lower jaw). Refer to the "Sensory Examination" section of this chapter and Chapter 10 for further discussion of sensory testing.

The corneal reflex assesses cranial nerve 5 (afferent) and cranial nerve 7 (efferent); this reflex is generally only checked in patients who are comatose to evaluate brainstem function.

Facial Strength (Assesses Cranial Nerve 7 and Its Central Nervous System Pathway)

Examination of facial strength is assessed by asking the patient to raise their forehead, close their eyes, and smile. During each of these maneuvers, the examiner should look for significant asymmetry or obvious weakness. Weakness affecting the entirety of one side of the face (ie, impaired forehead raise, eye closure, and lip/mouth movement on attempted smile) suggests dysfunction of cranial nerve 7 on that side, whereas weakness only affecting the smile suggests a central lesion affecting the contralateral cerebral hemisphere (or less commonly, the upper brainstem). For further discussion, see Chapter 11.

Hearing (Assesses Cranial Nerve 8 and the Ear)

Hearing can be assessed by asking the patient if they can hear the examiner's fingers rubbing together in each ear separately. This evaluates for asymmetries that could suggest ear or cranial nerve 8 dysfunction. Hearing loss is rarely neurologic in origin but can be seen with vestibular schwannoma and in rare neurologic conditions such as Susac syndrome and mitochondrial disease.

When a more detailed bedside assessment of hearing is needed, the Rinne and the Weber tests compare sound conduction through the external auditory apparatus (called *air conduction*) with sound through the auditory pathways embedded in the skull bones (called *bone conduction*).

The Rinne test is performed by asking the patient to compare the volume of a vibrating 512-Hz tuning fork placed first outside the patient's ear for 1 to 2 seconds, and then subsequently placed on the mastoid process on that same side. Typically, the sound from outside the ear (air conduction) will sound louder than when placed on the mastoid process (bone conduction); however, under conditions causing conductive hearing loss, the patient will hear the sound louder when placed over the mastoid process.

The Weber test is performed by holding a vibrating high-pitched (512 Hz) tuning fork on the center of the forehead and asking the patient if the sound is heard equally in both ears (the normal response) or whether it is louder on one side; lateralization to one side on the Weber test suggests conductive hearing loss on that side or sensorineural hearing loss on the opposite side.

Table 3.3 summarizes how the combination of examination findings of hearing (finger rub, Rinne, and Weber) can be used to determine whether hearing loss is conductive (eg, due to blockage through the external auditory canal) versus sensorineural (affecting the acoustic nerve).

Palatal Movement (Assesses Cranial Nerves 9 and 10)

The palate is assessed by evaluating the position of the uvula and palate at rest and when the patient says "ahh." A significant deviation of the uvula and palate to one side at rest or when the patient says "ahhh" suggests a lesion of cranial nerve 9 or 10 contralateral to the side to which the uvula and palate deviate.

Cranial nerves 9 and 10 can also be assessed using the gag reflex. This test should generally not be tested in an awake patient but is useful to assess brainstem function in a patient in coma.

Shoulder Shrug and Head Turn (Assesses Cranial Nerve 11)

Testing strength of head turning (sternocleidomastoid) and shoulder shrug (trapezius) evaluates cranial nerve 11. In practice, this nerve is only very rarely affected in neurologic disease (eg, spinal accessory nerve injury after cervical lymph node biopsy).

Tongue Movement (Assesses Cranial Nerve 12)

Tongue strength is examined by asking the patient to protrude ("stick out") their tongue. Unilateral tongue deviation suggests weakness on the side to which the tongue deviates (the tongue is pushed to the weaker side by the normal/stronger side). Tongue deviation can be caused by a lesion of cranial nerve 12 or, less commonly, as part of more extensive unilateral weakness also affecting the face and extremities in the setting of an upper motor neuron central nervous system lesion.

When evaluating for tongue fasciculations when motor neuron disease is suspected, the tongue should be observed relaxed on the floor of the mouth rather than protruded so that tremulousness of the tongue (which is often normal) is not mistaken for fasciculations.

THE MOTOR EXAMINATION

The examination of motor function includes the assessment of tone (eg, rigidity or spasticity), the assessment of muscle strength in the arms and legs, and observation for abnormal movements (eg, tremor, chorea, dystonia; see Chapter 13 for discussion).

Tone can be described as normal, decreased (flaccid), or increased (spasticity or rigidity). Assessment of tone is performed by passively moving the patient's relaxed limbs. Spasticity refers to an elevation in tone that is velocity dependent, leading to a "catch" when moving the limb rapidly (eg, when supinating the arm or extending the arm at the elbow). Lower extremity tone is generally assessed in the supine position.

TABLE 3.3	Summary of Examination Findings in Patients With Unilateral Sensorineural or Conductive Hearing Loss in the Left Ear				
Cause of hearing loss	**Hearing (L)**	**Hearing (R)**	**Rinne test findings (L)**	**Rinne test findings (R)**	**Weber test**
Sensorineural	Decreased	Normal	AC > BC	AC > BC	Lateralizes to R
Conductive	Decreased	Normal	BC > AC	AC > BC	Lateralizes to L

>, greater than; <, less than; AC, air conduction; BC, bone conduction; L, left; R, right.
Modified from Lewis SL. *Field Guide to the Neurologic Examination.* Table 18.1. Lippincott Williams & Wilkins; 2005.

TABLE 3.4   Function and Innervation of the Muscles of the Upper Extremities

Muscle	Function	Major root innervation[a]	Nerve innervation
Deltoid	Arm abduction	C5	Axillary
Biceps	Elbow flexion	C5, C6	Musculocutaneous
Brachioradialis	Elbow flexion	C6	Radial
Extensor carpi radialis	Wrist extension	C6, C7	Radial
Triceps	Elbow extension	C7, C8	Radial
Extensor digitorum	Finger extension	C7	Radial (posterior interosseous branch)
Flexor pollicis longus	Thumb tip flexion	C7, C8	Median (anterior interosseous branch)
Flexor digitorum profundus	Second and third fingertip flexion Fourth and fifth fingertip flexion	C7, C8, T1	Median Ulnar
Interossei	Finger abduction and adduction	C8, T1	Ulnar
Abductor pollicis brevis	Thumb abduction	C8, T1	Median

[a]Although muscles share root involvement from several adjacent root levels, this table lists the roots with the most important, clinically relevant innervation to the given muscle.
Modified from Lewis SL. *Field Guide to the Neurologic Examination.* Table 25.1. Lippincott Williams & Wilkins; 2005.

TABLE 3.5   Function and Innervation of the Muscles of the Lower Extremities

Muscle	Function	Major root innervation[a]	Nerve innervation
Iliopsoas	Hip flexion	L2, L3, L4	Femoral
Quadriceps	Knee extension	L2, L3, L4	Femoral
Adductors	Hip adduction	L2, L3, L4	Obturator
Hamstrings	Knee flexion	L5, S1	Sciatic
Tibialis anterior	Foot dorsiflexion	L4, L5	Fibular (peroneal)
Tibialis posterior	Foot inversion	L4, L5	Tibial
Extensor hallucis longus	Large toe dorsiflexion	L5	Fibular (peroneal)
Peroneus longus	Foot eversion	L5, S1	Fibular (peroneal)
Gastrocnemius	Foot plantar flexion	S1, S2	Tibial

[a]This table lists the roots with the most important, clinically relevant innervation to the given muscle.
Modified from Lewis SL. *Field Guide to the Neurologic Examination.* Table 26.1. Lippincott Williams & Wilkins; 2005.

The examiner rapidly lifts the patient's relaxed leg at the thigh and observes the response: if the tone is normal, the leg bends and the heel stays on the bed; if the tone is increased, the entire leg may come off the bed.

To assess for rigidity (a sign of parkinsonism; see Chapter 13), the patient's wrist and arm are passively rotated, observing for resistance throughout this movement, often accompanied by a "ratcheting" referred to as *cogwheel rigidity.*

Testing of muscle strength begins with observation for pronator drift. The patient is asked to hold their arms out and extended, with palms facing the ceiling (supinated), and then to close their eyes. Downward drift of the arm with pronation suggests subtle weakness of central nervous system origin.

Muscle strength testing should include an assessment of representative proximal and distal muscles of the upper and lower extremities (Tables 3.4 and 3.5). Each muscle should be tested against the examiner's resistance and graded on a scale of 0 to 5 (Table 3.6). Testing should compare left and right (testing each side independently), as well as proximal and distal. Particular patterns of weakness correlate with particular localizations (see Chapter 11).

TABLE 3.6	MRC Scale for Grading Muscle Strength

Grade	Definition
0	Complete paralysis of a muscle
1	Trace muscle movement
2	Muscle movement in the plane of the bed but that cannot overcome the resistance of gravity
3	Muscle movement against gravity but cannot overcome resistance applied by the examiner
4	Muscle movement against resistance applied by the examiner, but able to be overcome
5	Normal muscle strength

MRC, Medical Research Council.
Modified from Lewis SL. *Field Guide to the Neurologic Examination.* Table 24.1. Lippincott Williams & Wilkins; 2005.

THE SENSORY EXAMINATION

Sensory modalities that can be tested on examination include touch, pain (usually tested with a pin), temperature (usually tested with the cold metal of the tuning fork), vibration sense (tested with a 128-Hz tuning fork), and proprioception (testing the patient's ability to detect upward or downward movement of a joint with their eyes closed, eg, the big toe). Pain and temperature sensations are carried by one pathway (small fibers of peripheral nerves and spinothalamic tracts), and vibration and proprioception are carried by one pathway (large fibers of peripheral nerves and dorsal columns), so, generally, only one modality needs to be tested from each of these, which is usually pinprick for the former and vibration for the latter.

Touch is generally only used to compare between the left and right sides to evaluate for a unilateral central nervous system lesion.

Pain (pinprick) sensation is tested by evaluating whether the patient feels the sensation of a pin as sharp (as opposed to dull). This is particularly useful for mapping out a region of sensory change to determine whether the deficit corresponds to a particular nerve or root (see Figures 3.1 and 3.2 and Chapter 10), to assess sensation from distal to proximal to assess for a small-fiber neuropathy, or to evaluate for the level of a spinal cord lesion to see if there is preserved sensation

above a certain level on the back and absent sensation below it (called a *spinal level*).

Vibration sense is assessed by placing a 128-Hz tuning fork on a joint (usually the big toe) and asking the patient if they can feel the vibration and for how long compared to the length of time the examiner can feel it. If the patient cannot feel vibration at the big toe, the test is then repeated at successively more proximal joints to assess the extent of vibration loss (eg, ankle, mid-shin, knee). This is an excellent screening test for subclinical neuropathy and can be assessed to evaluate for the presence of a large-fiber neuropathy or dorsal column dysfunction (see Chapter 24). Dissociation between pain and vibration sensation (ie, one impaired and the other present in the same region) can be seen with spinal cord lesions and with neuropathies affecting either the small fibers or the large fibers rather than both fiber types.

THE CEREBELLAR (COORDINATION) EXAMINATION

Signs of cerebellar function include limb ataxia, gait ataxia, nystagmus, and dysarthria. Limb ataxia can be assessed by having the patient move their finger rapidly between their nose and the examiner's finger. Cerebellar ataxia causes inaccuracy and side-to-side tremor with these movements that is worse when approaching the patient's nose and the examiner's finger (although there is no tremor at rest or with a sustained posture with cerebellar lesions; see Chapter 13). A similar maneuver can be performed in the lower extremity by having the patient move their heel up and down the opposite shin in a straight line; again, side-to-side oscillation with inaccuracy with this movement suggests cerebellar ataxia. The patient can also be asked to follow the examiner's finger through a series of rapid movements in different directions as if "mirroring" the examiner. Patients with cerebellar dysfunction will often overshoot the target, called *past pointing*.

Another test for cerebellar dysfunction is to ask the patient to rapidly alternate, continuously tapping the palm of the hand against the thigh and the dorsum of the hand against the thigh. If this movement is clumsy and dysrhythmic, this is referred to as *dysdiadochokinesia*.

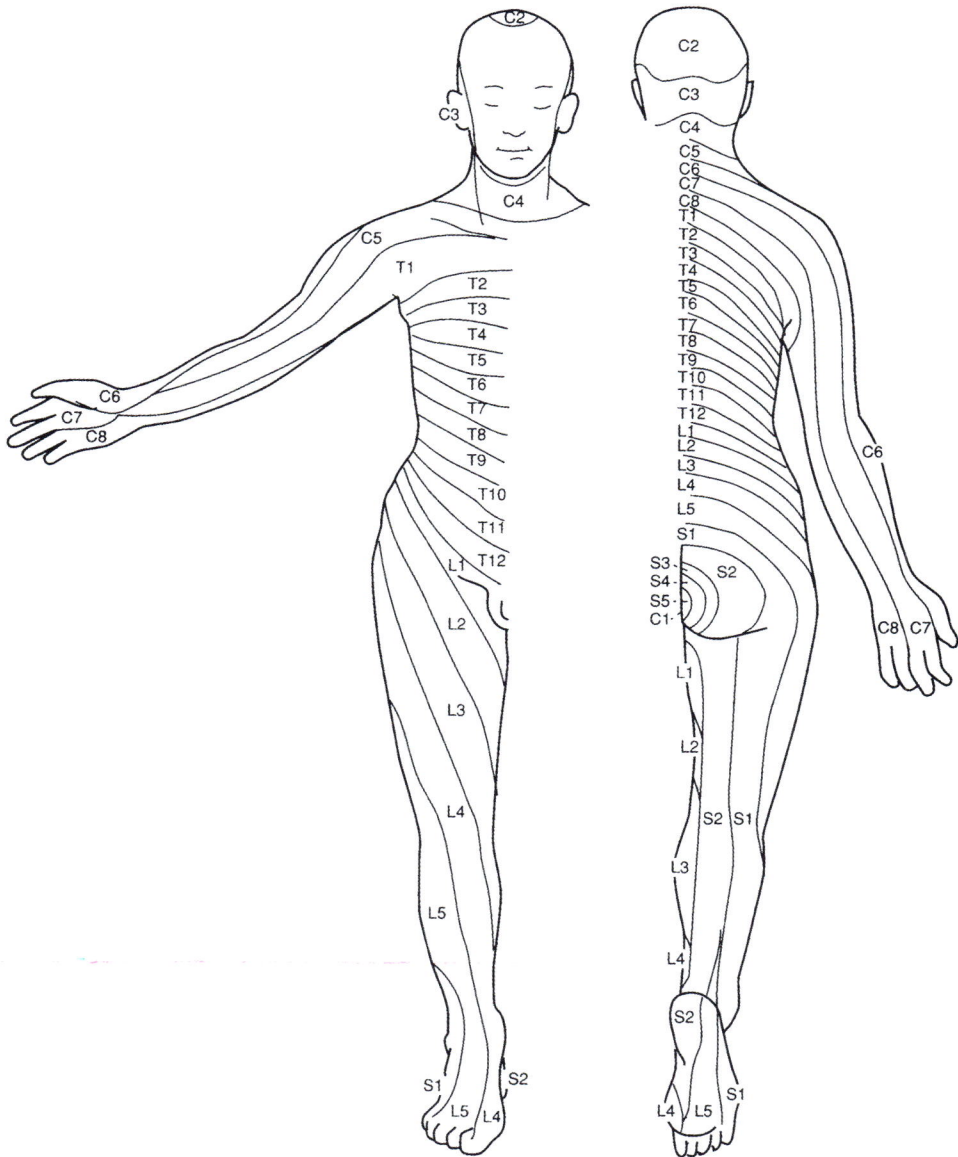

FIGURE 3.1 Dermatomes of the anterior and posterior body and extremities. (From Dudek RW. *High-Yield Gross Anatomy*. Williams and Wilkins; 1997.)

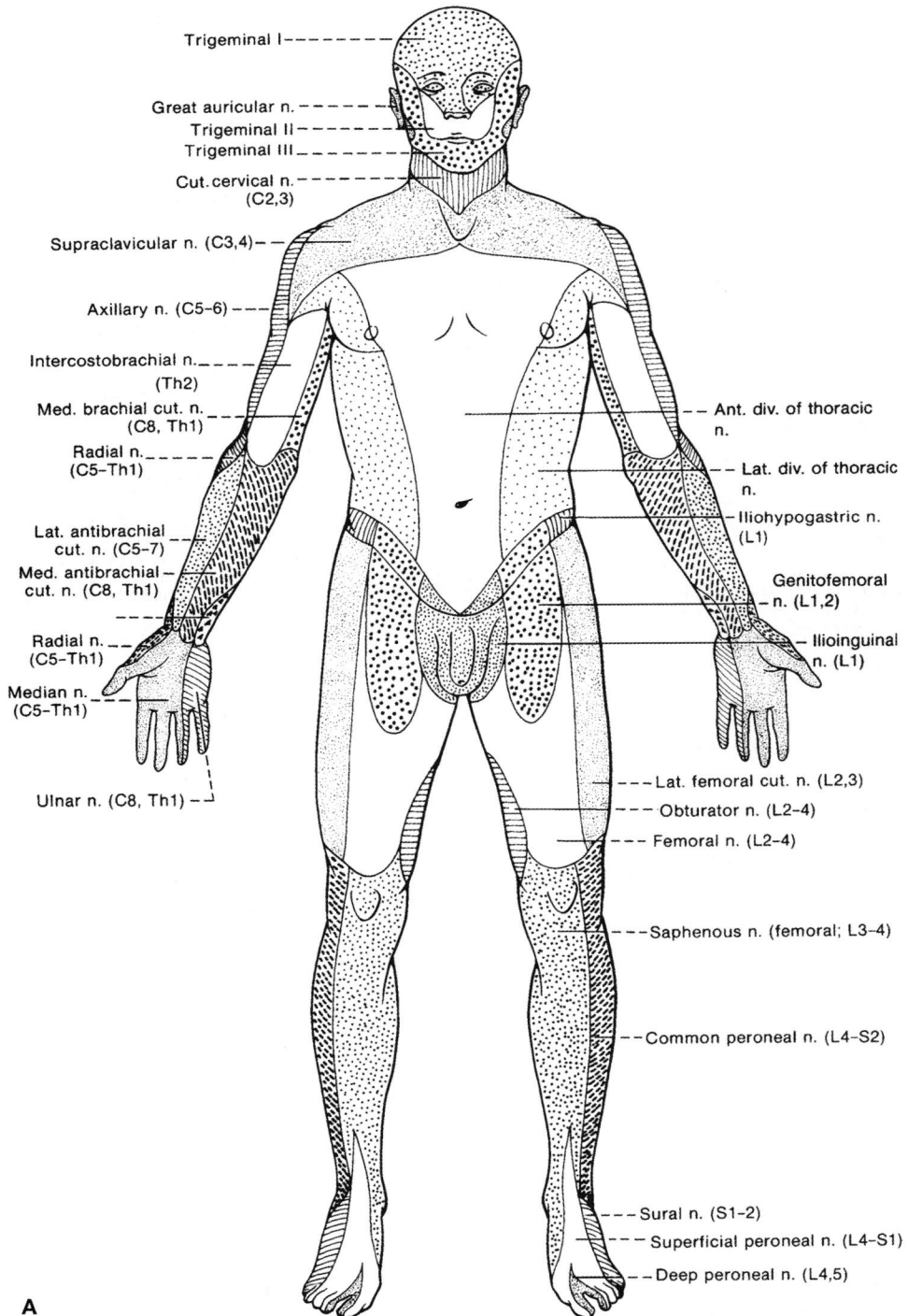

Trigeminal I

Great auricular n.
Trigeminal II
Trigeminal III
Cut. cervical n.
(C2,3)
Supraclavicular n. (C3,4)
Axillary n. (C5-6)
Intercostobrachial n.
(Th2)
Med. brachial cut. n.
(C8, Th1)
Radial n.
(C5-Th1)
Lat. antibrachial
cut. n. (C5-7)
Med. antibrachial
cut. n. (C8, Th1)
Radial n.
(C5-Th1)
Median n.
(C5-Th1)
Ulnar n. (C8, Th1)

Ant. div. of thoracic
n.
Lat. div. of thoracic
n.
Iliohypogastric n.
(L1)
Genitofemoral
n. (L1,2)
Ilioinguinal
n. (L1)
Lat. femoral cut. n. (L2,3)
Obturator n. (L2-4)
Femoral n. (L2-4)
Saphenous n. (femoral; L3-4)
Common peroneal n. (L4-S2)
Sural n. (S1-2)
Superficial peroneal n. (L4-S1)
Deep peroneal n. (L4,5)

A

FIGURE 3.2   A,B. The cutaneous distribution of the peripheral nerves. (From Haerer A. *DeJong's The Neurologic Examination.* Lippincott; 1992.)

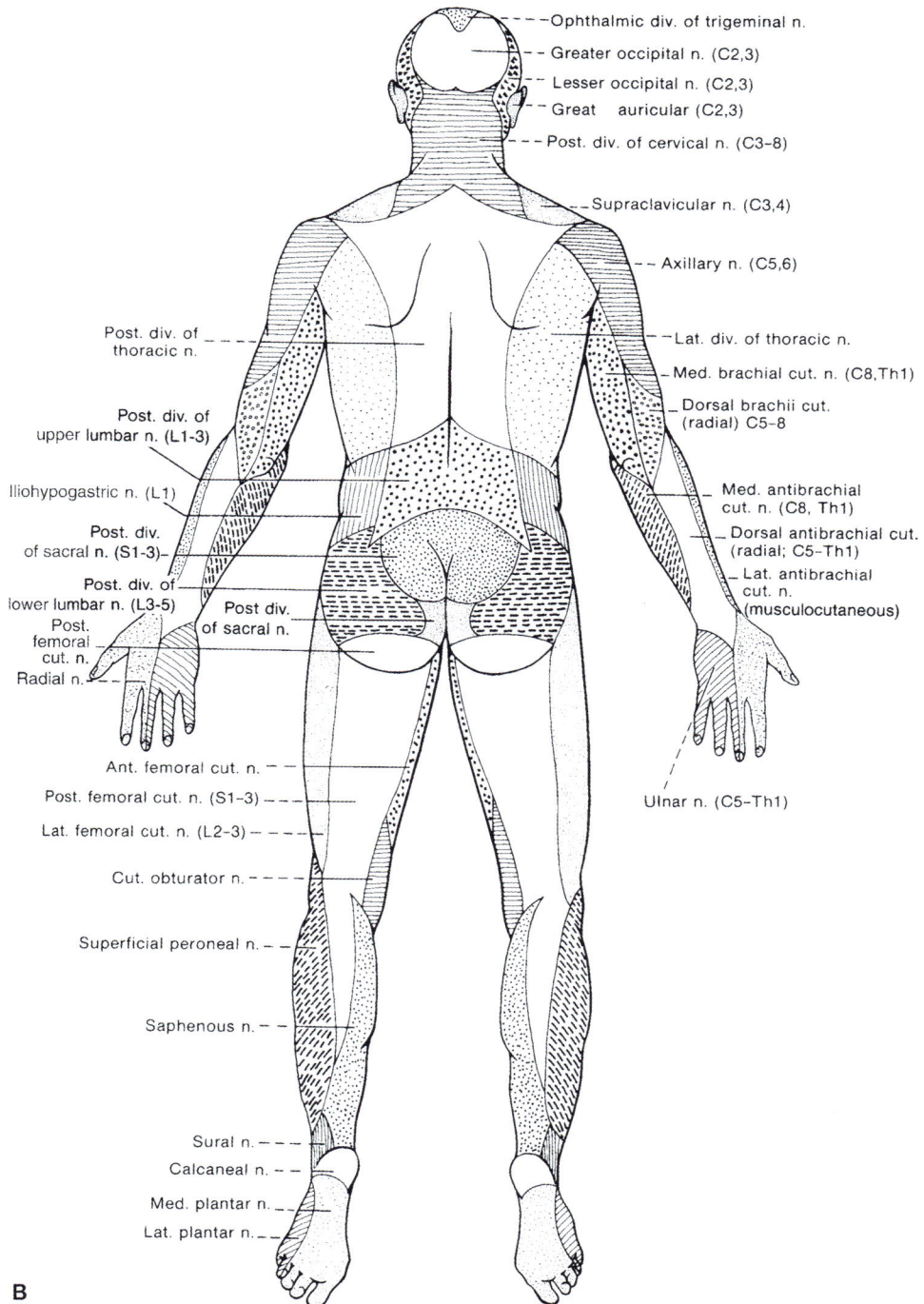

- Ophthalmic div. of trigeminal n.
- Greater occipital n. (C2,3)
- Lesser occipital n. (C2,3)
- Great auricular (C2,3)
- Post. div. of cervical n. (C3–8)
- Supraclavicular n. (C3,4)
- Axillary n. (C5,6)
- Lat. div. of thoracic n.
- Med. brachial cut. n. (C8,Th1)
- Dorsal brachii cut. (radial) C5–8
- Med. antibrachial cut. n. (C8, Th1)
- Dorsal antibrachial cut. (radial; C5–8)
- Lat. antibrachial cut. n. (musculocutaneous)
- Ulnar n. (C5–Th1)

Post. div. of thoracic n.

Post. div. of upper lumbar n. (L1-3)

Iliohypogastric n. (L1)

Post. div. of sacral n. (S1-3)

Post. div. of lower lumbar n. (L3-5)

Post div. of sacral n.

Post. femoral cut. n.

Radial n.

Ant. femoral cut. n.

Post. femoral cut. n. (S1–3)

Lat. femoral cut. n. (L2–3)

Cut. obturator n.

Superficial peroneal n.

Saphenous n.

Sural n.

Calcaneal n.

Med. plantar n.

Lat. plantar n.

B

FIGURE 3.2 (continued)

THE REFLEX EXAMINATION

The reflex examination assesses for the presence of hyperreflexia suggestive of an upper motor neuron (ie, central nervous system) lesion, or hyporeflexia suggestive of a lower motor neuron (ie, peripheral nervous system) lesion (see Chapter 11). Reflexes are tested using a moderately weighted hammer. To test a reflex, the limb being evaluated should be in a relaxed position; if the patient activates the joint, the reflex will not be able to be elicited. For example, the biceps reflex should be tested with the patient's arm in a relaxed, slightly flexed position, and the knee reflex should be tested with the patient seated and legs dangling over the examining table. The examiner should tap lightly on the tendon being evaluated. Reflexes are graded from 0 to 4+ (Table 3.7).

A Babinski sign should be assessed for by slowly stroking the plantar surface of the foot from the lateral heel to the base of the fifth toe and then medially to the base of the big toe. Extension of the big toe when the plantar surface is stimulated is a pathologic sign in adults indicating a lesion in the central nervous system.

Unilateral hyperreflexia suggests a spinal cord or brain lesion. Bilateral hyperreflexia suggests a spinal cord lesion (or rarely bi-hemispheric disease). Patients with subtle, symmetric, bilaterally brisk reflexes with no weakness, bowel/bladder dysfunction, or Babinski sign generally will not have an underlying lesion of significance (although they may have subclinical cervical stenosis).

Bilateral hyporeflexia suggests a polyneuropathy (see Chapter 24). Unilateral hyporeflexia can be seen with conditions affecting one or more specific roots or nerves (Table 3.8).

TABLE 3.7	Grading of Muscle Stretch Reflexes
Grade	**Definition**
0	Absent reflex
1+	Diminished reflex
2+	Normal reflex
3+	Brisk reflex with spread to adjacent reflexes
4+	Brisk reflex with accompanying clonus

Modified from Lewis SL. *Field Guide to the Neurologic Examination.* Table 37.1. Lippincott Williams & Wilkins; 2005.

TABLE 3.8	Spinal Root Levels Tested by the Muscle Stretch Reflexes
Reflex	**Root levels involved**
Biceps and brachioradialis	C5, C6
Triceps	C7, C8
Quadriceps	L2, L3, L4
Achilles	S1

Reflexes are commonly graded using the system described in Table 3.7. Modified from Lewis SL. *Field Guide to the Neurologic Examination.* Table 37.2. Lippincott Williams & Wilkins; 2005:125.

ASSESSMENT OF STANCE AND GAIT

The patient should be observed standing with their feet together. If they are able to do this, they should be asked to maintain this position with their eyes closed. If they lose their balance and take a step with their eyes closed, this suggests proprioceptive dysfunction (*Romberg sign*).

Gait requires coordinated functions of all previously tested functions of the nervous system: higher order cerebral control, strength, proprioception, and coordination. Gait dysfunction can, therefore, be seen with a lesion at any level of the nervous system or with multifocal disease. Evaluation of gait and particular patterns of abnormalities are discussed in Chapter 14.

ADDITIONAL BEDSIDE TESTS

Additional maneuvers may be performed in specific circumstances (eg, the Dix-Hallpike maneuver to evaluate for benign paroxysmal positional vertigo [see Chapters 9 and 22]), which are detailed in the chapters of Section 2.

SUMMARY

Although the neurologic examination has many components, with practice, it can be performed efficiently, providing a wealth of information about the functions of the central and peripheral nervous systems. Performing and interpreting the neurologic examination requires practice so that the range of normal findings and the patterns of abnormal findings can be appreciated. The results of the neurologic examination must always be interpreted in light of hypotheses about the localization and diagnosis from the clinical history. Based on the findings from the history and neurologic examination, the localization is often clear, and further diagnostic testing to assess the etiology of the patient's symptoms can be appropriately targeted. In Chapter 4, we discuss the use of neurodiagnostic tests such as neuroimaging, spinal fluid analysis, electroencephalography (EEG), and nerve conduction studies (NCS)/electromyography (EMG) in clinical practice.

REFERENCES

1. Folstein MF, Robins LN, Helzer JE. The mini-mental state examination. *Arch Gen Psychiatry*. 1983;*40*(7):812.
2. MoCA Cognition. https://mocacognition.com

Neurodiagnostic Testing

Aaron L. Berkowitz and Steven L. Lewis

INTRODUCTION

After completing the history and examination (see Chapters 2 and 3), the clinician will have determined the most likely localization and an initial differential diagnosis for the most likely etiology of the patient's presenting symptom(s). The localization and differential diagnosis together determine the next steps in diagnostic evaluation. In addition to serum laboratory tests to assess for systemic conditions, the main categories of neurodiagnostic tests are neuroimaging, cerebrospinal fluid (CSF) analysis, electroencephalography (EEG), and nerve conduction studies/electromyography (NCS/EMG).

This chapter discusses general principles regarding when to consider ordering these tests and some basic aspects of interpretation. Further details on which neurodiagnostic tests to order in which contexts can be found in the chapters of Section 2, and discussion of neurodiagnostic test findings in particular neurologic conditions can be found in the chapters of Section 3.

NEUROIMAGING

Background and Use in Clinical Practice

Computed tomography (CT) and magnetic resonance imaging (MRI) are most commonly used to evaluate the brain and spine. CT has the advantages of being able to be obtained rapidly, having minimal contraindications, and providing detailed imaging of bony structures. MRI provides superior resolution of anatomic detail of the brain, spinal cord, and nerve roots but requires more time to obtain, necessitates patient cooperation to lay still for long periods, and may be contraindicated in patients with certain types of implantable devices such as pacemakers.

CT is therefore the test of choice in emergent settings when evaluating for conditions such as subarachnoid hemorrhage, intracerebral hemorrhage, acute hydrocephalus, and in cases of head or spine trauma. Although CT can be normal in the initial hours after ischemic stroke, CT is the test of choice to exclude intracranial hemorrhage in the acute setting when deciding whether a patient is a candidate for thrombolysis or thrombectomy (see Chapter 16).

MRI of the brain is more sensitive than CT for the detection of small or subtle areas of pathology, such as metastases, small (or early) infarcts, microhemorrhages, or cortical malformations. MRI of the spine provides a more detailed visualization of intrinsic pathology of the spinal cord and nerve roots than CT (see Chapter 23). In the absence of contraindications to MRI, MRI (rather than CT) is the imaging modality of choice for nonemergent outpatient neuroimaging for the vast majority of conditions affecting the brain or spinal cord, given its much higher sensitivity for nervous system pathology, and the lack of exposure to ionizing radiation with MRI (which is present with CT). If a patient cannot undergo MRI, CT with contrast may provide additional information beyond noncontrast CT in evaluation for conditions such as tumor and abscess.

Unlike CT, MRI consists of a number of different sequences (including T1-weighted, T2-weighted, fluid-attenuated inversion recovery [FLAIR], diffusion-weighted imaging [DWI], apparent diffusion coefficient [ADC], and susceptibility-weighted imaging [SWI] and gradient recalled echo [GRE] sequences). Radiologists include all relevant sequences when an MRI is ordered based on the indication and differential diagnosis listed in the requisition, so specific sequences do not typically need to be specified by the ordering physician, only the region of the nervous system (eg, brain, cervical spine, thoracic spine, or lumbosacral spine) and whether or not contrast is to be given.

Both CT and MRI can be performed with contrast to provide further information about the imaging characteristics of particular lesions. Contrast is useful for the assessment of inflammatory, infectious, and neoplastic processes but is not typically needed in evaluation for structural conditions (eg, degenerative conditions of the spine [see Chapter 23] or patterns of brain atrophy in dementia [see Chapter 18]). In addition, both CT and MRI can be used to obtain angiographic images (CTA and MRA, respectively) of the head and neck to visualize the arterial supply and venous drainage of the nervous system to evaluate for conditions such as acute arterial occlusion in ischemic stroke, chronic cervical or intracranial arterial stenosis, aneurysms and other vascular malformations, and venous sinus thrombosis. Nuclear imaging, such as positron emission tomography (PET) and single-photon emission computerized tomography (SPECT), is increasingly used in the diagnosis of neurodegenerative disorders such as Alzheimer disease and Parkinson disease (see Chapters 18 and 19, respectively).

Basic Principles of Interpretation

Brain imaging should be assessed for the size and symmetry of anatomic structures to evaluate for areas of brain atrophy or expansion and ventricular enlargement (hydrocephalus) or compression. Areas of tissue abnormality are then classified on the basis of their imaging characteristics. Pathology on CT is characterized as hypodensity (darker) and hyperdensity (brighter). Pathology on MRI is characterized as hypointensity (darker) or hyperintensity (brighter), each of which has different significance depending on the MRI sequence being evaluated.

Hypodensity on CT can be seen wherever there is tissue degeneration (eg, prior stroke or trauma, chronic microvascular changes) or tissue edema (eg, infection, inflammation, neoplasm, or acute ischemic stroke) (Figure 4.1). Hyperdensity on CT can be caused by blood, calcification, or hypercellular tumors (Figure 4.2).

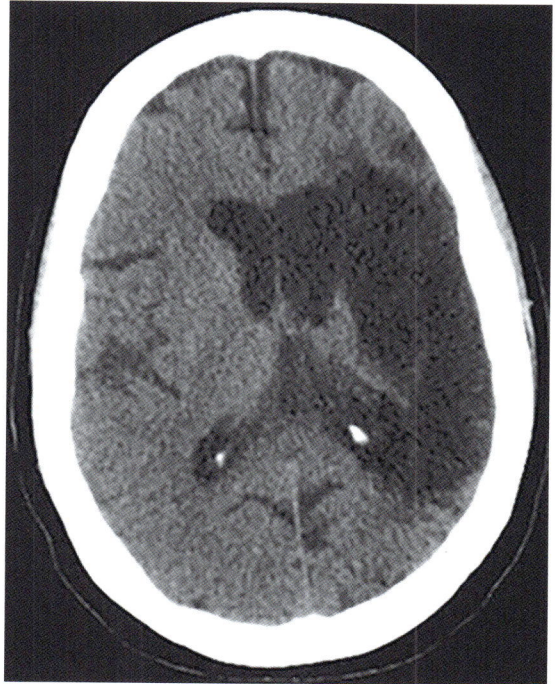

FIGURE 4.1 Axial computed tomography (CT) of the head showing a hypodensity in the left frontoparietal region consistent with remote left middle cerebral artery stroke.

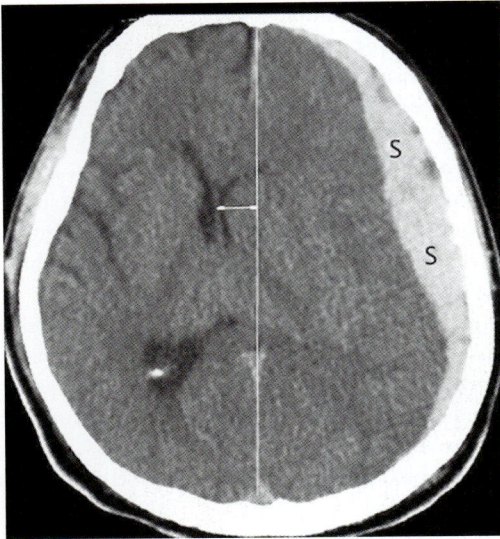

FIGURE 4.2 Axial computed tomography (CT) of the head showing a crescent-shaped hyperdensity overlying the left cerebral hemisphere consistent with subdural hematoma (S). There is also a midline shift from left to right due to the mass effect from the subdural hematoma. (From Thaler AI, Thaler, MS. *The Only Neurology Book You'll Ever Need.* Figure 4.2. Wolters Kluwer; 2022.)

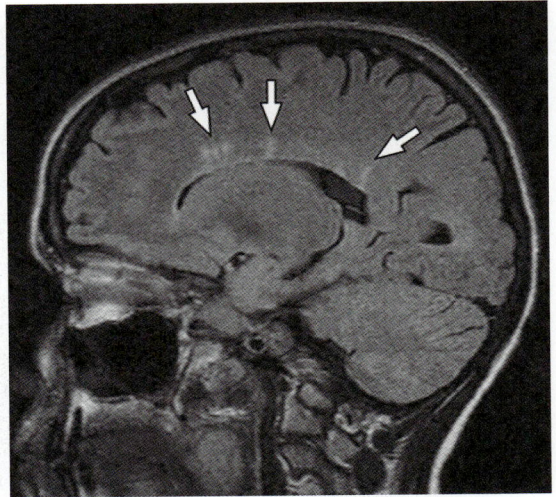

FIGURE 4.3 Sagittal magnetic resonance imaging (MRI) of the brain, fluid-attenuated inversion recovery (FLAIR) sequence, demonstrating multiple hyperintensities in the corpus callosum (arrows) in a patient with multiple sclerosis. (From Lee E. *Pediatric Radiology: Practical Imaging Evaluation of Infants and Children.* Wolters Kluwer; 2017.)

Most pathology on MRI is hyperintense on T2-weighted and FLAIR sequences (Figure 4.3). Additional signal characteristics that can be used to determine the etiology of pathology on T2-weighted and FLAIR sequences beyond distribution and morphology of the lesion(s) are the presence of contrast enhancement (on T1-weighted postcontrast sequences) (Figure 4.4), diffusion restriction (hyperintense on DWI and hypointense on ADC sequences) (Figure 4.5), and blood products (on SWI and GRE sequences).

MRI is such a sensitive test that incidental findings are common, such as small asymptomatic meningiomas, pineal cysts, isolated punctate white matter hyperintensities, small vascular anomalies, and degenerative changes of the spine that may be clinically irrelevant and pose minimal or no risk to the patient. Neuroradiology results must therefore always be correlated with the clinical presentation to avoid misdiagnosis, unnecessary further testing, and inappropriate treatment.

CEREBROSPINAL FLUID ANALYSIS

Background and Use in Clinical Practice

CSF can be obtained via lumbar puncture to aid in the diagnosis of immune-mediated, infectious, neoplastic,

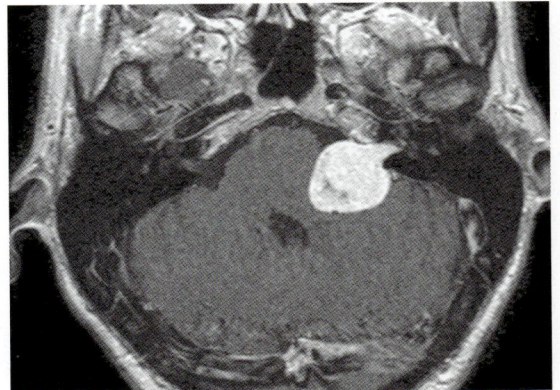

FIGURE 4.4 Axial magnetic resonance imaging (MRI) of the brain, T1-weighted postcontrast sequence showing a homogenously enhancing mass at the left cerebellopontine angle consistent with a vestibular schwannoma. (From Castillo M. *Neuroradiology Companion.* 4th ed. Fig 11750_30_06. Wolters Kluwer; 2011.)

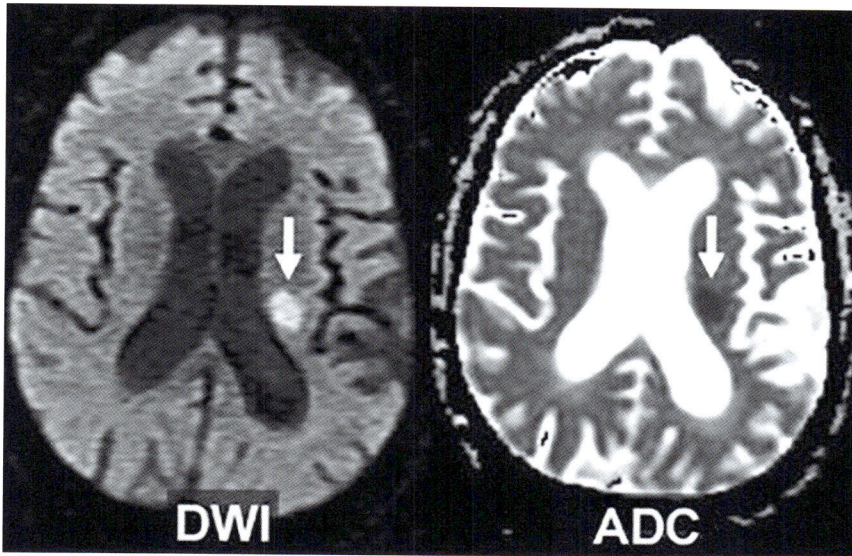

FIGURE 4.5 Axial magnetic resonance imaging (MRI) of the brain, DWI and ADC sequences, demonstrating a lesion in the left subcortical white matter that is hyperintense on DWI and hypointense on ADC (arrows) consistent with acute ischemic stroke. ADC, apparent diffusion coefficient; DWI, diffusion-weighted imaging. (From Klein J, Vinson EN, Brant WE, Helms CA. *Brant and Helms' Fundamentals of Diagnostic Radiology.* 5th ed. Wolters Kluwer; 2018.)

and degenerative diseases of the nervous system. Patterns of abnormalities of basic components (white blood cells, protein, and glucose) and CSF opening pressure can provide clues to the underlying etiology of neurologic disease. In addition, CSF can be evaluated for infection (Gram stain, culture, polymerase chain reaction [PCR], and antibody/antigen testing; see Chapter 21), immune-mediated conditions (eg, antibody panels for immune-mediated syndromes such as neuromyelitis optica, autoimmune encephalitis, and paraneoplastic conditions; see Chapters 20 and 26), malignant cells (cytology and flow cytometry; see Chapter 26), and biomarkers of neurodegenerative disease (eg, amyloid β-42 and tau in Alzheimer disease, real-time quaking-induced conversion [RT-QUIC] in Creutzfeldt-Jakob disease; see Chapter 18).

Basic Principles of Interpretation

Elevated CSF protein can be seen not only in immune-mediated neurologic disorders but also in patients with severe degenerative disease of the spine or diabetes. Elevated CSF protein with no or minimal elevation in white blood cells is called *albuminocytologic dissociation* and is a nonspecific marker of inflammation that can be seen in conditions such as Guillain-Barré syndrome and chronic inflammatory demyelinating polyradiculoneuropathy (CIDP). Elevated CSF protein accompanied by a significant elevation in white blood cells can be seen in immune-mediated and infectious conditions; these changes with normal CSF glucose suggest an immune-mediated or viral condition, whereas these changes with decreased CSF glucose suggest bacterial, fungal, or tuberculous infection (although decreased CSF glucose can also be seen in some viral infections, immune-mediated conditions, and in CNS malignancy). CSF protein can also be elevated in patients with spinal stenosis who do not have an inflammatory, infectious, or a neoplastic condition.

Elevated CSF protein and cell count can therefore provide evidence of inflammation as a result of an immune-mediated, infectious, or neoplastic condition, but do not provide a precise etiologic diagnosis. This information, in conjunction with the clinical syndrome and neuroimaging, can be used to guide further evaluation to determine the underlying diagnosis (eg, additional more specific CSF diagnostics).

ELECTROENCEPHALOGRAPHY

EEG uses scalp electrodes to evaluate cerebral electrical activity, serving as a sort of "ECG of the brain." EEG is most commonly performed as a 20- to 30-minute study in the outpatient setting to evaluate for abnormal brain electrical activity occurring between seizures that signifies a predisposition to seizures (called *interictal epileptiform discharges*). A single outpatient EEG is relatively insensitive for epileptiform discharges, but sensitivity increases when the test is repeated on multiple occasions, and the patient undergoes sleep deprivation prior to EEG. EEG is prone to artifact, the interpretation is dependent on the skill and experience of the neurologist reading the EEG, and epileptiform discharges can occur in a small percentage of the population who do not have epilepsy. Therefore, a single EEG should not be used to confirm or exclude the diagnosis of seizures or epilepsy in a patient in whom the etiology of the spell is not clear (eg, seizure, syncope, or psychogenic nonepileptic seizure; see Chapter 17), and the test should be repeated if there is uncertainty in the result.

EEG can also be obtained continuously during an inpatient admission to try to correlate clinical events with their electrophysiologic correlates. This is a highly effective way to distinguish seizures from nonepileptic events (eg, syncope, psychogenic nonepileptic seizures, paroxysmal movement disorders) and to detect nonconvulsive seizures in patients with altered level of consciousness. Ambulatory continuous EEG monitoring is also available to obtain longer periods of EEG data in the outpatient setting, ideally capturing the spells that are under evaluation to determine if they are seizures.

NERVE CONDUCTION STUDIES/ELECTROMYOGRAPHY

NCS uses electrical impulses and recording electrodes applied to the skin to evaluate conduction along peripheral nerves. EMG uses small needles inserted into muscles to evaluate muscular electrical activity. Both the NCS and the EMG components of the tests are typically performed when an NCS/EMG is ordered; the combined test is often simply referred to as an *EMG*. NCS/EMG studies are used for localization and diagnosis within the peripheral nervous system (see Chapters 24 and 25); for example, to distinguish radiculopathy from mononeuropathy (see Chapter 24), determine the site and severity of nerve compression (eg, to evaluate for carpal tunnel syndrome; see Chapter 24), determine whether a peripheral neuropathy is axonal or demyelinating (see Chapter 24), evaluate for disorders of the neuromuscular junction such as myasthenia gravis (see Chapter 25), and assess for changes suggestive of muscle disease (ie, myopathy; see Chapter 25).

NCS/EMG can be performed on any (or all) of the extremities, and different techniques are used depending on the differential diagnosis being investigated. Therefore, when ordering NCS/EMG, the precise clinical question should be placed in the consult so the electromyographer can plan the study accordingly.

When cervical or lumbosacral radiculopathy is suspected clinically, MRI of the spine is generally a more informative test than NCS/EMG since NCS/EMG cannot assess the dorsal (sensory) roots, although the EMG may be abnormal in patients with radiculopathy.

NCS/EMG may reveal subclinical conditions not related to the patient's presentation, such as mild carpal tunnel syndrome at the wrist, ulnar neuropathy at the elbow, or cervical or lumbosacral radiculopathy, and so results should be interpreted in the context of the patient's history and examination.

Performance and interpretation of NCS/EMG require highly specialized training. Reports should therefore be interpreted in light of the abovementioned considerations, and the study should be repeated if there is ambiguity of the result.

SUMMARY

Neurodiagnostic tests include neuroimaging, CSF analysis, and electrophysiologic tests of the brain (EEG) and peripheral nervous system (NCS/EMG). Determining which test(s) to order is based on the presumed localization, mechanism, and differential diagnosis of a patient's symptom(s) determined from the history and examination and must always be interpreted within the clinical context since incidental or ambiguous findings may be obtained. Further details about the tests discussed in this chapter can be found in the discussions of the approach to the evaluation of neurologic symptoms throughout Section 2 and the diagnosis of neurologic diseases in Section 3.

CHAPTER

5

Approach to the Patient With Cognitive Symptoms

Vijay K. Ramanan

INTRODUCTION

Cognitive symptoms such as memory difficulty are common in clinical practice. These symptoms may represent normal aging, primary neurologic disease, neurologic complications of a medical illness, or a psychiatric condition. Acute cognitive changes require an urgent search for acute neurologic conditions (eg, stroke, seizure, meningitis, encephalitis) or an acute toxic or metabolic precipitant. Chronic impairments in cognition may be due to reversible underlying medical etiologies (eg, vitamin B_{12} deficiency, hypothyroidism), psychiatric conditions (eg, depression), or may be caused by neurodegenerative disease (eg, Alzheimer disease, dementia with Lewy bodies, frontotemporal

dementia; see Chapter 18). The term *dementia* refers to the development of cognitive changes severe enough to affect activities of daily living (ADLs). The term *mild cognitive impairment* refers to cognitive changes that do not affect ADLs. Both dementia and mild cognitive impairment are syndromes that can have a variety of underlying etiologies. The goal of the evaluation of a patient with cognitive symptoms is to determine which cognitive domains are affected, the impact of the cognitive changes on the patient's life, and whether these symptoms are due to a reversible etiology or an underlying neurodegenerative disease.

COMMON CLINICAL PRESENTATIONS

Cognitive symptoms may be relayed by patients themselves or by their family, friends, or caregivers. It can often be helpful for patients or care partners to describe a few representative examples of observed cognitive symptoms. For instance, patients with memory symptoms may ask repeated questions or forget important details from recent events. The characteristics of these examples can help differentiate a memory deficit from a deficit in another cognitive domain.

For example, "forgetting" the names of objects could represent a language problem (aphasia); "forgetting" how to perform specific tasks or use objects may represent apraxia.

In some cases, patients report cognitive symptoms without objective deficits on bedside cognitive testing. In most patients, these subjective cognitive concerns are due to lifestyle or environmental factors (eg, stress) or personality traits (eg, introspection, heightened attentiveness, rumination, or worry) rather than medical or neurologic disease. However, close clinical follow-up is important since some subjective cognitive symptoms may reflect early signs of a neurodegenerative disease that are too subtle to detect with objective cognitive testing. When objective cognitive impairment is present on bedside testing, a thorough evaluation to identify its underlying cause(s) must be undertaken.

DOMAINS OF COGNITIVE FUNCTIONING

The principal cognitive domains include executive functioning, memory, language, visuospatial function, and praxis. These domains are supported by networks of functionally connected brain regions that may be affected by particular neurologic conditions.

Executive functioning includes attention (the ability to sustain focus), working memory (the ability to hold and manipulate information over a brief time interval), cognitive flexibility (the ability to shift between mental tasks or sets), and inhibitory control (the ability for reasoning to suppress automatic responses). These functions allow individuals to effectively plan, prioritize, multitask, and make decisions. In daily life, executive dysfunction may manifest with difficulties in utilizing devices or appliances, balancing checkbooks, maintaining hobbies, managing work tasks, or resisting scams. Executive function is subserved by circuits connecting the frontal lobes with regions throughout the brain. Conditions that can affect executive function include behavioral variant frontotemporal dementia (bvFTD), vascular dementia, and the dysexecutive variant of Alzheimer disease.

Memory refers to the ability to recall events, facts, and action sequences. In daily life, memory difficulties can manifest as asking repeated questions or lack of recall for recent conversations or life events. Memory is subserved by the limbic system, which includes the hippocampus, amygdala, cingulate cortex, and related structures. Memory can be impaired in Alzheimer disease, dementia with Lewy bodies, or other dementias, or more transiently in transient global amnesia and transient epileptic amnesia.

Language refers to the ability to communicate through speech (or sign language in individuals who are deaf) or writing. Difficulty with communication can be due to impairment in language (aphasia), impairment in speech articulation (dysarthria or speech apraxia), or as part of broader difficulties with mentation (cognitive communication deficits). In daily life, language difficulties can manifest as difficulties naming objects, finding the precise words to complete sentences, or mixing up yes/no or left/right answers to questions. Language is subserved by frontal and temporal regions in the left cerebral hemisphere in right-handed and most left-handed individuals. Aphasia is most commonly caused by stroke in the left middle cerebral artery territory but can also be seen in neurodegenerative conditions such as primary progressive aphasia.

Visuospatial function refers to the ability to perceive and process objects in space. Visuospatial functions are required for navigation, recognition of familiar people, and detection of objects within a visual field. In daily life, difficulties with visuospatial functioning can manifest as getting lost in familiar places or not attending to people or objects in one's field of view. Visuospatial functions are supported by the primary visual pathways (extending from the eyes to the occipital cortex) in connection with the parietal cortex. Visuospatial functioning is impaired in dementia with Lewy bodies, Alzheimer disease, and stroke in the posterior cerebral artery territory.

Praxis refers to the ability to plan and sequence skilled movements. Apraxia can manifest in daily life as difficulty dressing or utilizing tools despite preserved strength and coordination. Apraxia is typically seen with lesions of the parietal or frontal regions, and can be seen in Alzheimer disease, dementia with Lewy bodies, corticobasal syndrome, and stroke.

CLINICAL APPROACH

History

Ideally, the history from a patient with cognitive symptoms should include input from both the patient and a reliable collateral source who knows the patient well, such as a family member or caretaker. Key features of the history include determining the nature of the symptoms, their effect on the patient's ADLs, and the time course of symptom onset and evolution. The medical history should include background on education and occupation, current medications (with particular attention to sedating and psychiatric medications), coexistent psychiatric or sleep symptoms, and family history of cognitive disorders.

Elucidating the cognitive domain(s) affected can be challenging. Patients or care partners who report difficulty with memory should be asked about the types of information that are forgotten: forgetting recent conversations suggests short-term memory difficulties, forgetting how to use devices or appliances may reflect executive dysfunction or apraxia, and forgetting words could indicate aphasia. Reports of difficulties with communication should be further explored by requests for examples: challenges with object naming or spelling may indicate a language problem (aphasia), which often has a distinct differential diagnosis compared to changes in the sound and/or rate of speech (dysarthria or speech apraxia).

Inquiring when the patient last seemed to have normal mental functioning can help clarify the time course since mild earlier symptoms may be de-emphasized in the initial report in favor of more recent overt difficulties impacting daily life. Here, it can be helpful to prompt the patient and care partner to recall functioning around a specific time point (eg, 1 year ago, during a memorable trip, or near a major holiday). Using example hand gestures or drawings (eg, of a gradual trend downward, a sudden drop followed by stabilization, or variability with ups and downs) can help clarify the trajectory. Elucidating the time course of onset and evolution helps prioritize the differential diagnosis. Chronic progressive cognitive decline is highly suggestive of neurodegenerative disease, especially in older individuals. Transient or fluctuating symptoms should prompt consideration of metabolic, immune-mediated (primary autoimmune or paraneoplastic), or epileptic conditions. Abrupt onset (ie, seconds to days) of symptoms favors vascular etiologies, trauma, or systemic metabolic mechanisms. Subacute onset of dementia over months (referred to as *rapidly progressive dementia*) can be caused by systemic conditions, medications or toxins, immune-mediated conditions, Creutzfeldt-Jakob disease, and atypically rapidly progressive forms of neurodegenerative disease such as Alzheimer disease, dementia with Lewy bodies, and corticobasal syndrome.

Examination

The general medical examination can identify clues to a systemic disease that could cause or contribute to cognitive symptoms (eg, jaundice suggesting hepatic encephalopathy, proptosis or pretibial myxedema suggesting thyroid disease). A comprehensive neurologic examination should be performed to evaluate for focal features that may indicate a structural brain lesion causing cognitive changes (eg, neoplasm, chronic subdural hematoma), parkinsonism (which is common in dementia with Lewy bodies but can also be seen in other neurodegenerative dementias), apraxia (which is common in Alzheimer disease but can also be seen in other neurodegenerative dementias or with structural lesions), or myoclonus (which is common in Creutzfeldt-Jakob disease but can also be seen in other neurodegenerative dementias and metabolic disorders).

The patient's cognition and behavior can be observed in how they provide the history and their interpersonal interactions with staff and accompanying family members. When the patient presents for evaluation of cognitive concerns, standardized cognitive screening assessments can be used to provide insights into the presence, severity, and pattern of any cognitive impairment. Such tools also provide a baseline to follow up over time. Examples of screening tools include the Mini-Mental State Examination (MMSE), Short Test of Mental Status (STMS; also known as the *Kokmen*), and Montreal Cognitive Assessment (MoCA). The STMS is free to use (in contrast to the licensing/certification fees required for the MMSE and MoCA) but could be affected by cultural and language differences; the MoCA is available in multiple languages.

Compared to the widely used MMSE, the MoCA has better sensitivity, but the score should be contextualized in terms of the patient's years of education so as not to overdiagnose cognitive impairment. Nomograms exist for the estimated conversion of scores across some of these tools.[1,2] Abnormal scores on these tests in a patient with at least 12 years of education are MMSE ≤26/30, STMS ≤ 34/38, or MoCA ≤24/30. However, a highly educated individual may score above these cutoffs but still have cognitive impairment sufficient to cause a meaningful decline in job performance. More subtle deficits of this nature can be elicited by referring the patient for formal neuropsychological testing, which includes up to several hours of detailed assessments of the various domains of cognition.

Neuropsychological testing is particularly useful when the presence and/or severity of cognitive impairment cannot be clearly elucidated by the history and bedside examination. Neuropsychological testing can also provide more granular data on the domain-specific pattern of impairment, which can suggest particular diagnoses. For example, predominantly amnesia (short-term memory difficulty) is seen most commonly with Alzheimer disease, predominant aphasia is common in frontotemporal degenerative diseases, and prominent visuospatial dysfunction is common in dementia with Lewy bodies. However, neither cognitive screening assessments nor neuropsychological testing are sufficient to make etiologic diagnoses. The overarching goal of the history and examination is to define the syndrome in order to prioritize further investigations.

DIAGNOSTIC EVALUATION

Initial evaluation of patients with cognitive deficits should include laboratory testing for potentially reversible systemic etiologies and neuroimaging to evaluate for brain lesions or specific patterns of findings associated with particular neurodegenerative diseases. In addition, if the history suggests a potential sleep disorder, referral for a sleep study should be considered, and if the history suggests a potential psychiatric disorder, a psychiatry referral should be considered. Laboratory testing generally includes a comprehensive metabolic panel, complete blood cell count, vitamin B_{12} level (along with methylmalonic acid level if vitamin B_{12} level is borderline low), and thyroid-stimulating hormone. HIV and syphilis testing should be considered in patients at risk for these conditions. Brain imaging evaluates for subdural hematoma, mass lesion (eg, neoplasm), chronic sequelae of cerebrovascular disease (as can be seen in vascular dementia), or patterns of regional atrophy suggestive of neurodegenerative disease (see Chapter 18). Magnetic resonance imaging (MRI) of the brain is more sensitive than computed tomography (CT) for subtle abnormalities. If the diagnosis is unclear after this initial testing, nuclear imaging (eg, positron emission tomography [PET]) and/or cerebrospinal fluid (CSF) testing can be considered (discussed further in Chapter 18).

SUMMARY

Cognitive concerns are common among patients, and potential etiologies are diverse, including systemic, psychiatric, and neurologic conditions. A careful history and examination is important to determine the types of cognitive deficits present and possible etiologies. Evaluation should focus on both potentially reversible etiologies of cognitive changes and underlying neurologic diseases, targeted at the specific clinical syndrome and time course of symptom onset (Figure 5.1). Diagnosis and treatment of particular etiologies of cognitive impairment, such as neurodegenerative disease, are discussed in Chapter 18.

Define the Clinical Syndrome

History
- Descriptions and examples from patient and collateral source
- Symptom features: onset, duration, course, character, severity
- General level of functioning (eg, activities of daily living)

Examination
- Observations of comportment and interpersonal interactions
- General physical and neurologic examination
- Cognitive screening assessment (eg, MMSE, MoCA)

Evaluate for Etiology/Etiologies

Standard diagnostics
- Blood tests: CBC, CMP, vitamin B$_{12}$, TSH
- Structural neuroimaging: brain MRI (preferred) or head CT
- Symptom-based referrals (eg, Sleep Medicine, Psychiatry)

Advanced diagnostics
- Nuclear imaging (eg, fluorodeoxyglucose or amyloid PET)
- Cerebrospinal fluid testing (eg, neurodegenerative disease biomarkers, inflammatory markers, neural antibody panels)

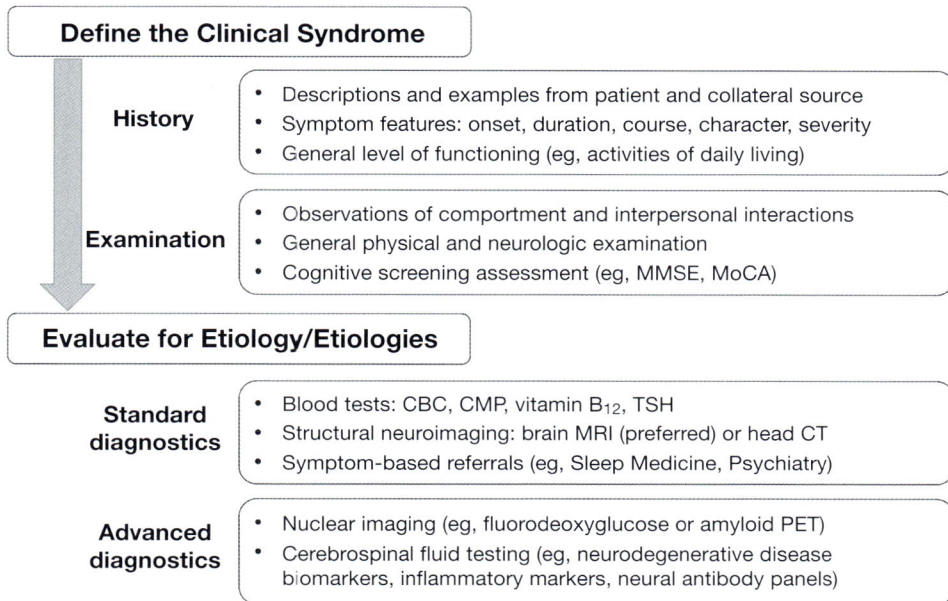

FIGURE 5.1 Framework for evaluating cognitive symptoms. CBC, complete blood count; CT, computed tomography; CMP, comprehensive metabolic panel; MMSE, Mini-Mental State Examination; MoCA, Montreal Cognitive Assessment; MRI, magnetic resonance imaging; PET, positron emission tomography; TSH, thyroid-stimulating hormone.

EDITORS' KEY POINTS

▶ The term *dementia* refers to the development of cognitive changes severe enough to affect ADLs. The term *mild cognitive impairment* refers to cognitive changes that do not affect ADLs.

▶ The goal of the evaluation of a patient with cognitive symptoms is to determine which cognitive domains are affected, the impact of the cognitive changes on the patient's life, and whether these symptoms are due to a reversible etiology or an underlying neurodegenerative disease.

▶ Standardized cognitive screening assessments can be used to provide insights into the presence, severity, and pattern of cognitive impairment and can also provide a baseline to follow up over time in patients with cognitive concerns.

▶ Initial evaluation of patients with cognitive deficits should include laboratory testing for potentially reversible systemic etiologies (eg, comprehensive metabolic panel, complete blood cell count, vitamin B$_{12}$ level, thyroid-stimulating hormone, and HIV and syphilis testing if indicated) and brain MRI to evaluate for causative brain lesions or specific patterns of atrophy associated with particular neurodegenerative diseases; CSF testing and nuclear imaging (eg, PET) can also be considered.

▶ The principal cognitive domains include executive function, memory, language, visuospatial function, and praxis. These domains are supported by networks of functionally connected brain regions that may be affected by particular neurologic conditions.

▶ Executive function refers to the ability to plan, prioritize, multitask, and make decisions and is subserved by circuits connecting the frontal lobes with regions throughout the brain.

▶ Memory refers to the ability to recall events and facts. Memory difficulties can manifest as asking repeated questions and a lack of recall for recent events. Memory is subserved by the limbic system, which includes the hippocampus, amygdala, cingulate cortex, and related structures.

▶ Language refers to the ability to communicate through speech or writing. Difficulty with communication can be due to either impairment in language (aphasia) or impairment in speech articulation (dysarthria or speech apraxia). Language difficulties can manifest as difficulties naming objects or finding the precise words to complete sentences. Language is subserved by frontal and temporal regions in the left cerebral hemisphere in right-handed and most left-handed individuals.

▶ Visuospatial functioning refers to the ability to perceive and process objects in space. Difficulties with visuospatial functioning can manifest as getting lost in familiar places or not attending to people or objects. Visuospatial functions are subserved by the primary visual pathways and the parietal cortex.

▶ Praxis refers to the ability to plan and sequence skilled movements. Apraxia can manifest in daily life as difficulty dressing or utilizing tools despite preserved strength and coordination and is typically seen with lesions of the parietal or frontal regions.

REFERENCES

1. Townley RA, Syrjanen JA, Botha H, et al. Comparison of the short test of mental status and the Montreal cognitive assessment across the cognitive spectrum. *Mayo Clin Proc.* 2019; *94*(8):1516-1523.

2. Tang-Wai DF, Knopman DS, Geda YE, et al. Comparison of the short test of mental status and the mini-mental state examination in mild cognitive impairment. *Arch Neurol.* 2003; *60*(12):1777-1781.

CHAPTER 6

Approach to the Patient With a Disorder of Consciousness

Sara C. LaHue

INTRODUCTION

Consciousness was defined by Plum and Posner as "the state of full awareness of the self and one's relationship to the environment."[1] Disorders of consciousness are classified by how severely they affect alertness and by the time course of symptom onset. The two most commonly encountered acute disorders of consciousness are delirium and coma. The *Diagnostic and Statistical Manual of Mental Disorders* (Fifth Edition; *DSM-5*) characterizes delirium as an acute, fluctuating disturbance in attention, awareness, and cognition distinct from one's baseline and not better explained by a preexisting neurocognitive disorder.[2] Coma is defined as unarousable unresponsiveness, meaning that a stimulus does not provoke a response or provokes only a reflexive response.[1] Acute deficits in consciousness whose severity falls between drowsiness and coma include obtundation and stupor, although overlap exists, and these terms should generally be avoided due to lack of precision. Acute disorders of consciousness, if persistent, can become subacute or chronic disorders of consciousness that include a minimally conscious state (characterized by severely impaired consciousness with evidence of preserved awareness of oneself or environment) and a persistent vegetative state (defined as intermittent wakefulness without awareness).[1] A number of other terms are often used to describe acute disorders of consciousness, including *encephalopathy, acute confusional state, acute brain failure*, and *altered mental status*, but these are considered nonspecific, and professional guidelines recommend against their use.[3]

Delirium and coma are clinical states with a broad differential diagnosis, including both medical and neurologic etiologies (Table 6.1). A systematic search for the underlying cause is therefore essential. Although delirium and coma are clinically distinct states that require different approaches to the bedside examination, there is significant overlap in the diagnostic evaluation of these two conditions.

TABLE 6.1	Common Precipitants of Disorders of Consciousness

Precipitant category	Example
Vascular	Posterior reversible encephalopathy syndrome (PRES)
	Stroke (ischemic or hemorrhagic; arterial or venous)
	Subarachnoid hemorrhage
Infectious	Neurologic (eg, cerebral abscess, encephalitis, meningitis)
	Systemic (eg, pneumonia, urinary tract infection)
Toxic	Intoxication or overdose
	Mediation use (prescription, over the counter, supplements)
	Toxins (eg, carbon monoxide, cyanide)
	Withdrawal
Traumatic	Fat embolism
	Posttraumatic encephalopathy
	Intracranial hemorrhage
Autoimmune	Acute disseminated encephalomyelitis
	Autoimmune limbic encephalitis
	Systemic lupus erythematosus
Metabolic	Electrolyte abnormalities (eg, hypo/hypernatremia, hypercalcemia, hypermagnesemia, hyperglycemic nonketotic coma)
	Endocrine abnormalities (eg, adrenal crisis, hypo/hyperglycemia, hypo/hyperthyroidism, pituitary apoplexy)
	Hyperammonemia
	Hypoxia, hypercarbia
	Uremia
	Vitamin deficiencies (eg, thiamine)
Iatrogenic[a]	Day/night dysregulation and sleep deprivation
	Limited mobility (eg, use of restraints, urinary catheters)
	New medications as part of clinical care, or polypharmacy (eg, anticholinergics, antihistamines, benzodiazepines, cephalosporin antibiotics, chemotherapy, immunotherapy, steroids)
	Pain
	Sensory deprivation (eg, hearing or vision impairments)
Neoplastic	Intracranial neoplasm (primary or metastatic)
	Paraneoplastic encephalitis
Neurodegenerative[b]	Creutzfeldt-Jakob disease
Seizure	Nonconvulsive status epilepticus
	Postictal state
	Status epilepticus

[a]Aside from new medications, these are more likely to cause delirium than coma.
[b]Other neurodegenerative diseases, such as Alzheimer disease, dementia with Lewy bodies, are considered to be predisposing factors to delirium as opposed to precipitating factors. While dementia is more likely to predispose to delirium rather than coma, late-stage dementia may lead to coma.
Reprinted from LaHue SC, Douglas VC. Approach to altered mental status and inpatient Delirium. *Neurol Clin.* 2022;40(1):45-57, with permission from Elsevier.

COMMON PRESENTATIONS AND SYMPTOMS

Delirium

Delirium in hospitalized adults is extremely common, diagnosed in approximately 20% of general medical patients, 50% of postoperative patients (making delirium the most common surgical complication in older adults), and 85% of critically ill patients.[4,5] There is also growing recognition that delirium is a prevalent complication of acute illness in children.[6] While the symptoms of delirium may be transient, delirium in adults is associated with numerous short- and long-term negative outcomes, including increased hospital length of stay, emergency department (ED) visits and hospital readmission, institutionalization, new and accelerated cognitive decline, and mortality.[7,8]

Despite its prevalence, delirium is often underdiagnosed due to its fluctuating course, potential subtlety of symptoms if superimposed on baseline dementia, and the frequent lack of hospital-wide systematic screening programs despite their documented benefits. One of the most widely used tools to screen for delirium is the Confusion Assessment Method (CAM).[9] The CAM assesses four fundamental features of delirium: (1) acute onset and fluctuating course, (2) inattention, (3) disorganized thinking, and (4) altered level of consciousness.[9] Delirium is diagnosed if patients have both one and two, as well as either three or four. Several versions of the CAM exist, including a validated version adapted for mechanically ventilated patients in the intensive care unit (CAM-ICU).[10] There are a variety of delirium assessment tools available depending on the patient population, training of the examiner, and time allotted for examination.[11,12]

Risk factors for delirium can be divided into predisposing and precipitating factors. A predisposing factor is one that precedes the onset of delirium by at least 1 month (eg, advanced age, dementia), whereas a precipitating factor is an acute or a subacute event occurring in the month prior to the onset of delirium (eg, acute illness, sleep deprivation, electrolyte imbalance).[13] In a systematic review of 315 delirium studies, 33 predisposing and 112 precipitating factors were associated with delirium in adults.[13] Given these large numbers, delirium prevention programs require a multipronged approach. For example, the first evidence-based delirium prevention model, the Hospital Elder Life Program (HELP), leverages a multidisciplinary team to enact a multicomponent, nonpharmacologic intervention centered on frequent reorientation, cognitively stimulating activities (especially social activities), sleep-wake cycle regulation, early mobilization, nutrition support, and adaptations for hearing or visual impairments.[14,15] Delirium is preventable in as many as 40% of cases with the use of such programs, which are also associated with reduced hospital length of stay, cost, and 30-day readmission for patients.[16,17] Although numerous clinical trials have tested pharmacologic interventions for delirium, there is currently no medication approved by the US Food and Drug Administration (FDA) for this purpose.

Coma

Coma must be distinguished from conditions such as locked-in syndrome, akinetic mutism, and psychogenic unresponsiveness. In locked-in syndrome, the patient is alert but appears comatose due to the inability to speak or move the limbs. This is most commonly caused by a vascular insult to the brainstem (specifically the pons) causing damage to the motor pathways while sparing upper brainstem projections that maintain consciousness. The pathways that control vertical eye movements and blinking are also often spared, and patients may be able to communicate through blinking or vertical eye movements. Therefore, any patient who appears comatose should be repeatedly asked to open and close their eyes and look up and down in order to screen for locked-in syndrome.

In akinetic mutism, an individual may be alert with intact cranial nerve functions but be unable to speak or move their limbs. The patient may appear awake, including reliably tracking the examiner with their eyes or looking toward a sound, but will not be able to follow commands, speak (mutism), or initiate purposeful movements (akinesia). Akinetic mutism can be due to damage to the prefrontal or premotor areas that are responsible for movement initiation, the thalamus, or cingulate gyrus, and may be seen in various conditions affecting these regions, including traumatic brain injury, stroke, delayed posthypoxic leukoencephalopathy, and Creutzfeldt-Jakob disease.

Psychogenic unresponsiveness is a diagnosis of exclusion. This diagnosis is made by demonstrating that both cerebral hemispheres and the reticular activating system within the brainstem are intact through a careful physical examination, and, if needed, brain imaging demonstrating no explanatory structural lesion and electroencephalogram (EEG) demonstrating wakefulness. Symptoms are varied and may include lack of response to verbal or noxious stimulation, sustained staring, eye closure with resistance to attempted eye opening by the examiner, and absence of movement despite normal tone and reflexes. Causes of psychogenic unresponsiveness include catatonia, fugue states, and functional neurologic disorders. In catatonia, sustained abnormal movements, including grimacing, posturing, rigidity, waxy flexibility, and oppositional paratonia (gegenhalten) in response to passive movement, may be observed.

Lastly, in patients who appear unable to open their eyes, it is important for the examiner to assess for apraxia of eyelid opening, which is the inability to initiate voluntary eyelid opening. This can be evaluated for by manually opening the patient's eyelids to look for preserved eye movements despite inability to open the eyes. Apraxia of eyelid opening can be seen in neurodegenerative conditions and after significant brain injuries (eg, stroke, traumatic brain injury), including in patients with retained alertness.

NEUROANATOMY AND PATHOPHYSIOLOGY

Consciousness and sleep-wake transitions are maintained by the ascending reticular activating system, a network of neurons that project from the upper brainstem diffusely throughout the cerebral hemispheres (bilateral thalami and cerebral cortex) through the neurotransmitters acetylcholine, dopamine, norepinephrine, histamine, and serotonin.

When coma is caused by a structural lesion, the two possible lesion localizations are (1) the upper brainstem (midbrain or pons) affecting the ascending reticular activating system and (2) the bilateral cerebral hemispheres. A unilateral hemispheric lesion can result in coma if it causes a mass effect on either the contralateral cerebral hemisphere or the brainstem (eg, herniation). Elevated intracranial pressure due to hydrocephalus can cause coma without a structural lesion in the brain parenchyma. Coma is also commonly caused by systemic conditions or toxic substances affecting cerebral metabolism and neuronal activity in networks supporting wakefulness.

CLINICAL APPROACH

An acute change in mental status is a medical emergency that warrants a rapid, systematic evaluation. The evaluation of patients with delirium and patients in coma overlaps substantially and so these are discussed together with mention of particular aspects specific to

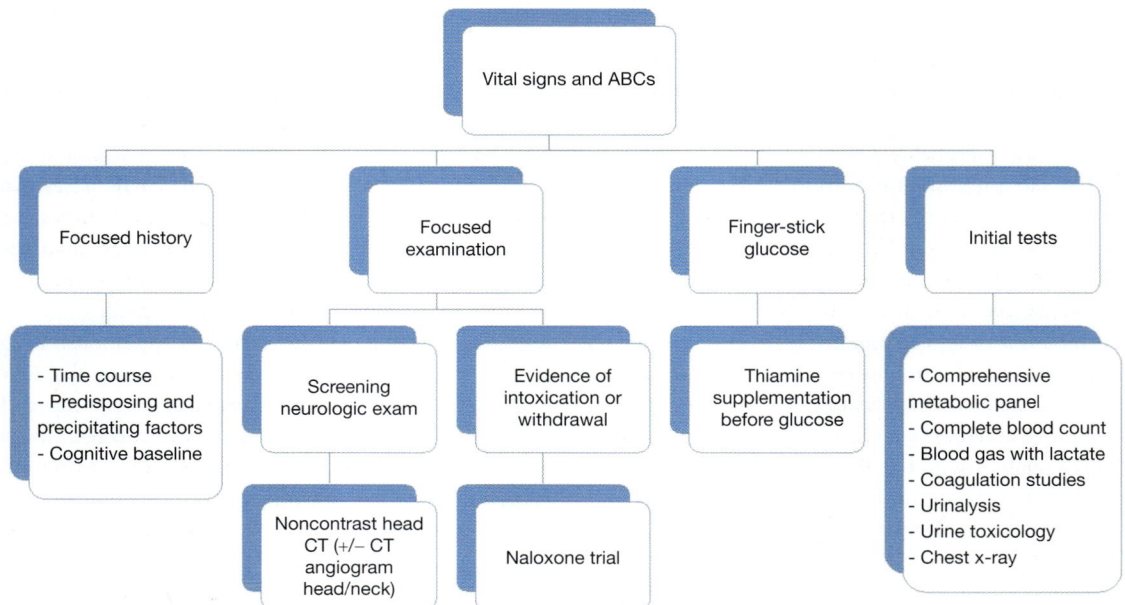

FIGURE 6.1 Initial evaluation of disorders of consciousness. ABC, airway, breathing, circulation; CT, computed tomography.

one or the other where relevant (Figure 6.1). A focused history detailing the specific timeline and context surrounding the change in mental status is key for formulating the differential diagnosis. However, the patient is unlikely to be able to provide the history, so the clinician must obtain collateral information from the patient's family, caregiver, other witnesses, and medical professionals, including the circumstances of the patient's acute change and any preceding symptoms, recent illnesses or trauma, prior medical history (including history of prior cognitive impairment), medications, and potential drug or toxic exposures.

The initial assessment of a patient with altered consciousness is centered on the identification and treatment of life-threatening conditions. The key components of this initial assessment are best described using the primary advanced cardiovascular life support (ACLS) survey mnemonic "ABCDE," which stands for: airway, breathing, circulation, disability (eg, neurologic assessment), and exposure (eg, examination). This primary survey should occur in tandem with obtaining an updated set of vital signs and evaluation for cardiac arrhythmia or hypotension (which may cause cerebral hypoperfusion), hypoxemia, hypothermia, or fever. Finger-stick blood glucose should be obtained to assess for hypoglycemia or hyperglycemia, both of which can cause altered consciousness. If hypoglycemia is discovered, intravenous thiamine supplementation should be administered before glucose repletion to reduce the risk of Wernicke encephalopathy, which can be caused by alcohol use disorder, malnutrition, bariatric surgery, and hyperemesis gravidarum. Naloxone should be administered if opiate overdose is possible, clues to which include pinpoint pupils and decreased respiratory rate. Opiate overdose is an important consideration for both patients presenting to the ED and hospitalized patients receiving opiates for perioperative pain control who are at risk for accidental iatrogenic overdose. In addition, screening laboratory tests should include a comprehensive metabolic panel, blood gas with lactate, complete blood cell count, coagulation studies, a urine sample for urinalysis and toxicology screening, a chest x-ray, and consideration of head CT (head CT should be obtained in all cases of coma; in cases of delirium, it should be considered if there are focal findings on the neurologic examination or no other provoking cause is apparent).

General Physical Examination

In addition to assessing adequate airway, breathing, and circulation, a focused general physical examination may reveal important clues to guide management. Examination of the head may reveal trauma, icteric sclera concerning for liver disease, or a tongue laceration suggestive of seizure. Resistance to passive neck flexion suggests meningeal irritation (meningismus), which can occur in meningitis and subarachnoid hemorrhage. Auscultation of the heart may reveal a murmur suggestive of endocarditis. Auscultation of the lungs may indicate infection or volume overload. Hyperventilation can be seen in sepsis or liver failure, Cheyne-Stokes respirations may be observed in the setting of heart failure or increased intracranial pressure, and hypoventilation may be seen in opiate overdose. An abdominal examination may reveal ascites or hepatomegaly signifying liver disease, which may result in hepatic encephalopathy. A skin examination may reveal jaundice concerning for liver disease, rash suggestive of meningitis or thrombotic thrombocytopenia purpura, abnormal bruising concerning for a coagulopathy or an injury, or puncture marks suggestive of intravenous drug use.

Neurologic Examination

The goal of the neurologic examination in patients with altered consciousness is to determine whether there are any focal findings to suggest an underlying structural brain lesion, such as deficits in particular cognitive domains, abnormal brainstem reflexes, or asymmetries in the motor, sensory, or reflex examination. In patients with altered consciousness due to a nonstructural systemic or toxic etiology, the neurologic examination usually lacks focal abnormalities.

Scales that measure levels of arousal allow for consistent communication between providers and trending clinical trajectories over time. The most commonly used score for arousal is the Glasgow Coma Scale (GCS; Table 6.2), which assigns a numeric value to the three categories of eye opening and motor and verbal responses.[18] The Full Outline of UnResponsiveness (FOUR) Score is an alternative scale with the addition of a brainstem reflex category.[19] In the ICU, the Richmond Agitation-Sedation Scale (RASS) is often

TABLE 6.2 Glasgow Coma Scale (GCS)	
Glasgow Coma Scale category	**Score**
Eye opening	
Spontaneous	4
Response to verbal command	3
Response to pain	2
No eye opening	1
Best verbal response	
Oriented	5
Confused	4
Inappropriate words	3
Incomprehensible sounds	2
No verbal response	1
Best motor response	
Obeys commands	6
Localizing response to pain	5
Withdrawal response to pain	4
Flexion to pain	3
Extension to pain	2
No motor response	1

used and provides a scale ranging from "unarousable sedation (−5)" to "combative (+4)." While helpful, these scales are distinct from diagnostic tools for delirium and are no substitute for a detailed neurologic examination to assess for subtle findings that may provide clues to a focal lesion or systemic condition. Here, we discuss strategies for examining a delirious adult, with an emphasis on mental status, followed by a systematic approach to examining a comatose adult.

Mental Status Examination

Evaluating a patient's level of arousal is a key aspect of the neurologic examination since the level of arousal will determine the patient's ability to participate in the rest of the neurologic examination. If a patient is alert, cognitive modalities such as attention, memory, and language can then be assessed (see Chapter 3). Inattention is one of the hallmarks of delirium and can significantly affect performance on other domains of the mental status examination. Common bedside tests of attention include reciting the months of the year backward, reciting a list of numbers spoken by the examiner forward and backward (digit span), and variations on a psychomotor vigilance test wherein the patient is read

a series of letters and asked to indicate (eg, by tapping) when the target letter (eg, "A") is spoken. Mild deficits in attention are unlikely to significantly impact an examiner's ability to perform a neurologic examination; however, moderate or severe attention difficulties may impair even attending to (and thus, correctly following) examination instructions, which can be challenging for the examiner and the patient. Inattention may also impair performance on memory and language testing. Both immediate and delayed recall will be affected if the patient is unable to attend to the stimulus they are being asked to retain. While inattention is less likely to affect object naming or verbal fluency, or result in paraphasic errors or neologisms, inattention may affect aspects of language, including repetition, comprehension, and maintaining linear speech content.

There are several strategies one can use to facilitate examining an inattentive patient who is unable to consistently follow commands. Important information can be gleaned by observing the patient in a calm and quiet environment, including the content of their spontaneous speech, whether the patient appears preoccupied with internal stimuli (which might suggest hallucinations), and whether they track stimuli appropriately or neglect one side. The overall symmetry of spontaneous face and limb movements, and the existence of abnormal movements, can also be observed. Strength and coordination can be further assessed through social graces (eg, shaking hands), or through classic games that involve hand clapping (eg, pat-a-cake). Examination maneuvers that involve touching the patient or potentially startling the patient (eg, blink to threat to check visual fields by rapidly moving the hand toward the eye) should be reserved for later in the examination because they may disturb the patient and affect their level of participation.

If the patient is unarousable to stimulation, it will not be possible to assess mental status in detail. In this case, the examiner should confirm that the patient does not open their eyes to verbal command or painful stimulus, nor does the patient provide a verbal response or move to command. If the patient is on sedation, this should be held (if possible), allowing for sufficient time for the medication effect to be eliminated depending on renal and hepatic function in order to obtain a neurologic examination that best reflects the abilities of the patient (as opposed to being clouded by medication effects). The examiner should also verify whether the patient is receiving, or has recently received, paralytics since this will affect all parts of the neurologic examination except for pupil reactivity. Once it is clear that the patient is comatose, a neurologic examination designed to be performed without the need for patient participation can be completed.

Cranial Nerve Examination

All cranial nerves can be assessed in a patient who is comatose except cranial nerves 1 (olfactory), 11 (accessory), and 12 (hypoglossal). Cranial nerves 2 and 3 are evaluated through the pupillary light reflex. Pupils that are abnormal in size but symmetric are often due to a toxic/metabolic etiology. For example, bilateral constricted ("pinpoint") pupils can be seen with opiate overdose, and bilateral dilated pupils can be seen with serotonergic, anticholinergic, or sympathomimetic drugs. Note that bilateral pinpoint pupils can also be seen in pontine lesions due to disruption of the oculo-sympathetic pathway ("pontine pupils"). Asymmetric pupillary size (anisocoria) can be caused by a lesion affecting cranial nerve 3 (eg, posterior communicating artery aneurysm, uncal herniation), a lesion affecting the oculosympathetic pathway (Horner syndrome), or asymmetric exposure to nebulizer treatment; for discussion of anisocoria, see Chapter 12.

Cranial nerves 3 (oculomotor), 4 (trochlear), 6 (abducens), and 8 (vestibulocochlear) can be tested by passive head movement (ie, the doll's eyes maneuver) to assess the vestibulo-ocular reflex: The eyes should move conjugately in the opposite direction of the head rotation. If the reflex is absent, the eyes will remain in the midline position and move in the same direction as the head is turned. The absence of the vestibulo-ocular reflex suggests brainstem dysfunction, which may be due to a lesion or from pharmacologic sedation. This test should not be performed in patients with cervical spine injury; in such cases, cold caloric testing (instilling cold water in the external auditory canal) can be performed (as long as the tympanic membrane is intact). Conjugate gaze deviation (deviation of both eyes to one side) could indicate stroke, seizure, or other focal brain pathology.

Cranial nerves 5 and 7 can be evaluated through the corneal reflex. The corneal reflex is assessed by stimulating the cornea, preferably with a droplet of saline to avoid potential injury from repetitive use of a cotton swab with serial assessment in patients who are comatose. The corneal reflex may be absent with sedation and in coma due to toxic/metabolic etiologies. Absence on one side only suggests a brainstem lesion at the level of the pons. Cranial nerve 7 can also be assessed by observing grimacing during noxious stimulation to evaluate for any asymmetry in facial movement.

Cranial nerves 9 and 10 can be evaluated by the gag reflex. In intubated patients, this can be assessed using an oral suctioning device. Since the gag reflex is a noxious stimulus, this maneuver may also trigger motor movements of the arms and legs, which can be observed for symmetry.

Motor Examination

For a patient who is comatose, the motor examination begins with observing for the presence and symmetry of spontaneous abnormal movements (eg, myoclonus), muscle bulk, and muscle tone. Multifocal, asynchronous muscle jerks (eg, myoclonus) may be caused by conditions such as uremia, hyperammonemia, medications (eg, cefepime, opiates, gabapentin), and hypoxic-ischemic injury due to cardiac arrest. Rhythmic movements may indicate seizure activity. Reduced muscle bulk may indicate malnutrition and risk for nutritional deficiencies that can cause encephalopathy, such as thiamine deficiency. Rigidity can be seen in neuroleptic malignant syndrome, whereas flaccid tone can be seen in limbs affected by peripheral nervous system disease, acute stroke, or acute spinal shock. Asymmetries in tone, movement, or reflexes are highly suggestive of a nervous system lesion.

Movements that are purposeful tend to cross to the other side of the body ("cross the midline"), may move toward a stimulus (so as to move the noxious stimulus away), or actively withdraw from a noxious stimulus. Reflexive movements to noxious stimulation ("posturing") can be divided into flexor (decorticate) and extensor (decerebrate). Flexor (decorticate) posturing refers to involuntary flexion of the arms, which often occurs due to dysfunction involving the cerebral hemispheres or the midbrain. Extensor (decerebrate) posturing refers to involuntary extension of the arms that may indicate dysfunction involving the brainstem below the level of the red nucleus (which is located in the midbrain). How the patient moves in response to pain (withdrawal, flexor posturing, extensor posturing, or no movement) is incorporated in both the GCS and FOUR scores.

DIAGNOSTIC EVALUATION

Additional testing is warranted if the cause of altered mental status is not determined by the initial history, physical examination, or basic laboratory results (Figure 6.2). Both delirium and coma are syndromes, not diseases, and require evaluation for the underlying etiology. The mnemonic VITAMINS will ensure that the most life-threatening etiologies are evaluated: vascular, infectious, traumatic/toxic, autoimmune, metabolic, iatrogenic, neoplastic/neurodegenerative, and seizure (Table 6.1). However, as these broad categories indicate, the workup for disorders of consciousness can become an overwhelming, expensive, and potentially invasive pursuit fraught with false positives and ambiguous results. Therefore, a focused systematic approach informed by clinical suspicion is essential to determine which patients may require

tests such as neuroimaging, lumbar puncture, EEG, and/or blood tests.

In an adult with delirium without any obvious focal neurologic findings on physical examination, it may be reasonable to initially focus the workup on blood and urine tests before pursuing head imaging. These include a comprehensive metabolic panel (with particular attention to glucose, sodium, and renal and liver function), complete blood cell count, blood gas with lactate, medication concentration levels, extended toxicology screen, and vitamin B_{12} level. Ammonia should be checked in patients with liver disease, evidence of liver enzyme abnormalities, or who use medications that are hepatically metabolized; hyperammonemia of unclear etiology may be due to a portosystemic shunt or a urease-producing bacterial infection. HIV and syphilis testing should be obtained if serostatus is unknown. In select patients, tests of thyroid and adrenal function may be warranted, in addition to other autoimmune screens for systemic lupus erythematosus (SLE) or Sjögren syndrome; in patients with known SLE, disease activity should be screened for with antinuclear antibodies, anti-double-stranded DNA antibodies, and complement levels.

Although patients may develop delirium due to myriad nonneurologic systemic etiologies, they could also have aphasia, amnesia, or neglect as the cause of their confusion, all of which are caused by focal

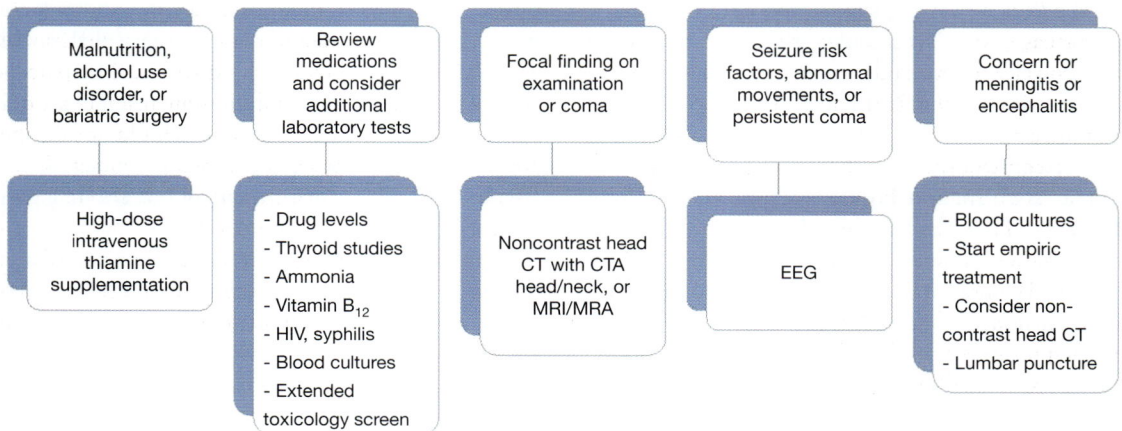

FIGURE 6.2 Subsequent evaluation for the etiology of disorders of consciousness. CT, computed tomography; CTA, computed tomography angiography, EEG, electroencephalography; MRA, magnetic resonance angiography; MRI, magnetic resonance imaging.

brain lesions that must be evaluated for and treated. Although most strokes present with focal deficits, strokes in certain regions (thalamus, inferior division right middle cerebral artery, posterior cerebral artery) or diffuse small emboli can present as confusion without clear focal features. Focal features may be hard to elicit on examination if the patient is confused, and performing an accurate and thorough neurologic examination in confused patients is challenging. For these reasons, a noncontrast CT of the head may be an appropriate component of the evaluation in patients with delirium, especially if initial blood and urine tests are unrevealing, or if the neurologic examination cannot be adequately performed.

When evaluating a comatose adult, urgent head imaging should always be obtained along with blood and urine testing. A noncontrast CT of the head is an appropriate initial screening test for abnormalities such as hydrocephalus, hemorrhage, or a large mass. CT angiography of the head and neck should also be obtained to evaluate for basilar artery thrombosis if clinically suspected. MRI of the brain should be pursued if an initial head CT and blood work do not reveal an obvious explanation for a patient's coma.

In a patient with delirium or coma of unclear etiology, EEG should be obtained to evaluate for nonconvulsive seizures. This is especially important for patients who are comatose, since not only can coma be caused by nonconvulsive status epilepticus but the conditions that may cause coma (eg, intracranial hemorrhage, encephalitis, metabolic derangements) can also cause nonconvulsive status epilepticus. Some patients with nonconvulsive status epilepticus have no clinical symptoms aside from impaired or fluctuating level of consciousness or coma, whereas others may exhibit subtle eye deviation, nystagmus, myoclonus of the face or limbs, or automatisms such as lip smacking. However, nonconvulsive status epilepticus can only be diagnosed by EEG. In addition to being used to detect nonconvulsive status epilepticus, EEG may also demonstrate findings consistent with a metabolic etiology for coma, such as generalized triphasic waves.

A lumbar puncture should be performed to evaluate for central nervous system infection if clinically indicated, and may also be abnormal in patients with inflammatory or neoplastic conditions of the central nervous system. If there is concern for subarachnoid hemorrhage and head CT is normal, lumbar puncture can be used to evaluate for blood in the cerebrospinal fluid. If there is concern for meningitis, empiric treatment should not be delayed while awaiting lumbar puncture. A head CT to evaluate for a structural lesion that could increase the risk of herniation should be obtained before pursuing a lumbar puncture in patients with altered mental status, focal neurologic deficits, seizure, immunocompromise, or age older than 60 years.[20] Note that an elevated cell count and elevated protein are not specific for infection and can be seen in inflammatory conditions; even decreased glucose can be seen in noninfectious conditions such as carcinomatous involvement of the meninges. The prevalence of autoimmune encephalitis is now approaching that of infectious encephalitis, so cerebrospinal fluid evaluation should also include tests that may indicate an inflammatory disorder such as oligoclonal bands, immunoglobulin G index (both in CSF and serum), and autoantibody panels.

SUMMARY

Disorders of consciousness, such as delirium and coma, are common and can be due to a multitude of life-threatening and reversible conditions. A detailed neurologic examination should be performed to evaluate for focal deficits that could indicate a neurologic etiology for the disorder of consciousness. Additional evaluation should include blood tests, urine toxicology, and neuroimaging, and, in some instances, EEG and lumbar puncture. Delirium should ideally be prevented, but if it arises, a comprehensive search for the cause and rapid treatment is essential to improve patient outcomes. Patients in coma should similarly be comprehensively evaluated for neurologic and systemic etiologies as well as followed with serial neurologic examinations to assess for emergence from coma.

FUNDING

Dr Sara C. LaHue is supported by R03AG074035 from the National Institute on Aging, A137420 from the Larry L. Hillblom Foundation, P30 AG044281 from the NIA to the UCSF Claude D. Pepper Older Americans Independence Center, the UCSF Bakar Aging Research Institute, and 2023-0240 from the Doris Duke Foundation.

EDITORS' KEY POINTS

▶ The two most common acute disorders of consciousness are delirium and coma.

▶ Delirium is an acute, fluctuating disturbance in attention typically seen in the setting of acute systemic illness or toxic-metabolic disorders.

▶ Coma is a state of unarousable unresponsiveness. When coma is caused by a structural lesion, the two possible lesion localizations are (1) the upper brainstem (midbrain or pons), affecting the ascending reticular activating system, and (2) the bilateral cerebral hemispheres. Coma is also commonly caused by systemic or toxic/metabolic conditions diffusely affecting the brain.

▶ Acute disorders of consciousness may evolve into chronic states such as a minimally conscious state (characterized by severely impaired consciousness with evidence of preserved awareness of oneself or environment) and a persistent vegetative state (defined as intermittent wakefulness without awareness).

▶ The initial assessment of a patient with altered consciousness is centered on the identification and treatment of life-threatening conditions that can cause irreversible brain dysfunction if not treated expeditiously.

▶ The goal of the neurologic examination in patients with altered consciousness is to determine whether there are any focal findings to suggest an underlying structural brain lesion, such as deficits in particular cognitive domains, abnormal brainstem reflexes, or asymmetries in the cranial nerve, motor, sensory, or reflex examinations.

▶ When evaluating a patient in coma, emergent head imaging (typically CT) is needed, along with blood and urine testing for systemic etiologies. Brain MRI should be performed if head CT and blood work do not reveal an obvious explanation for a patient's coma. In patients with delirium or coma of unclear etiology, EEG should be obtained to evaluate for nonconvulsive seizures. Lumbar puncture to evaluate for CNS infection should be considered if the patient has a fever, is immunocompromised, or if no etiology is determined on systemic and neuroimaging evaluation.

▶ Patients with locked-in syndrome are alert but appear comatose due to the inability to speak and quadriplegia. Locked-in syndrome is most commonly caused by a vascular insult to the brainstem (specifically the pons) resulting in damage to the motor pathways while sparing dorsal structures that maintain consciousness. Patients with locked-in syndrome may be able to communicate through blinking or vertical eye movements.

REFERENCES

1. Posner JB, Plum F, eds. *Plum and Posner's Diagnosis of Stupor and Coma.* 4th ed. Oxford University Press; 2007.
2. *Diagnostic and Statistical Manual of Mental Disorders.* DSM Library. Accessed February 1, 2022. https://dsm.psychiatryonline.org/doi/book/10.1176/appi.books.9780890425596
3. Slooter AJC, Otte WM, Devlin JW, et al. Updated nomenclature of delirium and acute encephalopathy: statement of ten societies. *Intensive Care Med.* 2020;46(5):1020-1022.
4. Marcantonio ER. Delirium in hospitalized older adults. *N Engl J Med.* 2017;377(15):1456-1466.
5. Gleason LJ, Schmitt EM, Kosar CM, et al. Effect of delirium and other major complications on outcomes after elective surgery in older adults. *JAMA Surg.* 2015;150(12):1134-1140.
6. Traube C, Silver G, Reeder RW, et al. Delirium in critically ill children: an international point prevalence study. *Crit Care Med.* 2017;45(4):584-590.
7. Goldberg TE, Chen C, Wang Y, et al. Association of delirium with long-term cognitive decline: a meta-analysis. *JAMA Neurol.* 2020;77(11):1373-1381.
8. Witlox J, Eurelings LS, de Jonghe JF, Kalisvaart KJ, Eikelenboom P, van Gool WA. Delirium in elderly patients and the risk of postdischarge mortality, institutionalization, and dementia: a meta-analysis. *JAMA.* 2010;304(4):443-451.
9. Inouye SK. Clarifying confusion: the confusion assessment method: a new method for detection of delirium. *Ann Intern Med.* 1990;113(21):941-958.
10. Ely EW, Inouye SK, Bernard GR, et al. Delirium in mechanically ventilated patients: validity and reliability of the confusion assessment method for the intensive care unit (CAM-ICU). *JAMA.* 2001;286(21):2703-2710.
11. De J, Wand APF. Delirium screening: a systematic review of delirium screening tools in hospitalized patients. *Gerontologist.* 2015;55(6):1079-1099.

12. Bellelli G, Morandi A, Davis DHJ, et al. Validation of the 4AT, a new instrument for rapid delirium screening: a study in 234 hospitalised older people. *Age Ageing*. 2014;*43*(4):496-502.

13. Ormseth CH, LaHue SC, Oldham MA, Josephson SA, Whitaker E, Douglas VC. Predisposing and precipitating factors associated with delirium: a systematic review. *JAMA Netw Open*. 2023;*6*(1):e2249950.

14. Inouye SK, Bogardus ST, Charpentier PA, et al. A multicomponent intervention to prevent delirium in hospitalized older patients. *New Engl J Med*. 1999(9);*340*:669-676.

15. Hshieh TT, Yang T, Gartaganis SL, Yue J, Inouye SK. Hospital elder life program: systematic review and meta-analysis of effectiveness. *Am J Geriatr Psychiatry*. 2018;*26*(10):1015-1033.

16. Inouye SK, Westendorp RGJ, Saczynski JS. Delirium in elderly people. *Lancet*. 2014;*383*(9920):911-922.

17. LaHue SC, Maselli J, Rogers S, et al. Outcomes following implementation of a hospital-wide, multicomponent delirium care pathway. *J Hosp Med*. 2021;*16*(7):397-403.

18. Teasdale G, Jennett B. Assessment of coma and impaired consciousness: a practical scale. *Lancet*. 1974;*2*(7872):81-84.

19. Wijdicks EFM, Bamlet WR, Maramattom BV, Manno EM, McClelland RL. Validation of a new coma scale: the FOUR score. *Ann Neurol*. 2005;*58*(4):585-593.

20. Hasbun R, Abrahams J, Jekel J, Quagliarello VJ. Computed tomography of the head before lumbar puncture in adults with suspected meningitis. *N Engl J Med*. 2001;*345*(24):1727-1733.

CHAPTER 7

Approach to the Patient With Transient Neurologic Symptoms

Elan L. Guterman and Megan B. Richie

INTRODUCTION

Patients commonly report transient neurologic symptoms that last minutes to hours and then resolve. These symptoms can include weakness, numbness, visual disturbances, dizziness, abnormal movements, alterations of consciousness, or altered cognition. Such symptoms may occur once or may be recurrent. The differential diagnosis for transient neurologic symptoms ranges from benign conditions such as benign paroxysmal positional vertigo and migraine to life-threatening conditions such as transient ischemic attack (TIA) and seizure. Given that the examination is usually normal after a spell (or between spells) of transient neurologic symptoms when a patient presents for evaluation, a detailed history is essential to characterizing the symptoms in order to guide the appropriate diagnostic evaluation. This chapter focuses on distinguishing between common causes of transient neurologic symptoms such as migraine, TIA, seizure, and syncope, as well as less common causes such as transient focal neurologic episodes associated with cerebral amyloid angiopathy.

CLINICAL APPROACH

History

The key elements of the history in a patient with transient neurologic symptoms are the type, distribution, duration, and frequency of the symptoms.

In taking a history from a patient with transient neurologic symptoms, clinicians should determine the primary symptom and whether symptoms occurred once or as recurrent spells. If the spells are recurrent, the clinician should determine whether the events are stereotyped, meaning that each occurrence is the same as previous occurrences. Recurrent, stereotyped spells are particularly suggestive of seizure. TIAs may recur but are rarely stereotyped since it would be improbable for the same vascular territory to be affected in the same way on several occasions unless there is a fixed distal stenosis. Migraines are generally recurrent and may be similar from event to event in an individual patient but can vary (eg, whether aura is present or not, type of aura). In patients who experience a combination of symptoms during an episode, it is useful to focus on the most prominent symptom to formulate an initial differential diagnosis, using the additional symptoms to refine the differential diagnosis.

For patients with transient motor, sensory, or visual disturbances, clinicians should determine whether the patient has experienced positive symptoms, negative symptoms, or both. Positive symptoms are defined by the presence of a finding that should normally be absent, whereas negative symptoms are defined as the absence of a neurologic function that should normally be present. For example, positive motor symptoms include twitching or jerking, whereas negative motor symptoms include weakness; positive sensory symptoms include tingling and burning, whereas negative sensory symptoms include numbness; positive visual symptoms include flashing lights or hallucinations, whereas negative visual symptoms include visual loss. Generally, transient positive neurologic symptoms occur in seizure and migraine, whereas transient negative neurologic symptoms occur in TIA, although this is not a perfect rule. Specific elements to characterize each type of transient neurologic symptom are detailed here and summarized in Table 7.1.

Transient Weakness

Transient weakness can arise from momentary disruption of the motor pathways anywhere along their course through the central and peripheral nervous system (see Chapter 11). The key aspects of the history are the distribution of the weakness and any associated symptoms beyond weakness.

Transient unilateral weakness suggests a process involving the brain, such as TIA, migraine, or seizure. Transient weakness due to a TIA commonly involves the face and arm, or face, arm, and leg; weakness may be accompanied by dysarthria or aphasia, depending on the region(s) of the brain affected by the TIA. Transient weakness due to a migraine is rare and most commonly accompanied by headache; migraine-associated weakness may precede headache and last through the period of headache. Transient weakness due to a seizure is typically postictal (Todd paralysis), occurring after the shaking, jerking, or twitching of the affected limb(s). Postictal weakness due to seizure can vary in length depending on the length of seizure activity but may last many hours after a prolonged seizure. The weakness of TIA is typically brief, lasting minutes to a few hours.

Focal weakness that comes on after activity (fatigable weakness) could suggest myasthenia gravis, particularly if weakness is of the eyes (causing diplopia) or eyelid(s) causing ptosis.

Transient bilateral weakness is generally less suggestive of a primary neurologic disorder than is transient unilateral or focal weakness. Many systemic conditions, such as infections, metabolic disorders, and endocrine disease, can cause a generalized feeling of weakness (asthenia) without impairment in muscular strength. Rare neurologic causes of transient bilateral weakness include transient spinal cord ischemia (usually due to aortic disease), metabolic myopathies (eg, glycogen storage disorders), and periodic paralysis (eg, hyperkalemic and hypokalemic periodic paralysis, both genetic conditions). Myasthenia gravis can cause fatigable bilateral weakness, but the eye muscles are almost always involved at presentation as described earlier.

Transient Sensory Symptoms

Like weakness, transient sensory symptoms can arise from momentary disruption of the sensory tracts anywhere along their course (see Chapter 10). Thus, like transient weakness, causes of transient numbness include TIA, migraine, and seizure. However, nerve root or nerve conditions can also cause episodic transient numbness or paresthesias in the affected region. TIA, migraine, and seizure typically cause unilateral sensory symptoms affecting the face, arm, and/or leg; radiculopathy and mononeuropathy typically cause focal sensory symptoms in one aspect of one limb; and polyneuropathy typically causes bilateral sensory symptoms most prominent in the distal extremities. Polyneuropathy-related sensory symptoms are most commonly persistent rather than transient but can wax and wane. TIA classically causes numbness (lack of sensation), whereas migraine and seizure usually cause positive sensory symptoms such as tingling. The sensory symptoms in TIA are often sudden and maximal at onset, whereas those of migraine and seizure tend to spread from one region to another over seconds to minutes. Transient sensory symptoms related to migraine and seizure are often distinguished by whether there is an associated headache (as typically occurs in migraine) and whether the symptoms are stereotyped (as occurs in seizure).

Transient focal neurologic episodes (formerly called *amyloid spells*) are a less common cause of transient sensory symptoms that occur in patients with cerebral amyloid angiopathy, a condition of the cerebral blood vessels in older individuals that predisposes to intracerebral hemorrhage. These episodes present as brief periods (minutes to hours) of spreading tingling, numbness, or weakness, or, less commonly, language disturbances. Cerebral amyloid angiopathy is diagnosed by the presence of cerebral microhemorrhages and/ or superficial siderosis (blood products in the cerebral sulci) on magnetic resonance imaging (MRI) sequences sensitive for blood (susceptibility-weighted images [SWIs] and gradient recalled echo [GRE] sequences).

Transient Visual Disturbances

Transient visual disturbances can be characterized as positive or negative: positive visual symptoms include flashing lights and hallucinations, whereas negative visual symptoms refer to visual loss.

Common causes of positive transient visual disturbances include migraine aura, focal seizures, and ophthalmologic disorders such as retinal detachment. Migraine auras are usually abstract, linear, or geometric in shape, and often appear monochromatic (black and white). Patients may describe seeing flashing lights, dots, zigzags, or cross-hatched lines that often arise in a single visual field (left or right) and grow or move across visual space, after which a typical migraine headache arises. The positive visual phenomena of focal seizures are often colorful, associated with motion across visual space, and can be geometric and simple (occipital lobe focus) or, rarely, more complex (temporal lobe focus). A critical clue that positive visual phenomena may be epileptic in origin is that spells of positive visual symptoms are stereotyped (patient reports seeing the same visual phenomenon on every occurrence) and restricted to a single hemifield (ie, left or right). Visual hallucinations due to neurologic disorders other than migraine and focal seizure can result from a wide range of conditions, including delirium, neurodegenerative dementia, narcolepsy, midbrain lesions (peduncular hallucinations), or vision loss itself (also known as *release hallucinations* or *Charles Bonnet syndrome*). The visual hallucinations associated with these disorders vary in appearance and can be complex (eg, of people or animals).

When patients describe transient visual loss in one eye, they may be describing loss of one visual field in both eyes (in which case the visual field deficit persists with either eye covered) or visual loss limited to a single eye (true monocular visual loss). Clinicians should, therefore, not only ask whether the visual loss was in one eye or both but also ask whether the patient covered either eye during the episode to determine whether the contralateral eye was also affected; in practice, however, this can be challenging to distinguish on history.

Transient monocular visual loss (visual loss limited to a single eye) suggests transient ischemia of the retina or optic nerve, whereas transient visual field loss suggests transient ischemia of the brain. Patients should be evaluated for vascular risk factors (hypertension, diabetes, hyperlipidemia, smoking), arterial disease of the head or neck (carotid disease) for monocular visual loss; carotid or vertebrobasilar disease for unilateral visual field loss, and cardiac conditions such as atrial fibrillation for monocular or unilateral visual field loss. In patients older than age 50 with transient monocular visual loss, erythrocyte sedimentation rate (ESR) and C-reactive protein (CRP) should also be obtained to evaluate for giant cell arteritis.

Transient visual loss in both eyes can occur with elevated intracranial pressure and, less commonly, due to transient ischemia of the bilateral occipital lobes. Increased intracranial pressure affects the optic nerves (causing papilledema), and patients may experience brief episodes of monocular or binocular visual obscurations, often described as temporary graying of vision that occurs with Valsalva or bending forward, both of which increase intracranial pressure. In addition to neurologic causes of transient visual loss, ophthalmologic causes should be considered and may require referral to an ophthalmologist for dilated funduscopic examination.

Transient Vertigo or Dizziness

Vertigo is an illusory sensation of movement (usually spinning) arising from vestibular dysfunction in the central nervous system, vestibulocochlear nerve (cranial nerve 8), or inner ear. Vertigo must be distinguished from the less specific symptom of dizziness that can also refer to lightheadedness, imbalance, or anxiety. Vertigo and dizziness should be characterized with respect to whether the symptom is acute or chronic, constant or episodic, and, if episodic, whether it is triggered or spontaneous (Table 7.2). The approach to dizziness and vertigo is discussed further in Chapter 9.

Transient Abnormal Movements

The differential diagnosis of transient abnormal movements includes epileptic seizures, psychogenic

TABLE 7.1	**Clinical Features and Evaluation of Transient Focal Neurologic Symptoms**					
				Key clinical features		
Etiology	**Onset**	**Recurrent**	**Stereotyped**	**Negative symptoms**	**Positive symptoms**	**Diagnostic evaluation**
TIA	Sudden	No[a]	No[a]	Weakness, numbness, vision loss, aphasia	Uncommon	• MRI brain without contrast (CT if MRI is not available) • Evaluate for vascular risk factors. • Vascular imaging of head/neck • Echocardiogram • Cardiac monitoring • Lipid panel • Hemoglobin A_{1c}
Seizure	Spreads	Yes	Yes	Weakness, numbness, loss of consciousness	Shaking, tingling, hallucinations	• Evaluate for provoking factors (see Chapter 17). • MRI brain with and without contrast • EEG
Migraine	Spreads	Yes	Variable	Weakness	Tingling	MRI brain with and without contrast if red flags (see Chapter 8)
Radiculopathy/ Compressive neuropathy	Variable; often possible to trigger	Yes	Yes	Numbness	Tingling, pain	Consider spinal imaging and/or EMG/NCS.
Syncope	Sudden	No	Variable	Tunnel vision, loss of consciousness		Cardiac evaluation with telemetry, echocardiogram, long-term cardiac monitoring
Ischemic causes of vision loss	Sudden	No	No	Monocular partial or complete vision loss	Headache, jaw pain (giant cell arteritis only)	MRI brain and orbit, ESR and CRP for patients older than 50, vascular imaging of the head and neck, echocardiogram, long-term cardiac monitoring

CRP, C-reactive protein; CT, computed tomography; EEG, electroencephalogram; EMG, electromyography; ESR, erythrocyte sedimentation rate; MRI, magnetic resonance imaging; NCS, nerve conduction study; TIA, transient ischemic attack.

[a] TIA may be recurrent if there is a significant vascular lesion (eg, carotid stenosis) or ongoing embolic etiology, and may be stereotyped if the culprit vascular lesion is distal, leading to recurrent ischemia in the same brain region(s).

nonepileptic seizures (PNES), and movement disorders (eg, tremor, myoclonus). Transient abnormal movements should be characterized by the type of movement (eg, shaking, jerking, twitching), which part(s) of the body are involved, whether the movements are unilateral or bilateral, whether there are any provoking factors that bring on the movements (eg, change in position of the affected body part or parts), and whether there is any associated alteration in consciousness. If spells are recurrent, it is critical to determine whether the episodes are stereotyped. If movements are not sufficiently frequent to be observed

in the clinic, patients or observers should be asked to record one or more videos of the abnormal movements for analysis by the clinician.

Seizures are typically recurrent, stereotyped episodes lasting at least 10 seconds, which may or may not be associated with alteration in awareness or complete loss of consciousness. The motor manifestations of seizures are typically rhythmic and synchronous, meaning that the involved regions of the body contract simultaneously. Focal seizures (most commonly due to focal brain lesions) may cause rhythmic jerking of one side of the body with preserved consciousness, whereas seizures that cause bilateral movements are always accompanied by loss of consciousness since bilateral movements indicate epileptic activity in both cerebral hemispheres. Such generalized seizures are also commonly associated with bladder and bowel incontinence, self-injury, and a postictal state of altered consciousness. Seizures are usually stereotyped, recurring with identical or similar manifestations in each instance. Seizures typically arise spontaneously without an associated trigger, although some seizure types may be triggered by an external stimulus such as flashing visual stimuli. For further discussion of seizures and epilepsy, see Chapter 17.

There are important exceptions to these general principles. Frontal lobe seizures have motor manifestations that differ from the classic rhythmic jerking associated with seizures from other areas of the brain, including asymmetric posturing of both arms and legs or complex movements such as bicycling movements of both legs, often associated with a brief change in mental status that rapidly normalizes. Hemifacial spasm is a disorder characterized by unilateral, stereotyped facial twitching that can easily be mistaken for focal seizure but is actually myoclonus caused by compression of the facial nerve (most commonly due to a vascular loop).

PNES represent a type of functional neurologic disorder, meaning that the condition is not due to a structural problem in the nervous system or other neurologic disease. Spells in a PNES resemble epileptic seizures but do not result from epileptiform brain activity. Spells in a PNES typically differ from epileptic seizures in that PNES spells are often variable in nature (as opposed to being stereotyped in epileptic seizures), movements are often asynchronous (as opposed to synchronous muscle contractions in seizure), complex (eg, back arching, side-to-side head movement, and pelvic thrusting, as opposed to rhythmic tonic-clonic movements in epileptic seizures), and waxing and waning (as opposed to rapid on-off or decreasing in intensity over the course of a seizure), and there is often forced eye closure (as opposed to the eyes remaining open in epileptic seizures) and a relatively rapid return to baseline after the event concludes (as opposed to a prolonged postictal state after an epileptic seizure). Spells in PNES are also typically longer than epileptic seizures, can be provoked by specific environmental situations,

commonly occur in the presence of witnesses, and do not respond to antiseizure medications. Finally, while most patients with PNES have a reduction in their level of awareness during an episode, some may still be able to interact during an episode and/or may retain some memory of the episode once it has terminated, neither of which occur with generalized epileptic seizures. Of note, some patients may have both epileptic seizures and PNES, often requiring inpatient video electroencephalographic (EEG) monitoring to diagnose the etiology of different spell types.

Movement disorders are generally relatively easily distinguished from seizures as they are more likely to be able to be observed directly in the clinic. The tremor of parkinsonism may be transient in that it only occurs with rest or sustained posture. An enhanced physiologic or essential tremor may occur only with movement. Tics are more complex movements preceded by an urge and followed by a sense of relief. These and other movement disorders are discussed in Chapters 13 and 19.

Rarer causes of episodic transient abnormal movements include paroxysmal dyskinesias and limb-shaking TIAs. Paroxysmal dyskinesias are a rare group of genetic disorders in which patients report spells of involuntary abnormal movements that may be triggered by sudden movement (paroxysmal kinesigenic dyskinesias) or other triggers (paroxysmal nonkinesigenic dyskinesias) such as alcohol, caffeine, and emotional upset. Limb-shaking TIAs are a rare type of TIA in which there is involuntary irregular shaking of the involved arm and/or leg on one side, usually accompanied by weakness of the same limb(s) and associated with high-grade stenosis of the carotid artery contralateral to the involved limb.

Transient Loss of Consciousness

Transient loss of consciousness is most commonly due to syncope or seizure. Rarer etiologies include vertebrobasilar TIA and transient ventricular obstruction due to a third ventricular mass (eg, colloid cyst). Since loss of consciousness results from global disruption of brain function, patients generally cannot recall these events, requiring collateral history from observers of the event to elicit clinical features (Table 7.3). In certain regions, health care providers may be legally mandated to report patients with loss of consciousness to

TABLE 7.2   Causes of Transient Vertigo and Dizziness

	Onset	Duration	Triggers	Associated symptoms
Brain-related causes				
TIA	Sudden	Minutes	None identified	Cranial neuropathies, numbness, speech disturbance
Migraine	Gradual	Minutes to hours	None identified	Headache (may also have visual or sensory aura)
Peripheral vestibular system-related causes				
BPPV	Sudden	Seconds to minutes	Turning head in particular direction	Nausea/vomiting, imbalance
Ménière disease	Sudden	Minutes to hours	Variable or no trigger	Hearing loss, tinnitus
Cardiac causes				
Orthostatic hypotension	Sudden	Seconds to minutes	Standing from a lying or sitting position	Tunnel vision, warmth
Cardiac arrhythmia	Sudden	Seconds	None, exertion	Palpitations, dyspnea

BPPV, benign paroxysmal positional vertigo; TIA, transient ischemic attack.

the government and the Department of Motor Vehicles to determine whether the patient's driver's license should be temporarily revoked.

Syncope and seizure are two of the most common causes of transient loss of consciousness. Clinicians should characterize the symptoms that occurred before, during, and after the episode to distinguish between the two. Before the loss of consciousness, patients with syncope will report a prodrome of lightheadedness, facial flushing, and/or tunnel vision, whereas patients with seizure either report no symptoms or a stereotyped aura such as a sense of déjà vu, fear, abnormal smell/taste, or nausea. During the loss of consciousness, patients with syncope typically have no movements or brief, convulsive movements lasting up to 10 seconds, whereas patients with seizure typically have prolonged convulsive movements lasting minutes. Syncope-related brief convulsive movements are frequently mistaken for seizure, so it is important to consider other aspects of the history that may help distinguish syncope from seizure. After the loss of consciousness, patients with syncope typically return to their normal mental status within seconds to minutes, whereas patients with seizure typically have a postictal period with a period of lethargy or drowsiness that can last minutes, hours, or even days.

There is a subset of patients with syncope due to a cardiac arrhythmia or structural heart disease who have no premonitory symptoms. Because cardiac arrhythmia and structural heart disease are both risk factors for sudden cardiac death, it is critical to consider these possibilities in any patient who presents with loss of consciousness and complete absence of a prodrome.

A TIA affecting the posterior circulation (vertebral arteries or basilar artery) can cause transient loss of consciousness due to hypoperfusion of the reticular activating system in the brainstem. This loss of consciousness may be accompanied by posturing movements that can be mistaken for seizure. Preceding or concurrent brainstem or cerebellar symptoms (eg, dysarthria, diplopia, vertigo, ataxia, weakness, or sensory loss) or other transient spells of such symptoms should raise concern for vertebrobasilar disease, and computed tomography (CT) angiography or magnetic resonance (MR) angiography of the head and neck should be performed.

Transient Alteration of Cognition

There are certain disorders that cause transiently altered cognition with preserved consciousness. These include PNES, transient focal neurologic episodes in cerebral amyloid angiopathy, dementia with Lewy bodies, and transient global amnesia. PNES can cause mental status changes lasting minutes to hours that are often accompanied by nonstereotyped, asynchronous movements, as described earlier. Transient focal neurologic episodes in patients with cerebral amyloid angiopathy can also present as isolated changes in mental status lasting up to 30 minutes. Dementia with Lewy bodies often causes episodes of inattention, confusion, or somnolence, during which families report the patient is staring blankly into space and having difficulty speaking for hours. Transient global amnesia causes acute-onset impairment in short-term memory characterized by repetitive questioning and lasting up to 24 hours (although typically <8 hours); episodes are often triggered by discrete precipitants such as a highly emotional event, sexual intercourse, or immersion in cold water.

Examination

Most patients with transient neurologic symptoms will be asymptomatic at the time of evaluation and have a normal neurologic examination. However, a detailed examination may reveal subtle focal findings suggestive of an underlying lesion, such as asymmetric reflexes, an upgoing toe (Babinski sign), a pronator drift, or a visual field deficit (see Chapter 3). It is also helpful to ask patients who have recurrent events to try to record them (or have a family member or caregiver record them) by video for clinicians to review. Clinicians can even instruct patients or family members to perform simple maneuvers, such as asking the patient to state their name or look in a particular direction to help further elucidate the level of awareness during the spell.

DIAGNOSTIC EVALUATION

Patients thought to have TIA should undergo evaluation for causes of stroke (see Chapter 16). This should include an MRI of the brain (since the clinical syndrome of TIA [ie, a brief focal neurologic deficit corresponding to a vascular territory] may be due to a small stroke with rapid recovery), imaging of the vasculature of the head and neck (CT angiogram or MR angiogram), echocardiogram, cardiac rhythm monitoring, and testing for vascular risk factors. If there is concern for seizure, brain imaging (preferably MRI) to evaluate for a lesion, laboratory tests for causes of provoked seizures, and an EEG should be obtained (see Chapter 17). In patients with presumed syncope, cardiac evaluation should be obtained.

TABLE 7.3	Clinical Features of Causes of Transient Loss of Consciousness				
	Trigger	**Duration**	**Symptoms**		
			Before	**During**	**After**
Syncope	Variable depending on type	Seconds to minutes	Lightheadedness, facial flushing, tunneling of vision; except cardiac arrhythmia where none identified	May have brief jerking or convulsive movements	Rapid return to baseline
Seizure	None	Minutes	Déjà vu, abnormal smell, head deviation, abnormal posturing	Stereotyped symptoms with a clear onset and offset without waxing/waning	Gradually resolving drowsiness, unilateral weakness, unilateral numbness, speech disturbance
Vertebrobasilar TIA	None	Minutes	May have preceding diplopia, dysarthria, vertigo	May have unilateral weakness and convulsive movements	Rapid return to baseline
Toxic or metabolic disturbance	Patient specific	Minutes to hours	Increasing systemic illness or toxidrome-specific symptoms	May have pupillary abnormalities (eg, pinpoint pupils with opiate toxidrome)	Waxing and waning improvement
PNES	Presence of witnesses, emotional stress	Minutes	Hyperventilation, palpitations, derealization, chest discomfort, dizziness, fear of dying, feeling of choking	Nonstereotyped, asynchronous, complex, waxing and waning	Rapid return to baseline

PNES, psychogenic nonepileptic seizures; TIA, transient ischemic attack.

SUMMARY

The cause of transient neurologic symptoms can be challenging to diagnose since patients are often asymptomatic at presentation. A detailed history can aid in distinguishing between common etiologies such as TIA, seizure, migraine, and syncope, and a careful examination should be performed to look for subtle signs of a focal lesion. When ambiguity remains, patients may be evaluated for multiple etiologies in parallel (eg, causes of both syncope and seizure) or even treated empirically for the most likely etiology in the setting of an indeterminate evaluation (eg, aspirin for a presumed TIA or antiseizure medications for presumed seizures).

EDITORS' KEY POINTS

▶ Common causes of transient neurologic symptoms include migraine, seizure, and TIA.

▶ Since the examination is typically normal after a spell (or between spells) of transient neurologic symptoms, a detailed history including type, distribution, duration, and frequency of the transient symptoms obtained from the patient and/or bystanders is essential to characterizing the spell(s) to guide the diagnostic evaluation.

▶ Transient visual disturbances can be characterized as positive (eg, flashing lights or hallucinations) or negative (ie, visual loss). Positive visual symptoms can be caused by migraine aura, focal seizures, and ophthalmologic disorders such as retinal detachment, whereas negative visual symptoms suggest an ocular problem or a problem along the visual pathway.

▶ Transient abnormal movements may be due to epileptic seizures or movement disorders (such as tremor or myoclonus). Transient abnormal movements should be characterized by the type of movement, which part(s) of the body are involved, whether the movements are unilateral or bilateral, whether there are any provoking factors, and if there is an associated alteration in consciousness.

▶ Seizures are typically recurrent and stereotyped (ie, the same symptoms/signs each time) and may or may not be associated with alteration in awareness.

▶ Transient loss of consciousness can be caused by syncope, seizure, or, rarely, vertebrobasilar TIAs. Collateral history from observers of the event is important to determine the etiology.

CHAPTER 8

Approach to the Patient With Headache

Jessica Ailani

INTRODUCTION

Headache is a common symptom seen in primary care clinics and emergency departments. The causes of headache are broadly divided into primary headache disorders and secondary headache disorders. Primary headache disorders are conditions such as tension-type headache, migraine, and cluster headache that are not caused by an underlying condition. Secondary headache disorders are those caused by an underlying condition, with a broad differential diagnosis, including intracranial processes (eg, meningitis, brain tumor), cranial processes (eg, conditions of the eyes, sinuses), or systemic illness (eg, giant cell arteritis) (Table 8.1). The diagnosis and treatment of primary headache disorders are discussed in Chapter 15. This chapter presents a practical approach for evaluating patients with headache.

COMMON PRESENTATIONS AND SYMPTOMS

The pain of a headache may be described as dull and aching pain (eg, tension-type headache, headache due to systemic illness), throbbing and pounding (eg, migraine headache), tingling and shooting pain (eg, trigeminal neuralgia or occipital neuralgia), or intense stabbing pain (eg, cluster headache). Patients may report pain involving the entire head (eg, tension headache) or on a particular side (eg, migraine, cluster, hemicrania continua, paroxysmal hemicrania) that may vary from person to person (eg, frontal, temporal, occipital, around the eye, from the neck to the front of the head). Patients may also describe associated features with their headache, such as

TABLE 8.1	Secondary Headache Disorders
Mechanism	**Cause**
Hydrocephalus	Obstruction of ventricular flow of cerebrospinal fluid (eg, mass lesion, meningitis, subarachnoid hemorrhage)
Infection	Meningitis, cerebral abscess, sinus disease, systemic infection
Inflammation	Giant cell arteritis, CNS vasculitis
Space-occupying lesion	Brain tumor, colloid cyst in the third ventricle, cerebral abscess
Vascular	Aneurysm rupture, cervical artery dissection, reversible cerebral vasoconstriction, intracranial hemorrhage, cerebral venous sinus thrombosis, hypertensive emergency
Extracranial	Ocular, sinus, dental, or cervical conditions

phonophobia and photophobia (eg, migraine, meningitis), visual obscurations (eg, migraine aura, elevated intracranial pressure), or autonomic symptoms such as tearing, redness of the eye, or nasal congestion (eg, cluster headache).

headache). Secondary headache can be elicited by direct stimulation of the meninges (eg, meningitis) or by indirect stimulation such as a mass lesion producing increased intracranial pressure triggering activation of the trigeminal pathway causing pain.

NEUROANATOMY AND PATHOPHYSIOLOGY RELATED TO HEADACHE SYMPTOMS

The brain itself has no pain receptors; however, other intracranial structures, such as the meninges and vasculature, are pain sensitive. The experience of headache is caused by activation of the trigeminal nerve, which transmits pain sensation from the face and pain-sensitive intracranial structures. Most headache pain is caused by non-life-threatening conditions that activate the trigeminal system either by a genetically sensitized pathway (eg, migraine and cluster headache) or via the myofascial system (eg, tension-type

CLINICAL APPROACH

The main goal of the history and examination in the evaluation of a patient with headache is determining whether the headache is due to a serious underlying illness (secondary headache disorder) or a primary headache disorder. Red flag features of the headache that raise concern for a secondary cause can be remembered by the mnemonic *SNNOOP 10*, shown in Table 8.2. Patients with red flags on history require neuroimaging. If the patient has no red flags, the goal of the evaluation is to characterize the headache to see which primary headache syndrome it most likely conforms to in order to guide treatment.

TABLE 8.2	SNNOOP10: Headache Red Flags	
S	Systemic symptoms (fever)	Infection, nonvascular intracranial disorder, carcinoid, pheochromocytoma
N	Neoplasm history	Metastasis, brain neoplasm
N	Neurologic deficit or dysfunction (altered mental status, abnormal exam)	Vascular or nonvascular intracranial disorder, brain abscess, other infection
O	Onset of headache, sudden or abrupt	Subarachnoid hemorrhage, cranial vascular disorder, cervical vascular disorder
O	Older age of onset (after 50)	Giant cell arteritis, neoplasm, cranial vascular disorder
P	Pattern change in headache	Neoplasm, cranial vascular or nonvascular disorder
P	Positional headache	Intracranial hypertension or hypotension
P	Precipitated by sneezing, coughing, or exercise	Posterior fossa malformation, Chiari malformation
P	Papilledema	Neoplasm, nonvascular cranial disorder, intracranial hypertension
P	Progressive headache and atypical presentations	Neoplasm, nonvascular cranial disorder
P	Pregnancy or puerperium	Cranial vascular disorder, postdural puncture headache, preeclampsia, cerebral sinus thrombosis, hypothyroidism, anemia, diabetes
P	Painful eye with autonomic features	Posterior fossa pathology, pituitary or cavernous sinus pathology, Tolosa-Hunt syndrome, ophthalmic causes
P	Posttraumatic onset of headache	Acute and posttraumatic headache, subdural hematoma, other headache attributed to vascular cause
P	Pathology of the immune system (eg, HIV)	Opportunistic infections
P	Painkiller overuse	Medication overuse headache

Adapted from Do TP, Remmers A, Schytz HW, et al. Red and orange flags for secondary headaches in clinical practice: SNNOOP10 list. *Neurology.* 2019;92(3):134-144.

History

In a patient who presents with a headache, the history begins with the open-ended question of asking the patient to describe their headaches. Features to note (or ask about if not mentioned in the patient's description) include location(s), quality (eg, pulsating, dull), onset (eg, sudden, indolent), associated symptoms (eg, fever, focal neurologic deficits, autonomic symptoms such as eye tearing and nasal congestion), exacerbating and alleviating factors, whether the headaches are new or have occurred previously, and, if they have occurred previously, whether there has been any change. Symptoms preceding and following the headache should also be asked about, including the presence of migraine aura (eg, flashing lights, visual obscurations, spreading paresthesias preceding or during the headache) or migraine prodromal symptoms (eg, nausea, dizziness, yawning, and/or cognitive or mood changes). The patient should also be asked about any medications they have taken in the past for headache and whether they were effective, the past medical history, and whether there is a family history of headache (migraine and cluster headache tend to run in families).

Red flags in the history concerning for a secondary headache include sudden onset (concerning for a vascular etiology such as subarachnoid hemorrhage or vascular dissection), headaches that are worse in the morning or awaken a patient from sleep (concerning for elevated intracranial pressure), headache associated with cough or exertion (also concerning for elevated intracranial pressure), a change in the quality, severity, or frequency in the headaches over time, new headache symptoms that had not been present previously (eg, a new aura in someone who has never had an aura, prolonged aura, or persistent aura), new headaches after age 50 (concerning for intracranial mass or giant cell arteritis), headache associated with fever (concerning for intracranial infection), headache associated with positional change (worse when supine suggests elevated intracranial pressure; worse when standing suggests low intracranial pressure), and headache associated with jaw claudication, scalp tenderness, and visual symptoms (concerning for giant cell arteritis). Contextual red flags include history of cancer (concerning for brain or leptomeningeal metastases),

immunocompromise (concerning for intracranial infection), and recent weight gain (concerning for idiopathic intracranial hypertension). The presence of any red flag in the history warrants neuroimaging to evaluate for a secondary cause of headache.

Features suggestive of a primary headache disorder include headaches remaining stable in quality, severity, and frequency over the years and particular characteristics diagnostic of specific primary headache disorders (eg, tension, migraine, cluster) discussed in Chapter 15.

Examination

A detailed neurologic examination to assess for any focal deficits and funduscopy to evaluate for papilledema (a sign of elevated intracranial pressure) should be performed in all patients with headache to determine whether there is concern for a secondary cause requiring neuroimaging. Additional features to evaluate include blood pressure, weight (elevated body mass index [BMI] could suggest idiopathic intracranial hypertension), and changes in temporal artery pulse or temporal artery tenderness (in older adults with new headache if giant cell arteritis is a concern).

DIAGNOSTIC EVALUATION

If there are no red flags on history or examination and the patient appears to have a primary headache disorder, no further diagnostic evaluation is indicated. The diagnosis of a primary headache disorder such as tension headache or migraine is based on the clinical history and a normal neurologic examination. Neuroimaging is needed if there are red flags on the history or examination; however, in practice, neuroimaging may also be performed if, after a discussion between the patient and provider, it is felt that neuroimaging would help in reassuring that there is no significant underlying structural condition (noting that imaging holds the risk of identifying incidental abnormalities that may require additional evaluation). Magnetic resonance imaging (MRI) of the brain is the study of choice as it provides a more detailed evaluation than computed tomography (CT) and no radiation is involved, although CT is preferred in emergent settings as it can be more rapidly obtained. Gadolinium contrast should be administered in patients with cancer or immunocompromise to evaluate for metastases or infectious lesions, respectively. Magnetic resonance (MR) venogram should be obtained if there is concern for venous sinus thrombosis (which is a differential diagnostic consideration in the evaluation for a patient with intracranial hypertension). Subtle radiologic signs suggesting elevated intracranial pressure include flattening of the posterior globe, protrusion of the optic nerve head into the vitreous, distension of the optic nerve sheath, empty or partially empty sella, and descent of the cerebellar tonsils. Many patients undergoing brain MRI, including those with migraine, have punctate foci of T2 hyperintensity in the subcortical white matter, which are nonspecific.

Erythrocyte sedimentation rate (ESR) and C-reactive protein (CRP) should be ordered if giant cell arteritis is a consideration. Lumbar puncture should be considered if there is concern for subarachnoid hemorrhage (eg, sudden-onset severe headache, also known as thunderclap headache) or meningitis (headache accompanied by fever and/or neck stiffness).

In patients with persistent headache despite an entirely normal evaluation, it is important to provide reassurance that no underlying structural etiology is present and that primary headache disorders can be effectively treated.

SUMMARY

Headache is a common chief concern with a broad differential diagnosis. The initial evaluation should screen for headache red flags that require further evaluation for an underlying secondary cause of headache with neuroimaging and other testing. If there are no red flags and the evaluation is normal, the history should determine the most likely primary headache syndrome (ie, migraine vs tension-type headache vs others).

The diagnosis and management of primary headache disorders are discussed in Chapter 15.

EDITORS' KEY POINTS

▶ Headaches can be classified as primary headache disorders (eg, tension-type headache, migraine headache, cluster headache) or secondary headache disorders (ie, a precise cause can be identified).

▶ Secondary headaches can be due to intracranial processes (eg, hemorrhage, tumor, meningitis, hydrocephalus), ocular processes, sinus disease, dental conditions, cervical disease, or systemic illness (eg, systemic infection).

▶ Red flags on the history that raise concern for a secondary cause of headache include sudden onset, progressive, worse with change in position (supine vs upright), change in headache quality or frequency in a patient with a history of prior headache, new onset in a patient older than 50 years, associated fever and/or focal neurologic deficits, and headache in a patient with cancer or immunocompromise.

▶ Patients with headache should be evaluated for features on examination that raise concern for a secondary cause of headache such as papilledema and focal neurologic deficits.

▶ Patients with headache red flags on history should undergo neuroimaging (CT for acute-onset headache; MRI for subacute presentation in the outpatient setting).

▶ In patients with no red flags on history and a normal examination who are thought to have a primary headache disorder, the history should characterize the headache with respect to quality, severity, frequency, and accompanying features so as to determine the precise headache type to guide treatment.

CHAPTER 9

Approach to the Patient With Dizziness

Justin L. Hoskin and Terry D. Fife

INTRODUCTION

Dizziness is a frequently encountered symptom in both the outpatient and acute care settings. Dizziness has a broad differential diagnosis, including both neurologic and medical conditions that range from life-threatening diseases such as stroke and cardiac arrhythmia to benign conditions such as benign paroxysmal positional vertigo (BPPV) and reversible medication side effects. Since many conditions that cause dizziness can have normal laboratory and radiologic evaluation, a structured approach to the history and examination is essential to diagnosis. An approach based on a combination of symptom description, timing, triggers, and associated symptoms is presented here. The specific vestibular disorders mentioned in this chapter are discussed in detail in Chapter 22.

HISTORY

Patients may use the term *dizziness* to describe a range of sensations, including vertigo (an illusory sense of motion, such as feeling like the room is spinning), lightheadedness, presyncope (a feeling of almost fainting, often needing to sit or lie down to prevent passing out), imbalance (a sensation of feeling unsteady with fear of falling), or brain fog (a feeling of cloudiness in thinking). Although the symptom of room-spinning vertigo is usually vestibular in origin, some patients with this sensation do not specifically describe spinning, and some patients with nonvestibular causes of dizziness may describe room spinning. Therefore, while the patient's description of the type of dizziness they are experiencing is an important aspect of the history, it is not sufficiently reliable to precisely determine the etiology. More specific elements in the history that are key to elicit are the timing (how often spells occur, how long they last) and triggers (factors that provoke the patient's dizziness). These elements, along with relevant physical examination maneuvers, are encapsulated in the TiTrATE (*Ti*ming, *Tr*iggers, *A*ssociated symptoms and *T*argeted *E*xamination) and ATTEST (*A*ssociated symptoms, *T*iming, *Tr*iggers, *E*xamination *S*igns, and *T*esting) frameworks, contained in helpful reviews on this topic.[1,2]

Description

A sense of room spinning is the most common description given in patients experiencing vestibular conditions affecting the inner ear or nervous system. A feeling of near-faintness as if one is passing out is the most common description given in patients with cardiovascular etiologies of dizziness, such as orthostatic hypotension. Some patients use the word "dizzy" to refer to unsteadiness or imbalance, for which there are many causes, only a few of which are vestibular. As described earlier, these descriptions are helpful to elicit but not specific and should not be relied on exclusively in determining the underlying etiology.

Timing

The patient should be asked about the timing of dizziness onset and evolution: Did the dizziness begin acutely or has it developed chronically? Is the dizziness constant or episodic? If the dizziness is episodic, how long do the symptoms last? Acute-onset continuous dizziness can be caused by posterior circulation stroke, vestibular neuritis, and intoxication. Chronic constant dizziness may be due to a structural lesion in the posterior fossa, medication side effect, or persistent postural-perceptual dizziness. Episodic dizziness can be due to BPPV, migraine, and Ménière disease. With regard to episode length, in BPPV, episodes of dizziness are brief, lasting seconds to minutes, whereas in migraine and Ménière disease, episodes last hours.

Triggers

If the patient reports episodic dizziness, they should be asked if there are any triggers that bring on the symptom. BPPV is triggered by changes in head position that can occur when rolling over in bed or when looking upward (eg, to reach for something on a high shelf). Orthostasis is triggered when the patient goes from supine or seated to standing. Spontaneous episodic dizziness (ie, dizziness with no trigger) can occur in migraine, Ménière disease, vertebrobasilar transient ischemic attack, and cardiac arrhythmia. Patients should also be asked about the timing of taking antihypertensive medications (which may cause or exacerbate orthostasis) and anti-hyperglycemic medications in patients with diabetes (which may cause episodic hypoglycemia). If dizziness is triggered by loud noises, this suggests rare otologic conditions such as superior semicircular canal dehiscence or perilymphatic fistula.

Accompanying Symptoms

Accompanying symptoms to inquire about include hearing loss, tinnitus, headache, and neurologic symptoms. Unilateral hearing loss accompanying dizziness suggests a problem in the inner ear. The combination of hearing loss, tinnitus, and ear fullness with episodic dizziness suggests Ménière disease. Headache accompanying dizziness suggests migraine. Neurologic symptoms (such as diplopia, numbness, weakness, or slurred speech) accompanying dizziness suggest a lesion in the posterior structures of the brain (brainstem and/or cerebellum)—acutely, this could indicate stroke or a demyelinating plaque, whereas chronically, it may suggest a neoplasm.

Putting It All Together

Based on the timing and triggers of the patient's dizziness elicited by history, most patients can be classified as having one of four clinical syndromes[3]:
- Episodic triggered vestibular syndrome: recurrent spells of dizziness that occur in response to a trigger
- Episodic spontaneous vestibular syndrome: recurrent spells of dizziness that occur spontaneously without a trigger
- Acute vestibular syndrome: acute-onset continuous dizziness
- Chronic vestibular syndrome: chronic dizziness lasting more than 3 months

Each syndrome has a particular differential diagnosis (Table 9.1); individual conditions are discussed in Chapter 22.

EXAMINATION

The examination of a patient who is dizzy should include a cardiovascular examination, neurologic examination, and particular neurovestibular examination maneuvers depending on the presenting syndrome.

General Examination

Patients with episodic dizziness triggered by a change in body position should have orthostatic vital signs checked. Orthostatic hypotension is defined as a sustained decrease in systolic blood pressure of

TABLE 9.1	Common Vestibular Syndromes With Definitions and Examples of Each	

Vestibular syndrome	Definition	Common etiologies
Episodic triggered vestibular syndrome	Recurrent spells of dizziness that occur in response to a trigger	• BPPV (trigger: change in head position) • Orthostatic hypotension (trigger: change in body position)
Episodic spontaneous vestibular syndrome	Recurrent spells of dizziness that occur spontaneously without a trigger	• Vestibular migraine • Ménière disease • Posterior circulation transient ischemic attack • Cardiac arrhythmia
Acute vestibular syndrome	Acute-onset, continuous vertigo	• Vestibular neuritis/labyrinthitis • Posterior circulation stroke • Alcohol or drug toxicity • Head trauma
Chronic vestibular syndrome	Chronic vertigo, lasting at least 3 mo	• Persistent postural perceptual dizziness • Bilateral vestibulopathy • Posterior fossa neoplasm • Mal de débarquement syndrome

BPPV, benign paroxysmal positional vertigo.
Reprinted from Bisdorff AR, Staab JP, Newman-Toker DE. Overview of the international classification of vestibular disorders. *Neurol Clin.* 2015;33(3):541-550, with permission from Elsevier.

20 mm Hg or of diastolic blood pressure of 10 mm Hg within 3 minutes of assuming an upright position. Delayed orthostatic hypotension occurs when this decline in blood pressure occurs after 3 minutes or more. With volume depletion or certain medication effects, the drop in blood pressure is often accompanied by at least a 20 beats per minute increase in heart rate; in patients with autonomic failure, there typically will not be a compensatory increase in heart rate. The patient's pulse should be checked for rate and rhythm to assess for cardiac arrhythmia.

General Neurologic Examination

Hearing can be assessed using a screening method such as a finger rub, tuning fork, or whispered voice to compare left and right. This method may be insensitive to subtle or bilateral deficits, so audiogram should be considered if the patient reports hearing loss. Unilateral hearing loss in a patient with dizziness suggests labyrinthitis or Ménière disease.

Patients with dizziness should be examined for any asymmetries in strength, sensation, or coordination with particular attention to evaluating for unilateral limb ataxia, which is associated with a lesion in the ipsilateral cerebellum. This can be assessed with finger-nose and heel-shin testing. Subtle ptosis and miosis (small pupil) along with acute-onset dizziness and ipsilateral ataxia suggests lateral medullary infarction.

Neurovestibular Examination

The most useful components of the neurovestibular examination depend on the clinical syndrome.

In patients with brief episodic dizziness triggered by head movement, BPPV can be diagnosed at the bedside with the Dix-Hallpike maneuver (Figure 9.1). In this test, the patient is asked to turn the head 45° to one side (eg, looking over the left shoulder) and is then rapidly taken from a sitting position to supine with the head hanging over the examination table in the examiner's hands. If there are no symptoms or signs elicited on one side after waiting a few seconds, the test is repeated with the patient looking over the other shoulder. When performing this maneuver on the affected side in a patient with BPPV, the patient will experience dizziness, and the examiner will observe nystagmus that is upbeating and torsional (rotatory) and occurs after a brief latency. Once diagnosed, this condition can also be treated at the bedside with the Epley maneuver (see Chapter 22).

In patients with the acute vestibular syndrome, the differential diagnosis is primarily between posterior circulation stroke and vestibular neuritis. Although magnetic resonance imaging (MRI) is very sensitive for stroke, it may not detect small strokes in the posterior circulation that may cause acute vertigo. A battery of three bedside tests can be used to distinguish between vestibular neuritis and posterior circulation stroke with

Dix-Hallpike maneuver

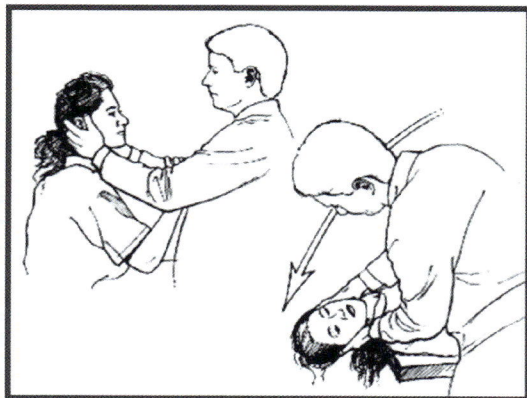

Dix-Hallpike right

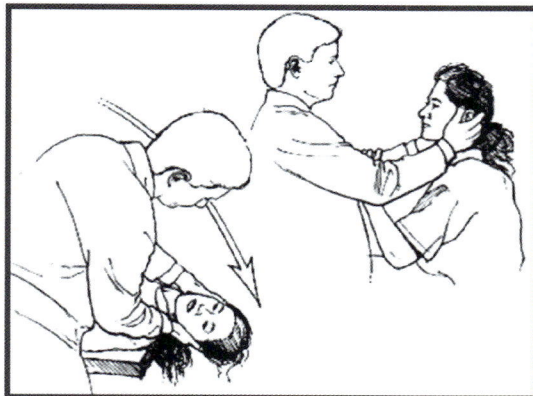

Dix-Hallpike left

FIGURE 9.1 Method for performing the Dix-Hallpike maneuver to evaluate for vertigo and nystagmus in the most common form of benign paroxysmal positional vertigo (BPPV), which involves the posterior semicircular canal. (Used with permission from Barrow Neurological Institute, Phoenix, Arizona.)

high sensitivity and specificity: the head impulse test, evaluation for nystagmus, and the test of skew, which can be remembered by the mnemonic HINTS (*h*ead *i*mpulse, *n*ystagmus, *t*est of *s*kew).[4]

The head impulse test assesses the vestibulo-ocular reflex, which is the ability of the patient's eyes to maintain fixation (eg, on the examiner's nose) while the head is turned briskly in different directions. In patients with a peripheral condition such as vestibular neuritis, this reflex will be impaired, causing a loss of fixation when the head is turned to the affected side, requiring the patient's eyes to make a "catch-up" movement to refocus on the target. In central etiologies of vertigo, such as stroke, the test result is normal. Note that a normal result on the head impulse test is concerning for a serious etiology in the context of the acute vestibular syndrome.

A distinction between two types of nystagmus should be sought in the acute vestibular syndrome. In patients with a unilateral peripheral condition such as vestibular neuritis, the fast phase of nystagmus will beat in only one direction, regardless of the direction of gaze. The direction of the fast phase beats away from the impaired side. In patients with a central etiology of vertigo, nystagmus is direction-changing: The fast phase beats to the left on left gaze and to the right on right gaze. Note that this pattern of direction-changing

nystagmus can also be caused by medications. Spontaneous upbeat, downbeat, or torsional nystagmus is also suggestive of a central etiology.

Skew deviation refers to vertical misalignment of the eyes due to vestibular dysfunction (central or peripheral). This may be apparent at rest but may require covering and uncovering each eye sequentially to evaluate for subtle vertical deviation when each eye is uncovered. The presence of skew suggests a central etiology of acute vertigo (although it is not universally present and can also be seen with peripheral etiologies).

In the acute vestibular syndrome, normal head impulse test, direction-changing nystagmus, or presence of skew deviation suggests stroke and requires urgent neuroimaging. An abnormal head impulse test, nystagmus in only one direction, and absence of skew suggest a peripheral etiology. When performed by specialist examiners, the HINTS examination may be more sensitive than MRI at detecting these posterior strokes,[4] but in day-to-day practice, it remains prudent to consider brain imaging in acute vestibular syndrome if the examiner is not experienced in assessing and interpreting these subtle clinical signs. These findings are summarized in Table 9.2.

Some conditions that cause dizziness may have a normal examination, such as vestibular migraine (even

TABLE 9.2	Summary of HINTS Examination Findings in Central versus Peripheral Etiologies of Acute Vertigo	
	Central etiology	**Peripheral etiology**
Head impulse	Normal—patient's eyes remain fixed with no catch-up saccade seen	Abnormal—corrective saccade (catch-up saccade) after rapid head turn to affected side
Nystagmus	Gaze-evoked and direction changing May be purely vertical or purely torsional	Unidirectional and horizontal Attenuates with fixation
Test of skew	Vertical skew deviation present with the cover-uncover test	No vertical skew

HINTS, head, impulse, nystagmus, test of skew.

during an attack) and Ménière disease between attacks. In such cases, the history guides the differential diagnosis and further evaluation.

DIAGNOSTIC INVESTIGATION

Often, a thorough history and examination are sufficient to diagnose the cause of a patient's dizziness. If dizziness is thought to be cardiac in etiology, electrocardiogram (ECG), prolonged cardiac monitoring, cardiology consultation, and/or echocardiogram should be pursued. In severe or unexplained orthostatic hypotension, autonomic testing should be considered. In patients with associated asymmetric hearing loss or concern for Ménière disease, audiogram should be performed, and MRI of the internal auditory canals to assess for vestibular schwannoma can be considered (although not commonly associated with vertigo). If there are focal neurologic signs on examination, MRI of the brain should be obtained. When there is concern for otologic etiologies, computed tomography (CT) of the temporal bone is the appropriate neuroimaging modality. In patients in whom the cause of dizziness remains unclear after extensive evaluation, vestibular testing with videonystagmography (VNG) can be considered. This test evaluates vestibular function by analyzing eye movements and nystagmus patterns under various conditions, including caloric testing.

SUMMARY

Patients with dizziness can have a wide variety of underlying etiologies that may be neurologic, otologic, cardiac, or medication induced. A history focused on the timing and triggers of dizziness classifies patients into one of four syndromes (Table 9.1). This classification, along with the physical examination, can often allow for a bedside diagnosis. The diagnosis and treatment of particular etiologies of dizziness mentioned in this chapter are discussed further in Chapter 22.

EDITORS' KEY POINTS

▶ The term dizziness may be used by patients to describe vertigo, lightheadedness/presyncope, or imbalance.

▶ The history should attempt to determine what the patient means by dizziness, but there the phenomenon described by the patient (ie, vertigo vs lightheadedness vs imbalance) does not correlate perfectly with the underlying condition.

▶ The history should determine whether the dizziness is acute or chronic, continuous or episodic, triggered or spontaneous (and if triggered what the provoking factor is), and whether there are any accompanying symptoms (eg, diplopia, headache, hearing loss, tinnitus, ear fullness). This helps classify dizziness into four broad categories—acute continuous, chronic continuous, episodic spontaneous, and episodic triggered—that are helpful in determining the underlying diagnosis.

▶ The examination of a patient with dizziness should include assessment for orthostasis, eye movement abnormalities, ataxia, and hearing loss.

▶ When a patient presents with acute continuous vertigo, the primary differential diagnosis is posterior circulation stroke versus vestibular neuritis.

REFERENCES

1. Newman-Toker DE, Edlow JA. TiTrATE: a novel, evidence-based approach to diagnosing acute dizziness and vertigo. *Neurol Clin*. 2015;33(11):577-599.

2. Edlow JA, Gurley KL, Newman-Toker DE. A new diagnostic approach to the adult patient with acute dizziness. *J Emerg Med*. 2018;54(4):469-483.

3. Bisdorff AR, Staab JP, Newman-Toker DE. Overview of the international classification of vestibular disorders. *Neurol Clin*. 2015;33(3):541-550.

4. Kattah JC, Talkad AV, Wang DZ, Hsieh YH, Newman-Toker DE. HINTS to diagnose stroke in the acute vestibular syndrome: three-step bedside oculomotor examination more sensitive than early MRI diffusion-weighted imaging. *Stroke*. 2009;40(11): 3504-3510. doi:10.1161/STROKEAHA.109.551234

CHAPTER 10

Approach to the Patient With Sensory Symptoms

Meabh O'Hare

INTRODUCTION

Sensory symptoms such as numbness and paresthesias are extremely common, arising from a wide range of underlying causes. Sensory symptoms can be caused by a lesion at any level of the nervous system. The distribution of sensory symptoms and other elements of the history and examination guide localization and the subsequent diagnostic evaluation.

NEUROANATOMY AND PATHOPHYSIOLOGY

Somatosensory signals are transmitted from the skin and joints by peripheral nerves. Peripheral nerves are made up of different types of sensory nerve fibers conveying different sensory modalities. Large-diameter myelinated fibers (large fibers) convey discriminative touch sensation, joint position sense, and vibration sense. Small-diameter unmyelinated fibers (small fibers) convey pain and temperature sensation. Groups of nerve fibers carrying sensory information from a specific body region form peripheral nerves, which travel proximally through the relevant plexus (brachial plexus for the upper extremity, lumbosacral plexus for the lower extremity) and then enter the spinal cord through the dorsal nerve roots. At each spinal level, dorsal nerve roots convey sensory information corresponding to a specific region of skin, called a dermatome. As seen in Figures 10.1 and 10.2, the dermatomal maps for individual nerve roots (Figure 10.1) are partially overlapping with, but distinct from, the cutaneous distribution of individual peripheral nerves (Figure 10.2). This is because each nerve contributes to more than one root, and multiple nerves contribute to each root. The distinction between root and nerve sensory maps is clinically helpful for the purposes of localization to a particular root or nerve, as discussed later.

Within the spinal cord, sensory signals ascend in different tracts depending on the sensory modality: Joint position and vibration sense signals travel in the dorsal columns (also called the posterior columns), whereas pain and temperature signals travel in the spinothalamic tracts (also called the anterolateral tracts). Both pathways cross to the contralateral side of the central nervous system, but at different levels: Vibration and proprioception signals from the dorsal columns cross in the lower brainstem, whereas pain and temperature signals destined for the spinothalamic tracts cross almost immediately after entering the spinal cord.

The trigeminal nerve (cranial nerve 5) transmits all sensory information from the face. Sensory signals from the trigeminal nerve arrive in nuclei of the brainstem, cross to the contralateral side, and then ascend alongside the somatosensory pathways from the body in the contralateral brainstem.

Ultimately, all sensory signals from one side of the body (including face, arm, torso, and leg) converge on the contralateral thalamus, and finally travel from there to the primary somatosensory cortex in the parietal lobe.

A lesion anywhere along this pathway can result in sensory symptoms. The site of the lesion along these pathways can be determined from the pattern of sensory symptoms and the presence of associated symptoms or signs (eg, weakness).

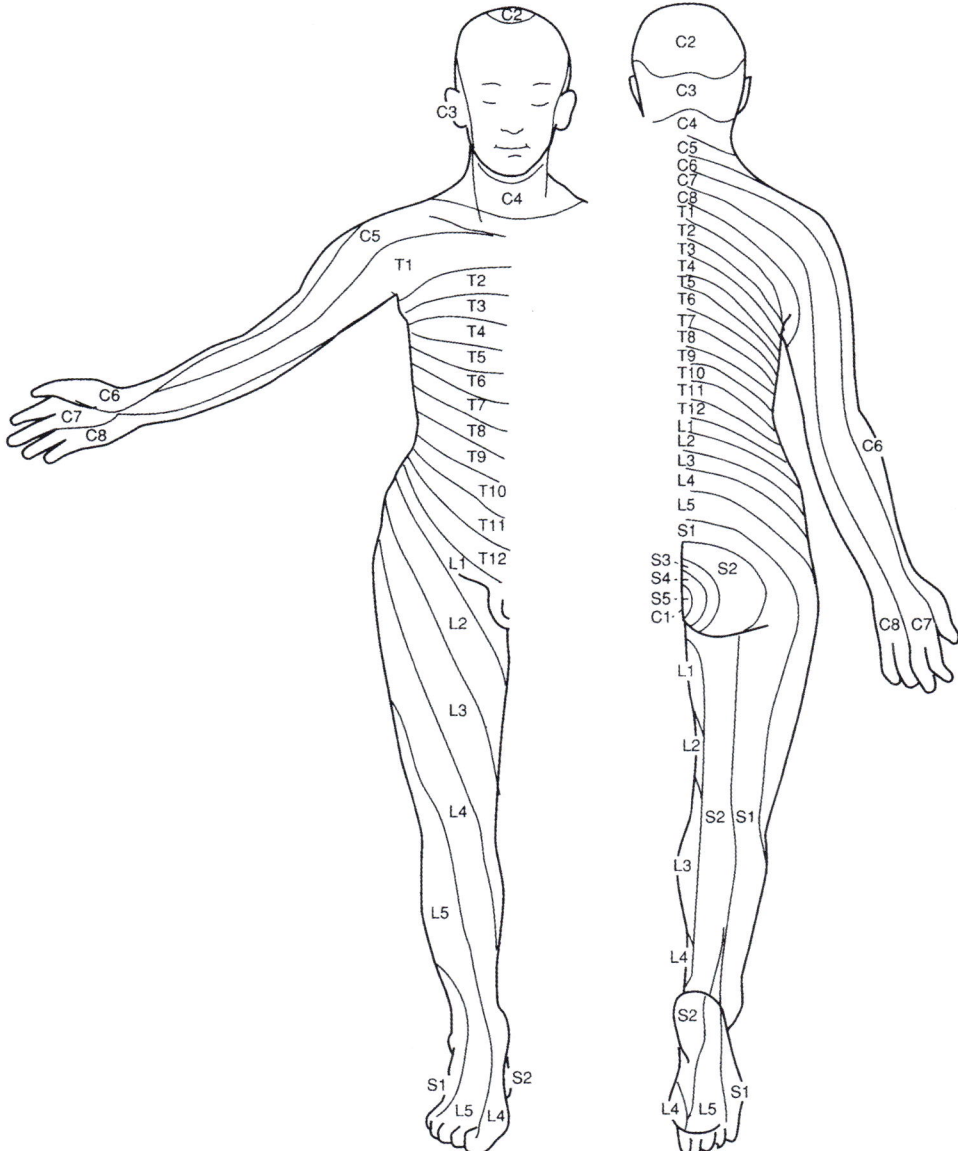

FIGURE 10.1 Dermatomes of the anterior and posterior body and extremities. (From Dudek RW. High-Yield Gross Anatomy, Williams and Wilkins 1997.)

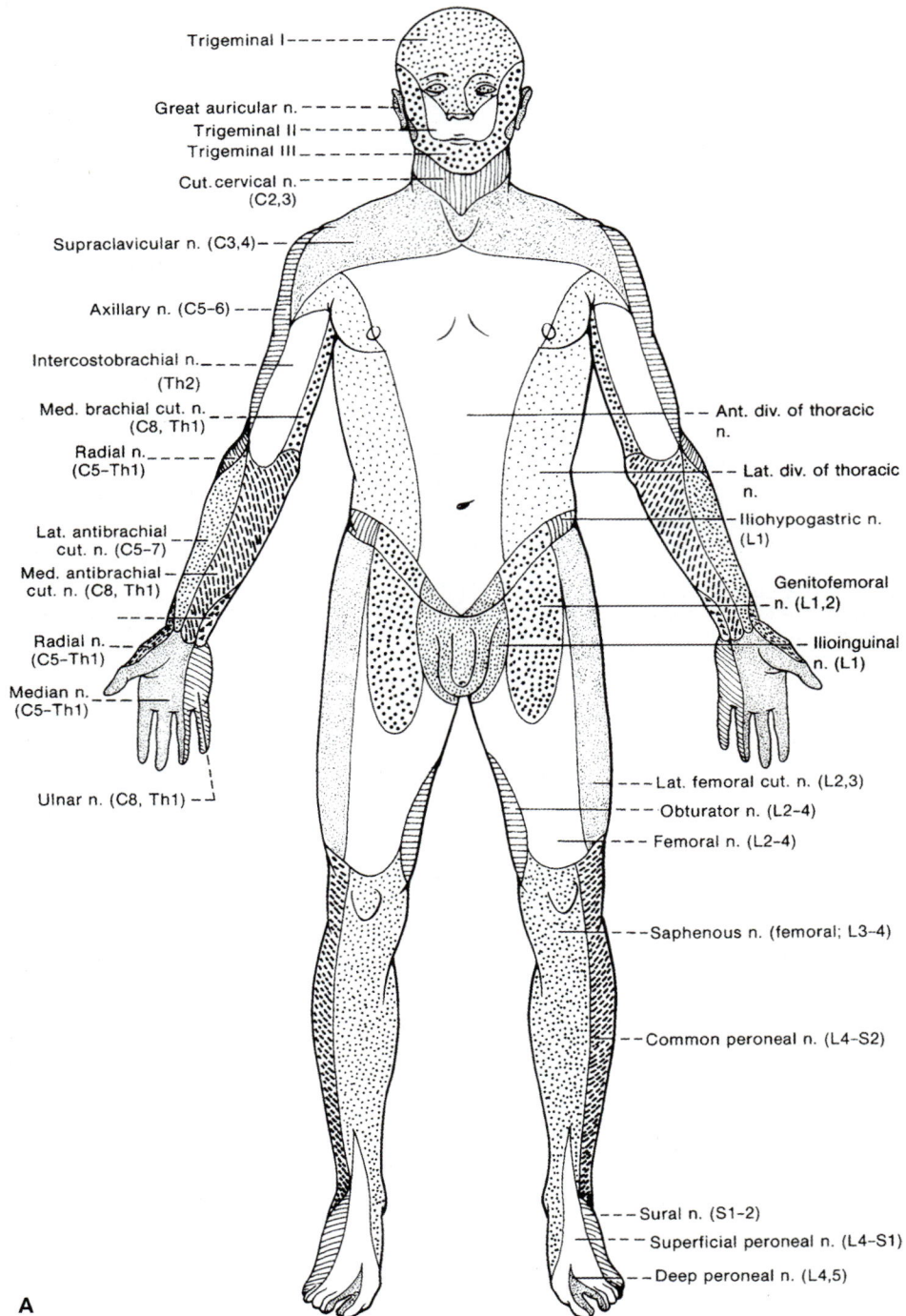

Trigeminal I

Great auricular n.
Trigeminal II
Trigeminal III

Cut. cervical n.
(C2,3)

Supraclavicular n. (C3,4)

Axillary n. (C5–6)

Intercostobrachial n.
(Th2)
Med. brachial cut. n.
(C8, Th1)
Radial n.
(C5–Th1)

Lat. antibrachial
cut. n. (C5–7)
Med. antibrachial
cut. n. (C8, Th1)

Radial n.
(C5–Th1)

Median n.
(C5–Th1)

Ulnar n. (C8, Th1)

Ant. div. of thoracic
n.

Lat. div. of thoracic
n.

Iliohypogastric n.
(L1)

Genitofemoral
n. (L1,2)

Ilioinguinal
n. (L1)

Lat. femoral cut. n. (L2,3)

Obturator n. (L2–4)

Femoral n. (L2–4)

Saphenous n. (femoral; L3–4)

Common peroneal n. (L4–S2)

Sural n. (S1–2)

Superficial peroneal n. (L4–S1)

Deep peroneal n. (L4,5)

A

FIGURE 10.2 A-B: The cutaneous distribution of the peripheral nerves. (From Haerer A. DeJong's The Neurologic Examination. Lippincott 1992.)

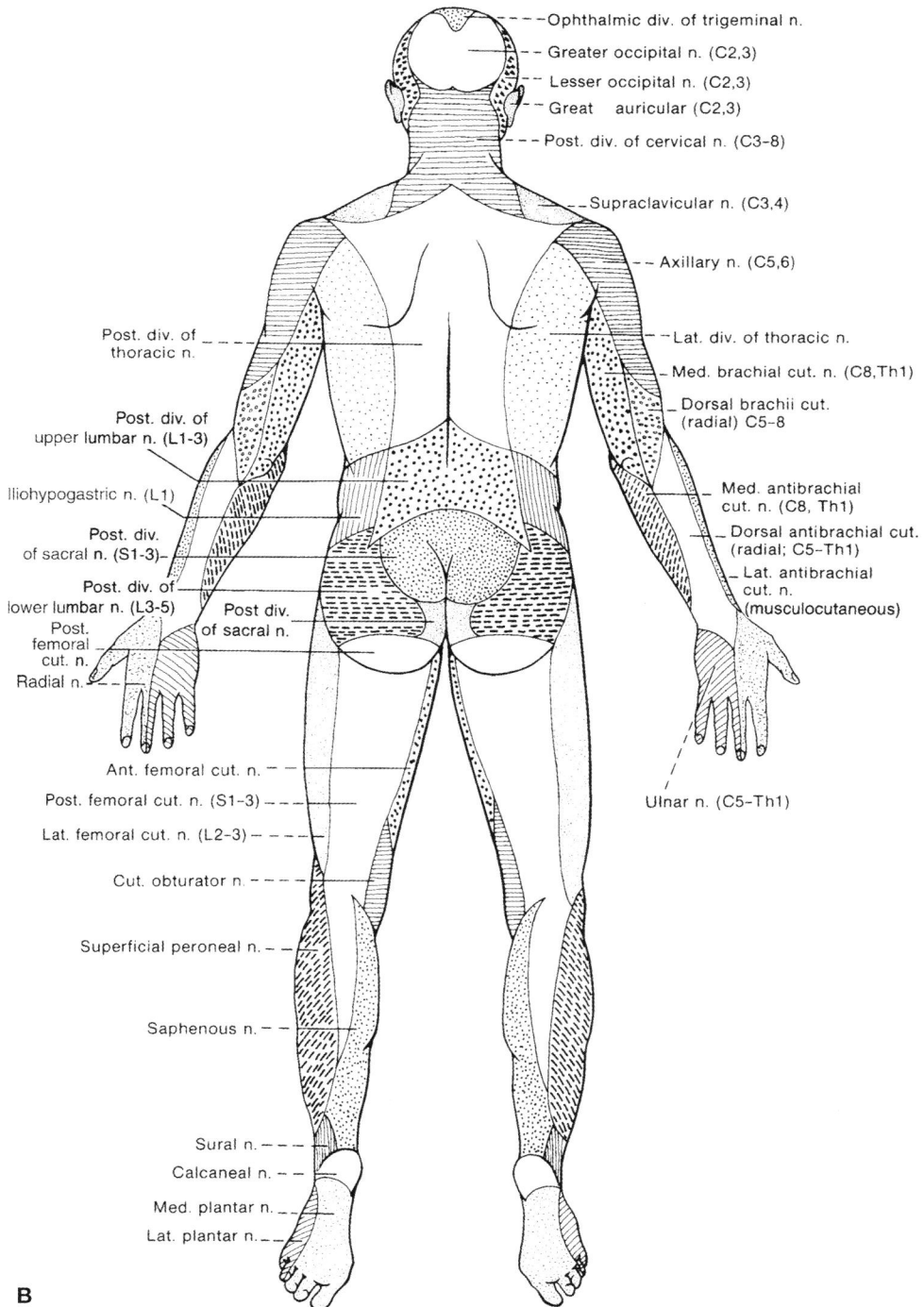

Ophthalmic div. of trigeminal n.
Greater occipital n. (C2,3)
Lesser occipital n. (C2,3)
Great   auricular (C2,3)
Post. div. of cervical n. (C3–8)
Supraclavicular n. (C3,4)
Axillary n. (C5,6)
Lat. div. of thoracic n.
Med. brachial cut. n. (C8,Th1)
Dorsal brachii cut. (radial) C5–8
Med. antibrachial cut. n. (C8, Th1)
Dorsal antibrachial cut. (radial; C5–Th1)
Lat. antibrachial cut. n. (musculocutaneous)
Ulnar n. (C5–Th1)

Post. div. of thoracic n.
Post. div. of upper lumbar n. (L1–3)
Iliohypogastric n. (L1)
Post. div. of sacral n. (S1–3)
Post. div. of lower lumbar n. (L3–5)
Post div. of sacral n.
Post. femoral cut. n.
Radial n.
Ant. femoral cut. n.
Post. femoral cut. n. (S1–3)
Lat. femoral cut. n. (L2–3)
Cut. obturator n.
Superficial peroneal n.
Saphenous n.
Sural n.
Calcaneal n.
Med. plantar n.
Lat. plantar n.

B

FIGURE 10.2 (*continued*)

COMMON CLINICAL PRESENTATIONS

Sensory symptoms can be classified as positive or negative, and both types of sensory symptoms may overlap in an individual. Positive sensory symptoms refer to abnormal spontaneous sensations (eg, paresthesias), which may be painful. Patients may describe "burning," "vibrating," "itching," "prickling," "tingling," or "electrical" sensations. Normal sensory stimuli may also be perceived as painful (allodynia)—for example, the light pressure of a bedsheet brushing over an affected body part may be extremely painful. As a result of allodynia, patients may be unable to wear tight-fitting clothing or footwear, or may be unable to tolerate walking barefoot. Positive sensory symptoms are usually worst at nighttime, presumably becoming more apparent because of the reduction in other competing sensory stimuli.

Negative sensory symptoms refer to a lack of normal sensation. This experience may be described by patients as part of the body feeling "numb," "dead," "swollen," or "like it has been injected with local anesthetic." Negative sensory symptoms involving the feet may cause the patient to feel like they are "walking on cement blocks," "wearing thick socks," "walking on cotton balls," or that their "socks are bunched up" under their toes. Lack of proprioceptive sensation can manifest as an unsteady gait or frequent falls, with unsteadiness worse in dim lighting or when the eyes are closed (eg, when rinsing shampoo in the shower).

The distribution of sensory symptoms is key to localizing the site of pathology within the nervous system. This localization allows for a differential diagnosis, which, in turn, guides the initial evaluation. Five common patterns should be recognized:

1. Length-dependent, symmetric, bilateral sensory symptoms
2. Non-length-dependent or asymmetric bilateral sensory symptoms
3. Focal sensory symptoms involving one limb
4. Hemibody sensory symptoms
5. Bilateral sensory symptoms below a sensory level

These patterns are discussed in detail here. If a patient's symptoms do not conform to one of these patterns, systemic etiologies (eg, hypocalcemia) or hyperventilation (eg, due to anxiety) should be

considered—in both, perioral and distal fingertip paresthesias are common.

Length-Dependent, Symmetric, Bilateral Sensory Symptoms

Length-dependent symptoms first involve the region innervated by the longest nerves in the body: the feet. Length-dependent symptoms begin in the feet and progress proximally in the lower extremities, not affecting the distal upper extremities (the fingertips) until they have reached the mid-shins in the lower extremities. Length-dependent symptoms are sometimes referred to as a "stocking and glove" distribution, which can be misleading as it implies that symptoms arise simultaneously in the feet and hands. A truly length-dependent pattern of symptom onset may ultimately involve both the hands and feet but will have begun in the feet and ascended in the lower extremities before affecting the hands (ie, a "stocking" distribution before a "stocking and glove" distribution).

A length-dependent, symmetric pattern of sensory symptoms (eg, numbness and/or paresthesias in both feet) is strongly suggestive of a polyneuropathy. Polyneuropathies may be caused by axonal or demyelinating pathophysiology involving peripheral nerves. The length-dependent pattern described here is characteristic of most axonal polyneuropathies (for further discussion of polyneuropathies, see Chapter 24).

Most polyneuropathies involve both small and large fibers. Some conditions, however, may cause a small-fiber neuropathy or a large-fiber neuropathy in isolation. Small-fiber neuropathies cause predominantly positive sensory symptoms (ie, painful paresthesias and allodynia). In addition, small-fiber nerves are required for the control of autonomic functions such as control of heart rate, blood pressure, sweating, and gut motility. Therefore, some patients with small-fiber neuropathy may also develop autonomic neuropathy, which can manifest as orthostatic hypotension, cardiac dysrhythmia, constipation, and loss of normal sweating. Patients with large-fiber neuropathies experience predominantly negative symptoms, with loss of discriminative touch and proprioception manifesting as numbness and gait imbalance. Muscle stretch reflexes require intact proprioceptive function, and so large-fiber neuropathy will also result in diminished or absent reflexes, especially distally. If there is concurrent motor fiber involvement, the patient may have distal weakness along with sensory loss.

The pattern described in this section—length-dependent, symmetric, bilateral sensory symptoms in the feet—is the most common pattern of sensory symptoms seen in the outpatient setting and is nearly always due to polyneuropathy. Less commonly, isolated sensory symptoms in the feet may be caused by radiculopathy affecting the bilateral L5 and S1 nerve roots (most commonly caused by degenerative disease of the lumbar spine). In lumbosacral radiculopathy, the sensory symptoms involving neighboring dermatomes overlap to produce a pattern of distal sensory loss that can mimic polyneuropathy. However, most patients with radiculopathies will also experience radicular pain (ie, pain radiating from the buttock into the lower extremity), which is often a helpful localizing clue (see "Clinical Approach" section). In addition, sensory symptoms caused by polyradiculopathies are often asymmetric, whereas sensory symptoms caused by polyneuropathy are usually symmetric.

Non-length-Dependent or Asymmetric Bilateral Sensory Symptoms

The presence of bilateral non-length-dependent symptoms (ie, simultaneously involving the upper and lower extremities both proximally and distally at onset) or asymmetric sensory symptoms can be caused by polyneuropathy due to demyelinating peripheral nerve pathophysiology, multiple mononeuropathies (ie, involvement of multiple individual nerves; sometimes referred to as mononeuropathy multiplex), sensory ganglionopathy (a rare condition affecting the dorsal root ganglia), polyradiculopathy (involvement of multiple nerve roots), or cervical spinal cord disease (affecting the upper and lower extremities together).

Although polyradiculopathy and cervical spine disease are relatively common due to degenerative disease of the spine, the demyelinating neuropathies, mononeuropathy multiplex, and sensory ganglionopathy are relatively uncommon. Therefore, a non-length-dependent and/or asymmetric pattern of sensory symptoms requires a more extensive diagnostic evaluation, as discussed later (see "Diagnostic Approach" section).

Focal Sensory Symptoms Involving One Limb

This pattern is most commonly caused by a lesion involving a single peripheral nerve (mononeuropathy) or a single nerve root (radiculopathy). These two localizations can be distinguished based on the distribution of sensory deficits within the limb, discussed in more detail later (see Figure 10.1 and "Sensory Examination" section). More extensive sensory symptoms isolated to one limb that span multiple nerve and root territories may be due to a lesion of a nerve plexus (ie, plexopathy; brachial plexopathy in the upper extremity, lumbosacral plexopathy in the lower extremity). Plexopathy typically presents with motor symptoms (ie, weakness) in addition to sensory symptoms.

Focal sensory symptoms in one limb can also be caused by a small central nervous system lesion, most commonly affecting the hand due to large representation of the hand in the brain. Simultaneous involvement of the hand and ipsilateral face (called a *cheiro-oral pattern*) localizes to the contralateral cerebral hemisphere.

Hemibody Sensory Symptoms

Sensory symptoms involving one side of the body suggest a lesion in the central nervous system: the brain or spinal cord. If symptoms involve the face, arm, and leg, the symptoms must be in the brain; if they involve the upper extremity, lower extremity, and torso only, they may be in the brain or spinal cord. The rarely encountered pattern of symptoms in the face on one side and the body on the opposite side localizes to the brainstem, although brainstem lesions are often accompanied by additional deficits beyond sensory loss (eg, cranial nerve palsies, ataxia).

Bilateral Sensory Symptoms Below a Sensory Level

A sensory level refers to the examination finding in which sensation is abnormal below a certain point on the torso but normal above this point. This finding strongly suggests a spinal cord lesion, with the lesion in the spinal cord at or superior to the sensory level. Particular types of spinal cord lesions can cause different patterns of sensory loss below the level of the lesion.

Hemicord lesions cause ipsilateral vibration sense and proprioception loss and contralateral pain and temperature loss below the level of the lesion (Brown-Séquard syndrome) due to the crossing of the spinothalamic tracts within the spinal cord; this syndrome is also associated with weakness ipsilateral to the lesion.

Spinal cord ischemia typically involves the anterior two-thirds of the cord, affecting the spinothalamic and corticospinal tracts but sparing the dorsal columns. This leads to a characteristic pattern of dissociated sensory loss in which there is loss of pain and temperature sensation below the level of the lesion but sparing of vibration sense and proprioception.

Subacute combined degeneration of the spinal cord (most commonly caused by vitamin B12 deficiency) causes loss of vibration sense and proprioception in the limbs with sensory ataxia due to involvement of the dorsal columns of the spinal cord, as well as upper motor neuron signs (eg, hyperreflexia, Babinski sign) due to involvement of the corticospinal tracts. The peripheral nerves may also be involved (myeloneuropathy), leading to lower motor neuron signs (hyporeflexia/areflexia) on examination, which may accompany upper motor neuron signs.

CLINICAL APPROACH

History

Clarifying the Nature of the Symptoms

Abnormal sensory experiences are subjective and can be difficult for patients to describe. The word "numbness" must be clarified to determine whether the patient is referring to sensory symptoms, weakness, or incoordination. Neuropathic pain (ie, pain from a neurologic condition) is typically burning, tingling, and/or electrical in nature and must be distinguished from the dull, aching pain of musculoskeletal or soft tissue etiology. In addition, patients may use the term "neuropathy" to refer to their sensory symptoms in general, even if the etiology is radiculopathy. The presence of radicular pain is suggestive of radiculopathy. This refers to pain that originates in the neck or shoulder and radiates down the arm (for cervical radiculopathy), or originates in the lower back or buttock and radiates down the leg (for lumbosacral radiculopathy). The latter is sometimes referred to as "sciatica" when it occurs in the leg (although the sciatic nerve is not usually involved, but rather the L5 or S1 root).

Clarifying the Distribution of Symptoms

The distribution of symptoms provides initial clues to the localization: hemibody symptoms suggest a lesion in the central nervous system (eg, a thalamic lesion), whereas symmetric length-dependent symptoms, focal symptoms limited to one limb, or asymmetric and/or non-length-dependent symptoms suggest a peripheral nervous system lesion. Given the important distinction between length-dependent and non-length-dependent processes, if patients have symptoms in both the upper and lower extremities, it is important to determine whether these arose simultaneously (non-length dependent) or whether symptoms in the feet preceded the development of symptoms in the upper extremities (usually length dependent).

Establishing the Time Course

The tempo of symptom onset and progression provides important clues to the etiology of the patient's symptoms. Chronic evolution of symptoms (over years) is seen in the vast majority of polyneuropathies (due to common etiologies such as diabetes) and radiculopathies (due to degenerative conditions of the spine). Subacute onset and progression (over weeks to months) can be seen in inflammatory polyneuropathies, multiple mononeuropathies, or sensory ganglionopathies. Acute onset and evolution of sensory symptoms (over hours to days) can be seen with inflammatory conditions such as Guillain-Barré syndrome or myelitis. Hyperacute symptoms (over seconds to minutes) can be caused by stroke, migraine, or seizure; stroke tends to cause negative symptoms (ie, numbness), whereas migraine and seizure tend to cause positive symptoms (eg, tingling).

Identifying Additional Symptoms

Radiating neuropathic pain from the neck down the arm or back/buttock down the leg suggests radiculopathy. Radicular pain may follow a classic dermatomal distribution suggesting a specific nerve root but may not perfectly correlate.

Bowel and/or bladder symptoms (retention or incontinence) suggest a lesion of the spinal cord or cauda equina (affecting sacral nerve roots).

Autonomic symptoms such as orthostatic hypotension, constipation, and loss of normal sweating can be seen in polyneuropathy.

Associated systemic symptoms such as weight loss, fevers, or night sweats may suggest a systemic inflammatory or neoplastic condition as the cause of the patient's sensory symptoms.

Inquiring About Risk Factors

Patients with sensory symptoms should also be asked about risk factors for polyneuropathy, such as diabetes, toxic exposure (eg, chemotherapy, heavy alcohol use, heavy metal exposure), or nutritional deficiency (eg, due to gastric bypass surgery, restricted diet).

Examination

Sensory Examination

The goal of the sensory examination is to determine the distribution of sensory deficits. After determining the distribution of sensory deficits, different sensory modalities can be tested (Table 10.1). It is not always necessary to test all modalities—for example, in a patient with focal sensory symptoms in one limb, demarcating the boundaries of the affected region using pinprick may be adequate. However, in patients with bilateral sensory symptoms, testing multiple modalities can determine whether the disorder preferentially involves large nerve fibers (vibration and proprioception), small nerve fibers (pain and temperature), or both (in cases of suspected polyneuropathy); or the spinothalamic tracts, dorsal columns, or both (in cases of suspected myelopathy).

In a patient with bilateral sensory symptoms, the goal of the sensory examination should be to determine whether the distribution of deficits is symmetric or asymmetric and whether the distribution is length dependent or non-length dependent. If the symptoms are limited to the lower extremities, a spinal level on the thorax should be sought by using a pin to identify a level on the back, chest, or abdomen below which sensation is diminished and above which it is normal.

In a patient with focal sensory symptoms involving one limb, the examination should clarify whether the distribution of symptoms fits better with a root or peripheral nerve distribution. For example, both carpal tunnel syndrome (ie, median neuropathy at the wrist) and C6 radiculopathy can cause sensory symptoms involving the thumb. However, the demonstration of a clear difference in sensation between the lateral and medial aspects of the fourth digit (impaired sensation on the medial aspect) is more suggestive of a median nerve lesion. Conversely, sensory loss extending proximal to the wrist along the lateral forearm would be more suggestive of a C6 radiculopathy (Figure 10.1). However, the examiner should not rely too heavily on typical dermatomal maps since there can be considerable interindividual variability.

In patients with a history of focal sensory deficits affecting one side of the body or one functional aspect of one limb (eg, the entire hand) but no objective signs in elemental sensory modality testing, subtle sensory processing deficits indicative of a cortical lesion should be sought. For example, a patient with a right parietal lesion may be able to sense tactile stimuli on their right and left side when tested separately, but when both sides are touched simultaneously, they may report sensing only the right side (called *extinction to double simultaneous stimulation*, a sign of neglect). Another cortical sign is agraphesthesia, in which the patient can detect tactile stimuli on the hand but is unable to identify more complex stimuli like a number being drawn by the examiner with their finger on the patient's palm.

Motor and Reflex Examination

Peripheral lesions involving sensory nerves or roots can also damage motor nerve fibers, causing associated lower motor neuron pattern weakness (ie, with associated atrophy, fasciculations, flaccid tone, and diminished or absent reflexes) in the distribution of the sensory symptoms. Typically, sensory symptoms predominate in the early and mild stages of neuropathy or radiculopathy, and the presence of motor deficits, therefore, indicates a more severe or advanced condition. For example, length-dependent peripheral neuropathies are typically associated with sensory symptoms, but in more chronic, advanced disease, wasting of the intrinsic foot muscles can be seen, associated with deformities such as pes cavus or hammer toes. These deformities are classically described in

TABLE 10.1	Suggested Methods of Testing the Sensory Modalities
Sensory modality	**Suggested method of testing**
Pain	Using a pin, find an area of normal sensation, typically the forehead. Demonstrate to the patient what the sharp pinprick sensation feels like. Then, test the affected region and ask if it feels the same or different. With distal sensory loss, determine the proximal extent by testing distal to proximal from the foot up the leg, asking when it starts to feel sharp.
Temperature	Use a cold object (eg, the cold metal of a tuning fork or reflex hammer). Again, demonstrate what that cold sensation feels like in an area of normal sensation before comparing to affected areas.
Vibration sense	Use a 128-Hz tuning fork. Demonstrate what vibration feels like in an unaffected area first (typically fingertips) and ask "can you feel that vibrating?" Then, test if the patient can feel vibration over more distal bony prominences, starting at the great toe. If vibration sense is absent at the big toe, move proximally to the ankle, tibial tuberosity, and knee, noting the first place where vibration is felt.
Proprioception	Test joint position sense at the metatarsophalangeal joint by holding the great toe by its sides (rather than holding over the nail) and moving it up and down. Demonstrate to the patient what you are doing ("I'm going to move your toe up and down; this is up, this is down"). Then, test if they can tell if the toe is up or down when their eyes are closed. If joint position sense is lost at the toe, assess at the ankle.
	Joint position sense in the hands can be tested similarly, substituting the abovementioned instructions for the big toe to the distal interphalangeal joint. In addition, patients with proprioceptive loss of the hands may exhibit subtle continuous movements of the fingers when their hands are outstretched and eyes are closed (called *pseudoathetosis*).
	Romberg sign: This is tested by having the patient stand with feet together and eyes closed. The sign is considered present if the patient loses their balance and takes a step. Patients with loss of proprioceptive sensation will sway significantly and may take a step when they close their eyes due to loss of the visual inputs they are reliant on for spatial awareness. Of note, patients with vestibular dysfunction may also exhibit a Romberg sign, as the ability to maintain a normal stance relies on a combination of visual, vestibular, and proprioceptive inputs.

hereditary forms of neuropathy (eg, Charcot-Marie-Tooth disease) but can be seen in any polyneuropathy with significant involvement of motor fibers.

Hyporeflexia or areflexia is commonly seen in peripheral nervous system conditions such as peripheral neuropathy, radiculopathy, and the rarer condition, sensory ganglionopathy.

On the other hand, central nervous system lesions affecting the corticospinal tracts cause weakness associated with hyperreflexia, spasticity, and clonus (upper motor neuron signs).

The reflexes are particularly helpful in patients presenting with gait instability and numbness in the bilateral lower extremities: Hyporeflexia or areflexia localize the problem to the peripheral nervous system, whereas hyperreflexia suggests a spinal cord lesion. An exception is acute spinal cord conditions in which there will be flaccid paralysis and areflexia in the period of spinal shock, with upper motor neuron signs emerging over weeks.

DIAGNOSTIC APPROACH

The diagnostic approach to sensory symptoms depends on their localization, which is largely determined from the pattern of symptoms described earlier.

Length-Dependent, Symmetric Sensory Symptoms

The majority of patients with chronic, length-dependent, symmetric sensory symptoms have polyneuropathy. Per the American Academy of Neurology practice guidelines, the highest yield screening tests evaluate for diabetes (fasting blood glucose or hemoglobin A_{1c}), vitamin B_{12} deficiency (vitamin B_{12} level), and paraprotein-associated disorders (serum protein electrophoresis [SPEP] with immunofixation).[1] These tests should be performed in all patients with suspected polyneuropathy. If these initial screening tests are unrevealing, further evaluation can be considered (see Table 10.2). However, in the majority of patients with mild, chronic, sensory-predominant, distal symmetric polyneuropathy, exhaustive laboratory testing is unlikely to be revealing, and many older patients have an idiopathic neuropathy. Patients with idiopathic peripheral neuropathy are often disappointed when an underlying etiology cannot be identified. However, they can be reassured that idiopathic neuropathy is typically a very indolent condition, with patients remaining stable or progressing only very slowly over many years. Patients are often specifically concerned

TABLE 10.2	Red Flag Features in Polyneuropathy

"Red flag" features in polyneuropathy presentations

Severe, disabling symptoms
- Frequent falls
- Requiring a walking aid
- Loss of fine motor skills

Acute/subacute time course
- Progressing over days (suggestive of Guillain-Barré syndrome)
- Progressing over weeks/months (suggestive of inflammatory, paraprotein-associated, or paraneoplastic neuropathies)

Motor involvement
- Prominent weakness +/− atrophy
- Motor deficits early in the disease course
- Motor > sensory deficits

Non-length dependent pattern
- Early involvement of hands
- Proximal sensory/motor symptoms

Systemic symptoms
- Weight loss
- Fevers, chills, night sweats
- Skin rash

that they will lose the ability to walk in the future, and should be counseled that this is very rarely seen as a consequence of idiopathic neuropathy.

However, some patients with length-dependent sensory symptoms will require a more extensive diagnostic evaluation. Identifying these patients requires recognition of specific red flag symptoms or signs suggesting a more extensive evaluation for a suspected polyneuropathy. These include rapid progression (over weeks to months rather than years), severe or disabling symptoms (eg, leading to early falls or requirement of mobility aids), predominant motor deficits out of proportion to sensory deficits, or concurrent systemic features such as weight loss (Table 10.2). Patients with a non-length-dependent pattern of symptoms also require more extensive evaluation (see subsequent section).

Patients with red flag symptoms or signs typically require more extensive laboratory testing (Table 10.3), nerve conduction studies and electromyography (NCS/EMG), and neurology consultation. NCS/EMG uses electrical stimulation and recording electrodes to study the peripheral nerves and nerve roots (NCS) and a needle electrode portion to assess the muscles (EMG) (see Chapter 3). It is helpful in determining the distribution, severity, and pathophysiology (ie, axonal vs demyelinating) of peripheral nervous system conditions.

Note that NCS/EMG only evaluates the large-fiber nerves, and so pure small-fiber neuropathies will have normal electrodiagnostic studies. Although skin biopsy is the gold standard test for diagnosis of small-fiber neuropathy (demonstrating reduced epidermal nerve fiber density), the diagnosis can often be made clinically.

Non-length-Dependent/Asymmetric, Bilateral Sensory Symptoms

A non-length-dependent and/or asymmetric pattern of sensory deficits usually requires NCS/EMG to distinguish between demyelinating polyneuropathy, multiple mononeuropathies, polyradiculopathy, and sensory ganglionopathy. A non-length-dependent and/or asymmetric pattern of sensory (and/or motor) symptoms is a red flag that should prompt a neurology referral.

Focal Sensory Symptoms Involving One Limb

Patients with clinically straightforward, mild cases of mononeuropathy or monoradiculopathy are often managed symptomatically and monitored clinically. For example, in suspected carpal tunnel syndrome, wrist bracing at night may resolve symptoms without the need for further diagnostic or therapeutic intervention (see Chapter 24); in radiculopathy without intractable pain or progressive weakness, a patient may be given analgesics and referred for physical therapy (see Chapter 24).

However, if symptoms of mononeuropathy or radiculopathy are severe, progressive, or include weakness, NCS/EMG can be helpful in confirming the localization and severity of nerve injury, particularly when operative intervention is being considered. Similarly, severe or progressive radicular symptoms may warrant magnetic resonance imaging (MRI) of the cervical or lumbosacral spine to determine whether a radiculopathy may be amenable to operative or interventional pain approaches.

Patients with sensory symptoms in one limb not clearly fitting an individual peripheral nerve or nerve root distribution may require NCS/EMG in order to accurately localize the lesion and/or MRI of the brain or spinal cord if a central nervous system lesion is under consideration.

TABLE 10.3 Diagnostic Testing in Suspected Polyneuropathy

Pattern of sensory deficits	Localization	Associated etiologies	Suggested evaluation
Length-dependent, symmetric, bilateral	Length-dependent polyneuropathy	Common: Diabetes, Vitamin B₁₂ deficiency, Toxic (eg, chemotherapy, alcohol), Idiopathic. Rare: other metabolic, inflammatory, nutritional, toxic, hereditary etiologies	Laboratory tests: HbA$_{1c}$, B$_{12}$ +/− methylmalonic acid, SPEP with immunofixation. CBC, renal, liver, and thyroid function. +/− expanded testing in selected cases: Inflammatory/autoimmune: ESR, CRP, ANA, SS-A, SS-B, RF, dsDNA, Sm, C3/4, TTG. Paraprotein: serum-free light chains, UPEP, cryoglobulins. Metabolic: oral glucose tolerance test. Nutritional: copper, B₁, B₆, vitamin E. Toxic: heavy metal screen. Infectious: hepatitis C, HIV. Hereditary: genetic testing
	Bilateral L5-S1 polyradiculopathies	Common: structural spine disease. Rare: infectious, inflammatory, neoplastic diseases of the nerve roots	+/− NCS/EMG. +/− MRI lumbar spine
Non-length-dependent +/− asymmetric, bilateral	Non-length-dependent polyneuropathy	Demyelinating/inflammatory neuropathies	NCS/EMG: key to correctly localize the pattern of deficits, characterize pathophysiology (demyelinating vs axonal), and guide further evaluation. Evaluation will depend on specific localization but, at a minimum, will include ESR, CRP, SPEP with immunofixation and serum-free light chains, and consideration of lumbar puncture
	Multiple mononeuropathies	Vasculitic neuropathy	
	Sensory ganglionopathy	Platinum-based chemotherapy, vitamin B₆ toxicity, Sjögren syndrome, HIV	B₆ level, SS-A, SS-B, HIV, +/− lumbar puncture
	Polyradiculopathy / Cervical myelopathy	Infectious, inflammatory, neoplastic. Commonly caused by structural spine disease	Consider MRI spine.
Focal sensory symptoms involving one limb	Mononeuropathy / Monoradiculopathy	Commonly caused by focal entrapment/compression. Commonly caused by structural spine disease	Consider NCS/EMG. Consider MRI spine.
	Plexopathy	Rare: seen in malignant infiltration, idiopathic inflammation (Parsonage-Turner syndrome), diabetes (diabetic amyotrophy, also known as diabetic lumbosacral radiculoplexus neuropathy), post-radiation, post-trauma	Consider MRI brachial or lumbosacral plexus.
Bilateral sensory symptoms below a sensory level	Myelopathy	Structural, inflammatory, infectious, neoplastic, vascular	MRI cervical +/− thoracic +/− lumbar spine
Hemibody sensory symptoms	Brain lesion (eg, thalamus; parietal cortex)	Stroke, Tumor, Migraine, Seizure	MRI brain and/or cervical spine (depending on whether the face is involved). Consider EEG if symptoms are positive.
	Hemicord syndrome	Commonly caused by penetrating trauma, may also be seen in inflammatory, demyelinating diseases	

ANA, antinuclear antibody; CBC, complete blood cell count; CRP, C-reactive protein; dsDNA, double-stranded DNA; EEG, electroencephalogram; ESR, erythrocyte sedimentation rate; MRI, magnetic resonance imaging; NCS/EMG, nerve conduction studies/electromyography; SPEP, serum protein electrophoresis; TTG, tissue transglutaminase.

Dedicated MRI of the brachial or lumbosacral plexus (sometimes referred to as *MR neurogram*) can be obtained in cases of suspected plexopathy.

Hemibody Sensory Symptoms

Brain imaging is indicated for patients with hemibody symptoms also involving the face, and spine imaging may be indicated if symptoms involve only the upper and lower extremity and torso on one side but not the face (although this pattern of face-sparing unilateral sensory loss can rarely be caused by a brain lesion). If hemibody sensory symptoms are episodic and positive, migraine or seizure should be considered depending on other history and examination features; EEG may be indicated if seizure is under consideration.

Bilateral Sensory Symptoms Below a Sensory Level

Patients with bilateral sensory symptoms and evidence of a spinal sensory level (with or without additional features such as bowel/bladder symptoms, weakness, or upper motor neuron signs) should be evaluated with MRI of the spine.

The extent of imaging depends on the distribution of symptoms. Sensory symptoms in the hands indicate that the lesion must involve the cervical spine, and therefore MRI of the cervical spine should be obtained. However, recall that a spinal level may indicate a lesion at or above that level; therefore, a spinal level on the torso, while suggestive of a thoracic cord lesion, could also be caused by a cervical cord lesion, thereby warranting MRI of both the cervical and thoracic spine.

If there is concern for a neoplastic, inflammatory, or infectious disease of the spine, MRI should be obtained with contrast. If purely structural disease is suspected (eg, degenerative spine disease), contrast is typically not required.

SUMMARY

Sensory symptoms can be caused by disorders involving any portion of the nervous system. The appropriate diagnostic evaluation is determined by the suspected localization, which is based on the distribution of symptoms and signs. The presentation most commonly seen in the outpatient setting is that of mild length-dependent sensory symptoms due to polyneuropathy, which is typically caused by conditions such as diabetes or vitamin B_{12} deficiency, or may be idiopathic. Additional evaluation and neurology referral should be pursued in patients with "red flags," including subacute time course, progressive symptoms, a non-length-dependent or asymmetric pattern of symptoms, and/or systemic symptoms.

EDITORS' KEY POINTS

▶ Sensory symptoms such as numbness and tingling can be localized on the basis of their distribution, analyzing whether symptoms are unilateral or bilateral, symmetric or asymmetric, proximal or distal (or both), and whether the face is involved.

▶ Symmetric, bilateral sensory symptoms in the feet suggest an axonal polyneuropathy and should be evaluated with hemoglobin A_{1c} (or fasting blood glucose), vitamin B_{12} level, and serum protein electrophoresis with immunofixation.

▶ Bilateral sensory symptoms that involve both the hands and feet at presentation, are both proximal and distal at presentation, or are asymmetric at presentation suggest a demyelinating neuropathy, mononeuropathy multiplex, polyradiculopathy, or sensory ganglionopathy.

▶ Focal sensory symptoms involving one limb are generally due to a mononeuropathy or radiculopathy.

▶ Sensory symptoms on one entire side of the body, including the face, localize to the brain and should be evaluated with brain imaging; if there are unilateral sensory symptoms and the face is not involved, the lesion may be in the brain or spinal cord.

▶ Bilateral sensory symptoms below a specific level on the torso localize to the spinal cord and should be evaluated with MRI of the spine.

REFERENCE

1. England JD, Gronseth GS, Franklin G, et al. Evaluation of distal symmetric polyneuropathy: the role of autonomic testing, nerve biopsy, and skin biopsy (an evidence-based review). *Muscle Nerve*. 2009;39(1):106-115.

Approach to the Patient With Weakness

Mark Terrelonge Jr

INTRODUCTION

Weakness is a common symptom with a broad differential diagnosis. Through the history and examination, a particular pattern of weakness can be elicited—focal or diffuse, unilateral or bilateral, proximal or distal. The pattern of weakness correlates with the most likely localization within the nervous system. The localization, in conjunction with other aspects of the history, guides the evaluation, which may include laboratory testing, neuroimaging, and/or nerve conduction studies and electromyography.

COMMON PRESENTATIONS AND SYMPTOMS

Weakness due to a neurologic etiology causes a true decrease in muscle power. However, patients may use the word "weakness" to describe fatigue or pain-limited movement, which are generally not caused by a neurologic condition. Patients may also use different words to describe the symptom of weakness, such as fatigue, stiffness, clumsiness, or numbness. Therefore, a key aspect in the evaluation of a patient presenting with weakness is determining whether the symptom is due to a loss of muscle strength.

The clinical presentation of weakness depends on the affected part(s) of the body. Weakness becomes apparent to a patient when they can no longer do a specific activity. Weakness in one or both hands can cause difficulty with writing, typing, or other manual skills. Weakness in one or both legs can cause difficulty walking. Proximal weakness in the legs makes it difficult to rise from a chair, while proximal weakness in the arms makes it difficult to reach for items on high shelves or pick up children or pets. Weakness of cranial nerve–innervated muscles of the face, larynx, and pharynx (known as bulbar weakness) can cause difficulty talking and swallowing and may cause drooling and aspiration. Weakness of the respiratory muscles can cause shortness of breath. Therefore, another key aspect of the evaluation of weakness is determining the affected region(s) of the body.

In this chapter, an approach to localization based on the pattern of weakness is presented.

NEUROANATOMY AND PATHOPHYSIOLOGY

Weakness can originate from pathology at any level of the neuraxis, including the brain, brainstem, spinal cord, anterior horn cell, nerve root, plexus, nerve, neuromuscular junction, or muscle (Table 11.1). The brain, brainstem, and spinal cord are components of the central nervous system, whereas the anterior horn cell, nerve root, plexus, nerve, neuromuscular junction, and muscle are part of the peripheral nervous system. The neurons of the motor pathway in the central nervous system are referred to as upper motor neurons, and the neurons of the motor pathway in the peripheral nervous system are referred to as lower motor neurons. Lesions of upper motor neurons and lower motor neurons both cause weakness, but they cause different accompanying findings on examination, as discussed later.

The cell bodies of the upper motor neurons are in the motor cortex of the frontal lobe on each side. The upper motor neurons for the limbs and torso travel in the corticospinal tracts, and the upper motor neurons for the cranial nerve–innervated muscles travel in the corticobulbar tracts. The axons of the corticospinal tracts traverse the subcortical white matter, brainstem, and spinal cord to synapse on the cell bodies of lower motor neurons in the spinal cord, whereas the axons of the corticobulbar tracts diverge from the corticospinal tracts in the brainstem to synapse on the cell bodies of lower motor neurons in the brainstem. The lower motor neuron cell bodies in the spinal cord send their axons through ventral roots, plexuses, and peripheral nerves to arrive at the neuromuscular junction and muscles of the body and extremities. The lower motor neuron cell bodies in the brainstem send their axons through cranial nerves to arrive at the neuromuscular junction and muscles of the head and neck (Figures 11.1 and 11.2).

After traversing the brain and brainstem, the corticospinal tracts cross (decussate) to the contralateral side at the cervicomedullary junction (the interface between the brainstem and spinal cord) such that upper motor neurons from the left side of the brain/brainstem travel in the right side of the spinal cord, and upper motor neurons from the right side of the brain/brainstem travel in the left side of the spinal cord. This means that lesions of the brain or brainstem cause contralateral weakness of the limbs, whereas lesions of the spinal cord or in the peripheral nervous system cause ipsilateral weakness. Similarly, lesions in the corticobulbar tract in the brain (or brainstem before the level of decussation to the corresponding cranial nerve nucleus) cause contralateral weakness in the associated cranial nerve–innervated muscles, whereas brainstem or cranial nerve lesions cause ipsilateral deficits.

PATTERNS OF WEAKNESS

The pattern of weakness provides important clues to the localization. Key aspects of the pattern of weakness are the distribution of weakness (unilateral,

TABLE 11.1	Neuraxis Lesions That May Cause Weakness	
Nervous system level	**Term for disease/ disorder at level**	**Example diseases**
Brain/brainstem		Stroke Neoplasm Demyelinating disease
Spinal cord	Myelopathy	Structural/degenerative disease of the spinal column Neoplasm Demyelinating disease
Spinal root	Radiculopathy	Structural/degenerative disease of the spinal column Herpes zoster
Anterior horn cell	Motor neuron disease	Amyotrophic lateral sclerosis West Nile virus Poliomyelitis
Brachial and lumbar plexus	Plexopathy	Brachial neuritis (also known as *neuralgic amyotrophy*) Diabetic amyotrophy (also known as *diabetic radiculoplexus neuropathy*) Neoplastic infiltration
Peripheral nerve	Neuropathy	Carpal tunnel syndrome Diabetic neuropathy Guillain-Barré syndrome
Neuromuscular junction	Neuromuscular junction disorder	Myasthenia gravis Lambert-Eaton myasthenic syndrome Botulism
Muscle	Myopathy	Inflammatory myopathy (eg, dermatomyositis) Toxic myopathy (eg, statin induced) Inherited myopathy (eg, muscular dystrophy)

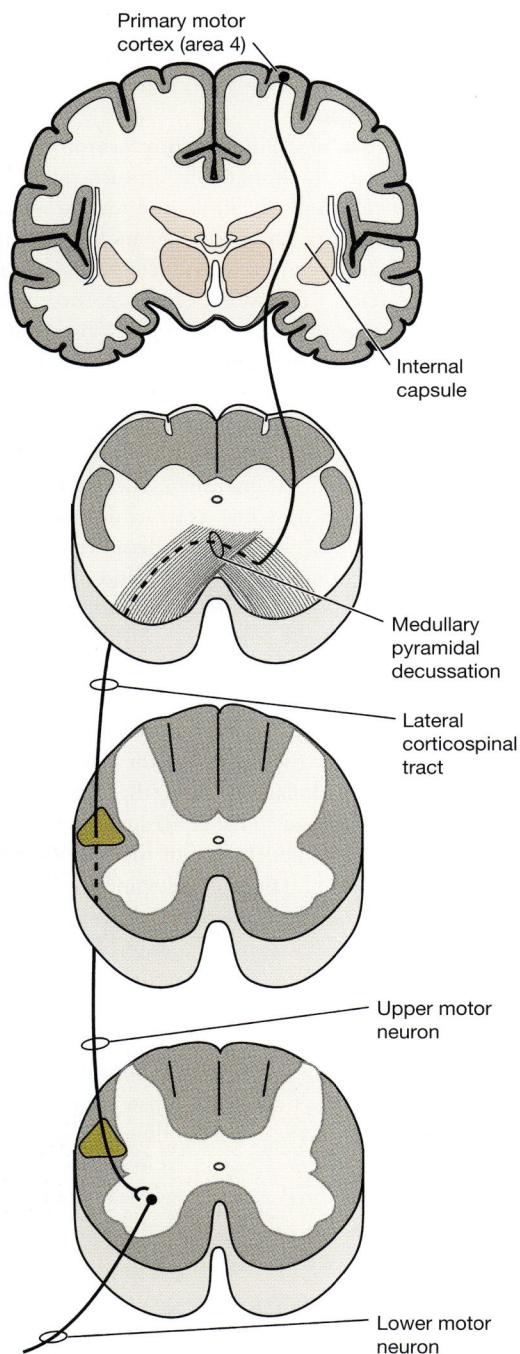

FIGURE 11.1 The corticospinal tract. (From Rhoades RA, Bell DR. *Medical Physiology.* 6th ed. Wolters Kluwer; 2022.)

bilateral, proximal, and distal) and whether the associated findings localize to the upper or lower motor neurons. When describing weakness, the suffix *-paresis* refers to diminished strength, whereas *-plegia* refers to complete paralysis. Common patterns of weakness include hemiparesis/hemiplegia (weakness on one side of the body), monoparesis/monoplegia (weakness in one limb), paraparesis/paraplegia (weakness in both legs), quadriparesis/quadriplegia (weakness of all four limbs), proximal limb weakness, distal limb weakness, generalized weakness, facial weakness, and respiratory weakness. Many of these patterns can be caused by either upper motor neuron lesions or lower motor neuron lesions, which can be distinguished on examination as discussed later (Table 11.2).

Hemiparesis

The term *hemiparesis* refers to weakness on only one side of the body. It can affect the face, arm, and/or leg. Hemiparesis involving the face, arm, and leg signifies a lesion in the contralateral brain or upper brainstem (above the mid-pons). Hemiparesis of the arm and leg that spares the face may be caused by a lesion of the contralateral medulla, ipsilateral cervical spinal cord, or, rarely, the contralateral brain. A common cause of hemiparesis/plegia is stroke.

Monoparesis

The term *monoparesis* refers to weakness of only one limb. The term can be used to describe weakness of part of the limb or the whole limb. Monoparesis is most commonly caused by lower motor neuron lesions involving individual peripheral nerves, nerve roots, or, less commonly, the brachial or lumbosacral plexus. However, a small brain lesion can also affect a single limb (eg, a stroke in the hand knob of the motor cortex, a small internal capsule stroke, or an anterior cerebral artery stroke affecting the leg region of the motor cortex), and a lesion of the thoracic or lumbar spinal cord can cause ipsilateral leg weakness.

Paraparesis

The term *paraparesis* refers to weakness of both legs with normal arm strength. Paraparesis is most

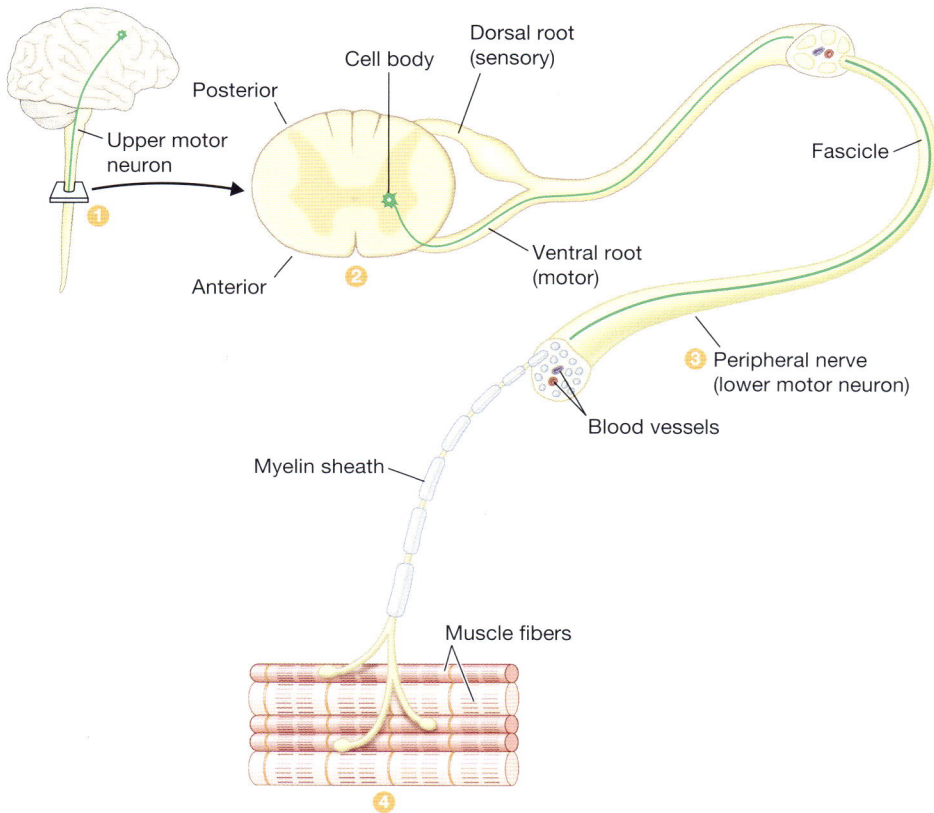

FIGURE 11.2 The motor pathway from the central nervous system (upper motor neurons) in the brain and spinal cord (1 and 2) to the peripheral nervous system (lower motor neurons) in the ventral roots, peripheral nerves (3), neuromuscular junction, and muscle (4). (Modified from Plowman S, Smith D. *Exercise Physiology for Health Fitness and Performance.* 5th ed. Wolters Kluwer; 2017.)

commonly caused by lesions of the spinal cord or cauda equina (the lumbosacral nerve roots in the spinal canal en route to the lumbosacral plexus). Examples of spinal conditions that can cause paraparesis include thoracic spinal epidural hematoma or abscess and transverse myelitis. Paraparesis can also be seen early in Guillain-Barré syndrome, a rapidly progressive radiculoneuropathy often starting in the legs before ascending to the arms, face, and respiratory muscles. Very rarely, paraparesis can be caused by a midline cranial lesion affecting the bilateral leg areas of the motor cortex (eg, parasagittal meningioma, bilateral anterior cerebral artery strokes).

Quadriparesis

The term *quadriparesis* refers to weakness in all four limbs sparing the muscles of the head and neck. Quadriparesis can be caused by a lesion of the cervical spinal cord or can be due to a process affecting the peripheral nervous system diffusely such as peripheral neuropathy, motor neuron disease, neuromuscular junction disease, or muscle disease.

Proximal Limb Weakness

Proximal limb weakness refers to weakness of the muscles around the shoulder girdle, proximal arm, hip girdle, and proximal legs. Bilateral proximal weakness

TABLE 11.2	Weakness Patterns and Likely Localizations
Weakness pattern	**Likely localization**
Hemiparesis	Contralateral brain or brainstem Ipsilateral cervical spinal cord
Monoparesis	Mononeuropathy Nerve root Plexus (Rarely, small brain lesion)
Paraparesis	Spinal cord Cauda equina Neuropathy (Rarely, superior, midline brain lesion)
Quadriparesis	Cervical spinal cord Neuropathy Neuromuscular junction Myopathy
Proximal limb weakness	Myopathy Neuromuscular junction (Border zone/watershed stroke)
Distal limb weakness	Neuropathy
Generalized weakness	Neuropathy Myopathy Neuromuscular junction Anterior horn cell Systemic illness
Facial weakness	Contralateral brain Ipsilateral brainstem Mononeuropathy (cranial nerve 7)
Respiratory weakness	Neuromuscular junction Neuropathy Anterior horn cell Neuromuscular junction Myopathy

is most commonly seen in muscle disease (myopathy). Neuromuscular junction disorders can also present with significant bilateral proximal weakness. Unilateral proximal weakness can be seen in brachial or lumbosacral plexus lesions. Strokes in the border zone/watershed region between the anterior cerebral arteries and middle cerebral arteries can cause a "person in a barrel" syndrome, leading to proximal limb weakness with preserved distal strength.

Distal Limb Weakness

Symmetric, bilateral, distal limb weakness is most commonly due to peripheral neuropathy. Asymmetric or unilateral distal limb weakness is usually due to a mononeuropathy or radiculopathy, although it can rarely be caused by a partial plexus lesion.

Generalized Weakness

Generalized weakness without other neurologic signs can be caused by diffuse peripheral nervous system disease or may be due to a systemic etiology.

Facial Weakness

Unilateral facial weakness without involvement of the arm and leg is most frequently caused by a lesion of cranial nerve 7, the most common cause being Bell palsy (idiopathic cranial nerve 7 palsy). Facial weakness that is accompanied by arm or leg weakness or other cranial nerve signs signifies a lesion in the brain or brainstem. Lower motor neuron facial weakness (due to a lesion of cranial nerve 7) affects the entire face: inability to raise the eyebrow, close the eye, or smile on the affected side. Upper motor neuron facial weakness (due to a lesion of the brain or upper brainstem) causes only weakness of the lower part of the face: inability to smile on the affected side with spared eyebrow raise and eye closure. Bilateral facial weakness can be seen in myasthenia gravis, inflammatory neuropathies such as Guillain-Barré syndrome or neurosarcoidosis, infectious neuropathies such as Lyme disease, and hereditary myopathies such as facioscapulohumeral muscular dystrophy.

Respiratory Muscle Weakness

Respiratory weakness can occur in neurologic conditions such as Guillain-Barré syndrome, myasthenia gravis, myopathies, and motor neuron disease. Patients may notice dyspnea at rest or on exertion, orthopnea, or weak cough. On examination, the clinician may note accessory muscle use for breathing.

At the bedside, breath counting can be used to help estimate lung function, particularly in patients with neuromuscular weakness. In the single breath count test, a patient takes a deep breath and then counts numbers aloud in their normal speaking voice and pace without taking another breath, ideally at a rate of about two numbers per second. The provider notes the highest number the patient can reach before needing to take another breath. Values above 30 are generally reassuring, although this depends on the speed at which patients count. Trending this value over time is more valuable than a single measurement.

In addition, patients with neuromuscular weakness usually have hypercarbic respiratory compromise rather than hypoxemic respiratory failure. A normal pulse oximetry measurement may therefore be falsely reassuring of a patient's respiratory status in neuromuscular disease.

CLINICAL APPROACH

History

The history should first attempt to determine whether the patient has true neurologic weakness (ie, loss of strength) or rather fatigue or pain causing the perception of weakness. For example, a patient with fatigue due to a systemic etiology or depression may describe weakness but report no trouble with lifting heavy objects or performing activities of daily living. The distribution of weakness should be elicited by asking which parts of the body are affected and how activities of daily living are impacted (Table 11.3). For example, difficulty chewing/swallowing or speaking would suggest weakness of cranial nerve–innervated muscles, difficulty reaching for objects on a high shelf or washing one's hair would suggest proximal upper extremity weakness, difficulty rising from a chair would suggest proximal lower extremity weakness, and difficulty writing or using one's phone would suggest distal upper extremity weakness. Although a patient may report severe weakness in one limb as the main symptom, the clinician should inquire about possible less prominent weakness in other limbs or muscles of the head and neck.

As with any symptom, determining the time course of onset and evolution is key to differential diagnosis. Sudden-onset focal weakness suggests stroke. Rapidly evolving generalized weakness over days to weeks can be seen in Guillain-Barré syndrome or botulism. Subacute weakness evolving over months can be seen in inflammatory neuropathies and inflammatory myopathies. Chronically evolving weakness can be seen with many causes of peripheral neuropathy, radiculopathy, myopathy, and motor neuron disease. Fluctuating and fatigable weakness can be seen in myasthenia gravis, which often causes symptoms greater after activity or later in the day. Episodic weakness can be seen in periodic paralysis. These conditions are discussed in Chapters 24 and 25. Preceding events should also be asked about: Trauma could lead to subdural or epidural hematoma, vertebral fracture with spinal cord compression, or peripheral nerve injury; infection often precedes Guillain-Barré syndrome or myelitis.

Associated symptoms accompanying weakness can also provide clues to the localization. A brain lesion may cause changes in speech, language, or vision. A brainstem lesion may cause diplopia, dysarthria, or dysphagia; these symptoms can also occur with conditions of the neuromuscular junction. Conditions affecting the nerves or nerve roots may cause accompanying numbness or paresthesias. Conditions affecting the spine may cause neck or back pain along with bladder or bowel dysfunction.

The history generally provides a clear picture of the distribution of weakness, leading to an initial hypothesis about localization to be tested with the examination.

Examination

The goal of the examination is to establish the pattern of weakness with respect to distribution (ie, unilateral, bilateral, proximal, and distal) and whether there are

TABLE 11.3	Weakness Localization and Activity Impairment
Weakness location	**Activity impairment**
Proximal arm weakness	• Difficulty brushing or washing hair • Difficulty reaching for high objects
Distal arm weakness	• Loss of grip strength • Frequent object dropping • Slow or clumsy typing and texting
Proximal leg weakness	• Difficulty climbing stairs • Difficulty rising from a low chair
Distal leg weakness	• Tripping over feet while walking • Rolling over ankle while walking
Facial weakness	• Difficulty with whistling • Food or liquid falling out of mouth while eating
Respiratory weakness	• Shortness of breath at rest • Orthopnea • Weak cough

upper or lower motor neuron signs. For a discussion of specific physical examination maneuvers and techniques, see Chapter 3.

Initial observations on the distribution of weakness may be made while taking the history. For example, a patient with proximal weakness may be unable to sit up in the chair, a patient with unilateral weakness may have more spontaneous movement of the contralateral limb, and a patient with respiratory muscle weakness may be short of breath.

Although both upper and lower motor neuron lesions cause weakness, they cause unique accompanying examination signs. Upper motor neuron signs on examination include increased muscle tone (spasticity), hyperreflexia, slow finger and foot tapping, pronator drift, a pyramidal distribution of weakness (see later), and Babinski sign (extension of the big toe when the plantar surface of the foot is stimulated). Lower motor neuron signs include decreased muscle tone (hypotonia), hyporeflexia or areflexia, significant muscle atrophy (except for neuromuscular junction disease), and fasciculations (Table 11.4).

Weakness due to an upper motor neuron lesion affects particular muscle groups, causing a pattern of weakness referred to as *pyramidal*: In the upper extremity, extensors are weaker than flexors, whereas in the lower extremity, flexors are weaker than extensors. Therefore, a patient with pyramidal pattern weakness

of the arm will be stronger in elbow flexion (biceps), wrist flexion (flexor carpi radialis and ulnaris), and finger flexion (flexor digitorum superficialis and profundus) but weaker in elbow extension (triceps), wrist extension (extensor carpi radialis and ulnaris), and finger extension (extensor digitorum). Of note, the commonly used technique of testing grip strength (a test of finger and wrist flexion) could miss pyramidal pattern weakness—testing finger and wrist extension is more sensitive. In the lower extremity, the patient with pyramidal pattern weakness will be stronger in knee extension (quadriceps) and ankle plantar flexion (gastrocnemius) but weaker in hip flexion (iliopsoas), knee flexion (hamstring), and ankle dorsiflexion (tibialis anterior).

Pronator drift is a sign of subtle upper motor neuron weakness. To look for pronator drift, a patient is asked to stretch out their arms in front of them with palms upward and close their eyes. If there is upper motor neuron weakness, the arm will pronate (rotate inward) and drift downward. Downward drift without pronation is nonspecific.

When evaluating for lower motor neuron changes, assessing for atrophy is critical. Asymmetric atrophy is most easily appreciated. While atrophy of the most proximal muscles is often the easiest to recognize, assessing for distal atrophy is also important, especially in the evaluation of neuropathies. In the hands, the thenar muscles and interossei muscles are the first to atrophy in neuropathic conditions. In the feet, the extensor digitorum brevis on the lateral dorsal surface may be atrophied.

Fasciculations, or brief involuntary twitches of muscle fibers, may be seen in some neuropathies and are one of the hallmark features of motor neuron disease. Fasciculations without associated weakness are usually benign, particularly when they occur in commonly used muscles such as the calves, interossei, or eyelids. Motor neuron disease often causes fasciculations more diffusely in the chest, back, limbs, and tongue. Notably, motor neuron disease frequently affects the lower cranial nerves, causing dysarthria, tongue weakness, tongue atrophy, and/or tongue fasciculations. Tongue strength can be tested by having the patient press the tongue on the inside of the cheek against resistance from the examiner's finger on the

TABLE 11.4	Upper Versus Lower Motor Neuron Findings on Neurologic Examination	
Sign	Upper motor neuron lesion	Lower motor neuron lesion
Bulk	Normal	Atrophy frequently present
Tone	Increased	Normal or decreased
Finger/foot tapping	Slowed	Normal, but may be limited by weakness
Reflexes	Increased	Decreased or absent
Fasciculations	Absent	May be present
Weakness pattern	Pyramidal	Variable depending on lesion
Babinski sign	Present (extensor response/ upgoing big toe)	Absent (flexor response/ downgoing big toe)

cheek. Tongue fasciculations are occasionally confused with tongue tremulousness. Fasciculations are best appreciated with the tongue resting at the bottom of an open mouth and will appear like a "bag of worms" moving below the surface. Tongue tremulousness will be more regular and rhythmic and lack the random, quick movement seen with fasciculations.

If a neuromuscular junction disorder such as myasthenia gravis is under consideration and strength testing does not demonstrate weakness, the patient can be asked to perform repetitive movements such as raising their arm above their head or going from sitting to standing repeatedly, and then the examiner can reassess strength to see if weakness has been induced by this, signifying fatigability.

The motor and reflex examination should be complemented by the other components of the complete neurologic examination. Abnormalities on the mental status examination suggest a brain lesion. Cranial nerve deficits could suggest a lesion of the brainstem, cranial nerves, neuromuscular junction, or muscle. Myasthenia gravis frequently causes ocular symptoms such as ptosis or gaze palsy. The ankle dorsiflexors and plantar flexors are extremely strong muscles that can support the entire weight of the body. Therefore, weakness in these muscles may be hard to elicit with simple strength testing but may be apparent when the patient walks: Difficulty with toe walking may be a sign of gastrocnemius weakness, while difficulty with heel walking implies dorsiflexion weakness. Evaluation of gait is discussed in Chapter 14.

In sum, with respect to the signs seen on examination with lesions at different levels of the nervous system:

- **Brain**: Weakness is usually contralateral to the lesion in the face, arm, and/or leg and follows a pyramidal distribution. Other upper motor neuron findings such as slowed finger and/or foot taps, pronator drift, increased tone, and hyperreflexia may be present.
- **Brainstem**: Weakness is usually seen on the ipsilateral face and contralateral body, depending on the site of the lesion. Additional cranial nerve findings, including extraocular movement abnormalities, dysarthria, or vertigo, may be present. Upper motor neuron findings may accompany limb weakness.
- **Spinal cord**: Weakness on the ipsilateral side of the lesion is usually present and follows a pyramidal distribution. Like brain and brainstem lesions, upper motor neuron findings may be seen in affected limbs. Sensory findings and bowel/bladder dysfunction may also be present.
- **Radiculopathy**: Weakness follows a specific pattern based on the muscles a particular nerve root innervates. Shooting pain and dermatomal numbness frequently occur with radiculopathy. If severe, atrophy of involved muscles may be seen. Hyporeflexia or areflexia of a specific root level may be seen (eg, absent patellar reflex in L4 radiculopathy).
- **Neuropathy**: Weakness is usually distal and accompanied by sensory changes and hyporeflexia or areflexia. Atrophy may be seen with chronic neuropathy, and fasciculations in affected regions may be present.
- **Anterior horn cell/motor neuron disease**: Weakness may begin focally and spread or may be diffuse at presentation. The most common motor neuron disease is amyotrophic lateral sclerosis (ALS), which affects both upper and lower motor neurons, causing mixed signs on examination. Fasciculations and atrophy are common. Sensory signs and symptoms are absent.
- **Neuromuscular junction**: Weakness may be proximal or generalized but is rarely only distal. The most common neuromuscular junction disorder is myasthenia gravis, which frequently affects the eye muscles at presentation. There is no atrophy, fasciculations, nor sensory signs or symptoms. In Lambert-Eaton myasthenic syndrome, reflexes may be decreased.
- **Myopathy**: Weakness is usually proximal and symmetric and does not have associated sensory signs or symptoms. Reflexes are usually normal until the muscles are too weak to generate the reflex. Atrophy may be present. Fasciculations are not seen. Neuromuscular junction and muscle disease are discussed in Chapter 25.

The examination generally determines the localization, which guides further testing for etiology affecting the implicated part of the nervous system.

DIAGNOSTIC EVALUATION

If the localization of weakness is in the central nervous system (brain, brainstem, or spinal cord), computed tomography (CT) or magnetic resonance imaging (MRI) should be performed to determine the underlying etiology. CT is often obtained in the emergency room for sudden-onset neurologic symptoms referable to the brain or may be used in patients who cannot undergo MRI. MRI is more sensitive for subtle pathology.

In the peripheral nervous system, evaluation depends on the localization (Table 11.5). For radiculopathy,

MRI of the cervical or lumbar spine should be performed. For peripheral neuropathy, evaluation depends on neuropathy phenotype and patient context and may include serum tests and/or cerebrospinal fluid analysis (see Chapter 24). Evaluation for causes of neuromuscular junction disorders and muscle disease is discussed in Chapter 25. When the localization within the peripheral nervous system is unclear, nerve conduction studies and electromyography can assist in determining the likely site(s) of pathology within the nervous system. Additional indications for nerve conduction studies and electromyography include assessing for the severity of a lesion to aid treatment decisions (eg, to assess the severity of median neuropathy in carpal tunnel syndrome to determine whether the patient is a surgical candidate) or to monitor a disease's progression.

TABLE 11.5	Localization of Weakness and Diagnostic Testing	
Localization	**Initial testing**	**Secondary testing**
Brain/brainstem	CT/MRI brain	Lumbar puncture
Spinal cord	CT/MRI cervical or thoracic spine	Lumbar puncture
Spinal root	CT/MRI cervical, thoracic, or lumbar spine	Lumbar puncture
Anterior horn cell	ALS mimic laboratory tests (see Chapter 24) NCS/EMG	Lumbar puncture Genetic testing
Plexus	NCS/EMG	MRI plexus
Nerve	Reversible neuropathy laboratory tests (see Chapter 24) NCS/EMG	Serum rheumatologic tests Lumbar puncture (acute and subacute) Genetic testing
Neuromuscular junction	Acetylcholine receptor antibodies NCS/EMG	Anti-MuSK antibodies Anti-voltage-gated calcium channel antibodies (for Lambert-Eaton myasthenic syndrome) Single-fiber EMG Botulinum toxin testing
Muscle	CK Aldolase	NCS/EMG Biopsy Genetic testing Inflammatory myopathy antibody panel

CK, creatine kinase; CT, computed tomography; MRI, magnetic resonance imaging; MuSK, muscle-specific kinase; NCS/EMG, nerve conduction study/electromyography.

SUMMARY

Using a systematic way of assessing for weakness increases the chance of correctly localizing and identifying the cause of a symptom of weakness. Using the history to characterize the weakness helps give plausible localizations from which it may originate. The examination adds additional information and is crucial for differentiating between upper motor neuron and lower motor neuron pathway dysfunction. Using both the localization and time course of symptoms helps determine the correct testing to not only confirm the localization but also determine the etiology so as to provide effective treatment of the underlying cause.

EDITORS' KEY POINTS

▶ Weakness can be caused by pathology at any level of the neuraxis, including the central nervous system (CNS—brain, brainstem, and spinal cord) or the peripheral nervous system (PNS—anterior horn cell, nerve root, plexus, nerve, neuromuscular junction [NMJ], or muscle). The neurons of the motor pathway in the CNS are called upper motor neurons, and the neurons of the motor pathway in the PNS are called lower motor neurons.

▶ The most likely localization of weakness within the nervous system can be determined by the pattern of weakness (eg, focal or diffuse, unilateral or

▶ bilateral, proximal or distal) and the presence of upper motor neuron or lower motor neuron findings on examination.

▶ Weakness in the face, arm, and/or leg on one side most commonly localizes to the contralateral brain hemisphere; upper motor neuron findings such as pyramidal pattern weakness, increased tone, and hyperreflexia may be present.

▶ Weakness on one side of the face and the opposite side of the body localizes to the brainstem (ipsilateral to the side of facial weakness, contralateral to the side of body weakness).

▶ Bilateral weakness accompanied by bowel/bladder dysfunction and upper motor neuron signs localizes to the spinal cord.

▶ Weakness in one particular aspect of one limb can be caused by a nerve root lesion or mononeuropathy. Shooting (radicular) pain and dermatomal numbness frequently occur with radiculopathy. Hyporeflexia or areflexia affecting the reflex innervated by the involved root(s) or nerve(s) may be seen on examination.

▶ Distal, symmetric weakness accompanied by distal sensory changes and hyporeflexia or areflexia is most commonly due to a polyneuropathy.

▶ Weakness that begins focally and spreads to other regions accompanied by both upper and lower motor neuron signs raises concern for ALS.

▶ Fluctuating weakness involving the eyes (causing ptosis and/or diplopia) and proximal extremities suggests myasthenia gravis, a neuromuscular junction disorder; myasthenia gravis can also involve the larynx, pharynx, and respiratory muscles.

▶ Proximal symmetric weakness with no sensory signs or symptoms suggests a muscle disorder (myopathy).

▶ Diagnostic investigation for the cause of weakness depends on the likely localization and may include neuroimaging (typically MRI) of the suspected region in the brain or spine, and nerve conduction studies and electromyography to evaluate the PNS (nerve roots, nerves, neuromuscular junction, and muscle).

CHAPTER 12

Approach to the Patient With Visual Symptoms

Sashank Prasad

INTRODUCTION

When evaluating a patient with new visual symptoms, the clinician must determine whether the problem is ocular or neurologic. Although visual symptoms are commonly caused by ocular pathology, countless neurologic disorders can also present primarily with visual symptoms, including vascular, neoplastic, infectious, and inflammatory conditions of the optic nerve or brain. This chapter describes a practical approach to the history and examination in patients with visual loss, double vision, anisocoria, ptosis, and oscillopsia in order to guide the initial diagnostic evaluation and appropriate referral to an ophthalmologist or a neurologist.

VISUAL LOSS

Neurologic disorders can impair vision if they affect the optic nerves, the optic chiasm, the optic tracts and radiations, the visual cortex in the occipital lobes, or visual processing areas in the parietal or temporal lobes (Figure 12.1). Ophthalmologic causes of vision loss include conditions that affect the cornea, the intraocular lens, the vitreous, and the retina.

History and Examination in Patients With Visual Loss

When a patient reports blurred vision or visual loss, the first step is to identify whether the symptoms affect one eye (monocular visual loss) or both eyes (binocular visual loss). If the patient has not already checked on their own, the clinician should assess this by having the patient cover one eye at a time (Figure 12.2). Visual symptoms that affect only one eye, with normal vision in the other eye, localize to the eye or optic nerve (Figure 12.2A). Vision loss in both eyes may be caused by a disease affecting both eyes or both optic nerves, but it is important to recognize which patterns of binocular visual loss suggest a lesion in the optic chiasm or cerebral hemisphere. One pattern of visual loss that signifies a neurologic cause is a homonymous visual field deficit, in which impaired vision is confined to the same part of the visual field for each eye, respecting the vertical midline. For example, a right homonymous hemianopia refers to the inability to see the right side of the world with both eyes (Figure 12.2B). Homonymous deficits occur with lesions in the brain that involve the visual pathways (ie, optic tracts, optic radiations, and the visual cortex in the occipital lobe). Of note, patients with a homonymous visual field deficit may report having a problem in one eye, but a careful history and

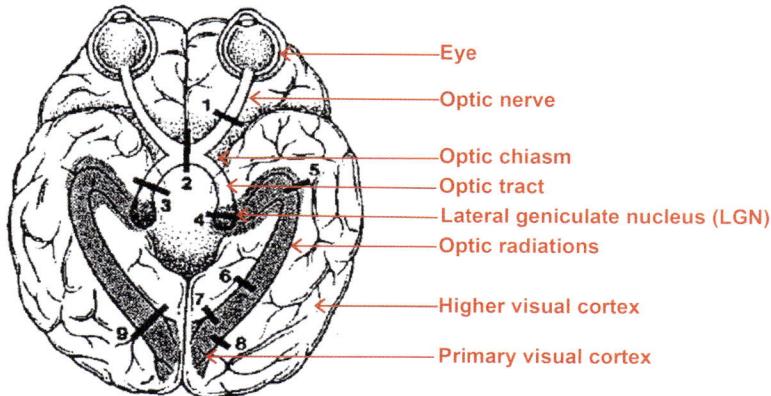

FIGURE 12.1 The visual pathways of the brain. Lesions at different locations cause different visual field deficits: lesion of the optic nerve (1) causes monocular visual loss; lesion of the optic chiasm (2) causes bitemporal hemianopia; lesion of the optic tract (3), lateral geniculate nucleus (4), or both optic radiations (9) cause a contralateral homonymous field deficit; lesion of the optic radiations (5, 6, 7, 8) causes a contralateral quadrantanopia. See text for explanation.

examination discloses the binocular nature of the visual deficit and allows correct localization to the visual pathways of the brain. This distinction is critical for pursuing appropriate triage and diagnostic evaluation.

Monocular Visual Loss

Monocular visual loss occurs due to a condition affecting the eye or optic nerve. In patients experiencing monocular vision loss, physical examination maneuvers

Monocular visual loss in the right eye

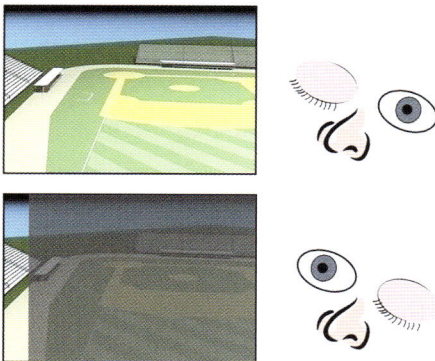

Right homonymous visual field loss

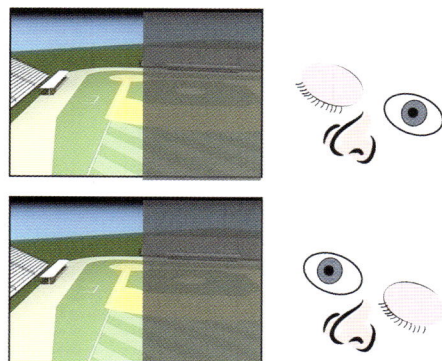

A

B

FIGURE 12.2 Distinguishing monocular visual loss from a homonymous visual field deficit. A. With monocular visual loss in the right eye, the patient will have normal vision with the left eye and reduced vision with the right eye. B. However, with a right homonymous visual field deficit, the patient will have reduced vision of the right side of the world with *both* the right and left eyes when tested separately.

that can distinguish whether the abnormality is in the eye or in the optic nerve include pinhole testing, assessment of color vision, the pupillary light reflex, and funduscopy.

Pinhole testing. If visual acuity improves when looking through a pinhole (Figure 12.3), the visual impairment is likely related to refractive error, and the cause is probably ocular. However, if the visual acuity does not improve when looking through a pinhole, an optic nerve condition should be considered.

Color vision testing. Testing color vision is another way to distinguish ocular conditions from abnormalities of the optic nerve. Impaired color vision (dyschromatopsia) is a feature of many optic nerve conditions, whereas color vision tends to be relatively preserved in most ocular conditions. Color vision can be assessed by asking the patient whether colored objects are equally vivid and bright when checking with each eye separately. Special color testing cards (including versions available for smartphones) can also be used, in which the patient is asked to identify a numeral that

can only be seen if the ability to distinguish colors is preserved (Figure 12.4).

Pupillary light reflex. Normally, when light is shined into either eye, both pupils constrict. When the light is swung from one eye to the other eye, both pupils should stay constricted. However, if there is a dysfunction of the optic nerve on one side, both pupils will dilate when the light is swung into that eye, and both pupils will constrict when the light is swung back to the normal eye (Figure 12.5). This is called a relative afferent pupillary defect and localizes most commonly to the optic nerve. Thus, the swinging flashlight test can provide objective evidence of optic nerve dysfunction by comparing the function of one optic nerve relative to the other.

Fundus examination. The fundus examination is an important part of the evaluation of patients with visual symptoms, allowing for visualization of the optic nerve (the optic disc), retina, and macula to assess for pathology in any of these structures. Some newer ophthalmoscopes such as the PanOptic offer improved visualization of the fundus without the need for

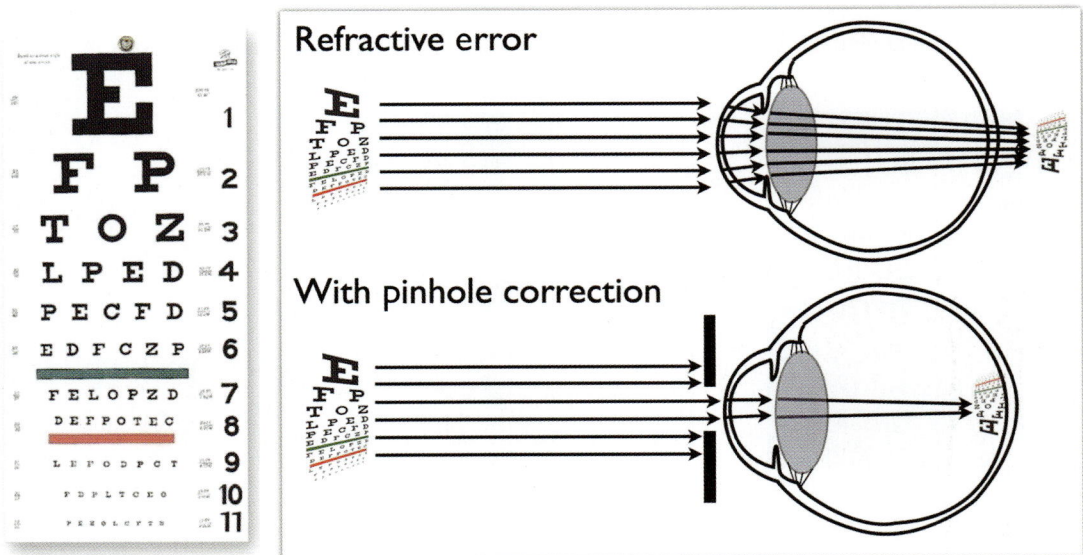

FIGURE 12.3 Use of a pinhole to determine the likely localization of reduced visual acuity. When reduced visual acuity is due to refractive error, the eye does not properly focus the image onto the retina. When viewing through a small pinhole, only focused beams of light enter the eye and the image on the retina is clear. Therefore, reduced acuity that improves with a pinhole suggests refractive error, whereas reduced acuity that does not improve with pinhole suggests conditions affecting the retina or optic nerve.

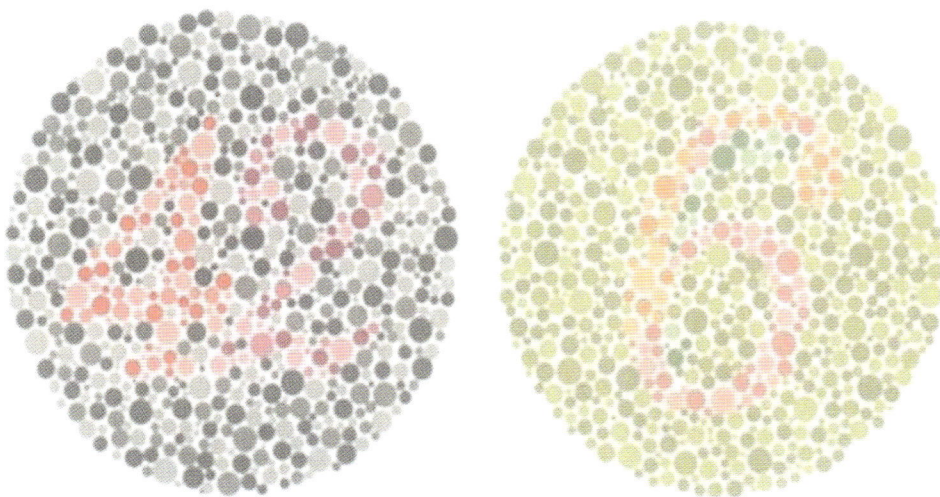

FIGURE 12.4 Ishihara color plates to assess color vision. To identify the numeral in each color plate, an individual must be able to distinguish the colors of the small circles in the testing plates.

pharmacologic dilation (Figure 12.6) compared to standard direct ophthalmoscopes, but detailed funduscopic examination generally requires ophthalmology referral.

Conditions Affecting the Optic Nerve (Optic Neuropathy)

Vision loss that is due to a condition affecting the optic nerve is typically characterized by reduced visual acuity that does not improve with pinhole, reduced color vision, and the presence of a relative afferent pupillary defect. The optic disc appearance may or may not be abnormal, depending on the precise location of the optic nerve abnormality. The differential diagnosis for an optic nerve condition depends on the tempo of onset of the visual deficits, the presence or absence of pain and other neurologic deficits, and the remainder of the medical history.

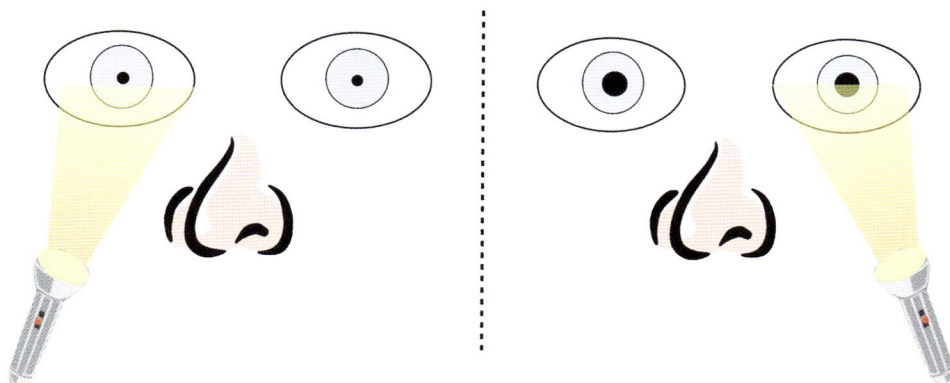

FIGURE 12.5 Left relative afferent pupillary defect identified by the swinging flashlight test. When the light is shined into the right eye, both pupils constrict, but when the light is swung and shined into the left eye, both pupils dilate. This abnormality in the pupillary light reflex indicates that there is likely a problem with the function of the left optic nerve.

Standard direct ophthalmoscope

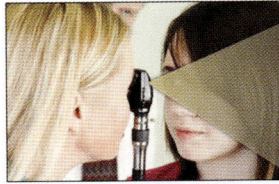

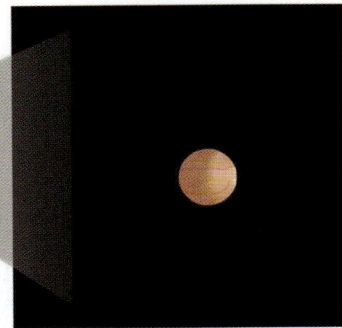

5° view

Panoptic direct ophthalmoscope

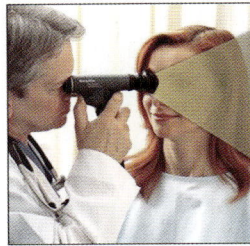

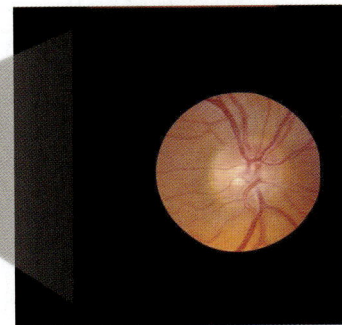

15° view

FIGURE 12.6 View of fundus with standard and PanOptic direct ophthalmoscopes. A standard direct ophthalmoscope offers only a 5° view, allowing visualization of only part of the optic disc. A PanOptic ophthalmoscope offers a 15° view, allowing visualization of the entire optic disc.

Optic Neuritis

Optic neuritis refers to inflammation of the optic nerve. It most commonly occurs in the setting of demyelinating disease (eg, multiple sclerosis, neuromyelitis optica spectrum disorder, and myelin oligodendrocyte glycoprotein [MOG]-associated disease; see Chapter 20), but can also be caused by systemic conditions such as sarcoidosis and infections such as Lyme disease and syphilis. Optic neuritis typically causes visual impairment that progresses over a few days and is commonly accompanied by pain with eye movement. The visual impairment can range from relatively mild to complete blindness. Patients will have reduced color vision and a relative afferent pupillary defect, although the fundus examination is usually unremarkable since the inflammation is occurring more posteriorly in the optic nerve.

Magnetic resonance imaging (MRI) of the orbits in optic neuritis usually shows abnormal enhancement of the optic nerve, indicative of the inflammatory process. It is important to note that MRI of the brain does not provide adequate imaging of the optic nerve because of orbital fat adjacent to the optic nerve that also appears bright; MRI of the orbit utilizes a fat-suppression imaging technique that is superior for visualizing optic nerve pathology (Figure 12.7). Therefore, when ordering MRI to assess the optic nerve, MRI of the orbits should be specifically requested. In this circumstance, obtaining MRI of the brain without MRI of the orbits could lead to an important diagnostic radiologic finding being missed.

For patients with optic neuritis thought to be related to demyelinating disease, intravenous (IV) corticosteroid treatment can improve the rate of recovery of

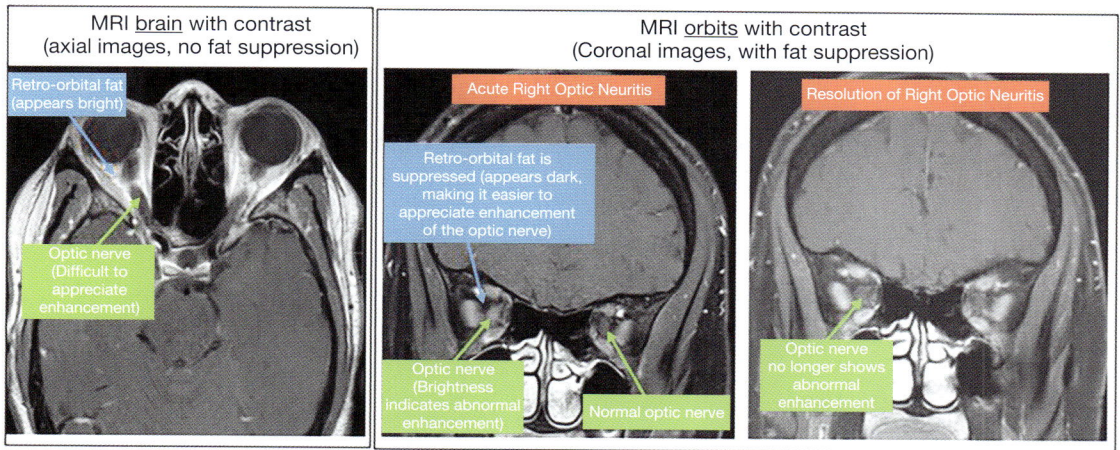

FIGURE 12.7 MRI of the brain compared to MRI of the orbits. With MRI of the brain, retro-orbital fat appears bright, making it difficult to identify the presence of abnormal contrast enhancement of the optic nerve. With MRI of the orbits, an imaging technique called "fat suppression" makes the retro-orbital fat appear dark so that the abnormal contrast enhancement of the optic nerve can be identified. MRI, magnetic resonance imaging.

vision, although it does not significantly impact the final visual outcome.[1] When optic neuritis occurs in the context of multiple sclerosis, the clinical features and/or neuroimaging will demonstrate additional inflammatory NS lesions disseminated in space and time. In these cases, referral to a neurologist should be made for discussion of the risks and benefits of the long-term disease-modifying immunomodulatory therapies that can reduce the risk of future relapses (further discussed in Chapter 20). Appropriate additional diagnostic evaluation for optic neuritis depends on the specific clinical context, but may include serologic testing for infections (eg, Lyme, *Bartonella*, HIV), anti-AQP4 and anti-MOG antibodies, and lumbar puncture (including assessment for oligoclonal bands). For bilateral and/or severe cases of optic neuritis, a diagnosis of neuromyelitis optica spectrum disorder (NMOSD) should be suspected. Patients with NMOSD with significant visual loss may require treatment with plasma exchange in addition to IV corticosteroids (See Chapter 20).

Papilledema

Papilledema refers to optic nerve swelling caused by elevated intracranial pressure. Patients with elevated intracranial pressure often experience headaches that are worse when supine and transient visual obscurations (eg, brief graying out of vision when changing posture for example, when bending over). Initially, patients with papilledema may have mild constriction of peripheral vision with spared visual acuity and color vision. However, with increasingly severe papilledema, significant vision loss including reduced acuity can occur.

Patients with papilledema should be evaluated with MRI and magnetic resonance venogram (MRV) of the brain to determine the cause of elevated intracranial pressure (eg, tumor or other mass lesion, obstructive hydrocephalus, or venous sinus thrombosis). MRI in patients with elevated intracranial pressure may also demonstrate subtle, nonspecific features including flattening of the pituitary gland (partially empty sella), distension of the optic nerve sheath, and flattening of the globe (Figure 12.8).

In patients with suspected elevated intracranial pressure and no clear etiology on neuroimaging, lumbar puncture is critical to identify whether the cerebrospinal fluid (CSF) constituents are abnormal. Several infectious, inflammatory, and neoplastic conditions can involve the meninges and present with elevated intracranial pressure. In addition, lumbar puncture allows measurement of the CSF opening pressure. Care must be taken to perform this test accurately, with the patient relaxed while the pressure is measured, to avoid

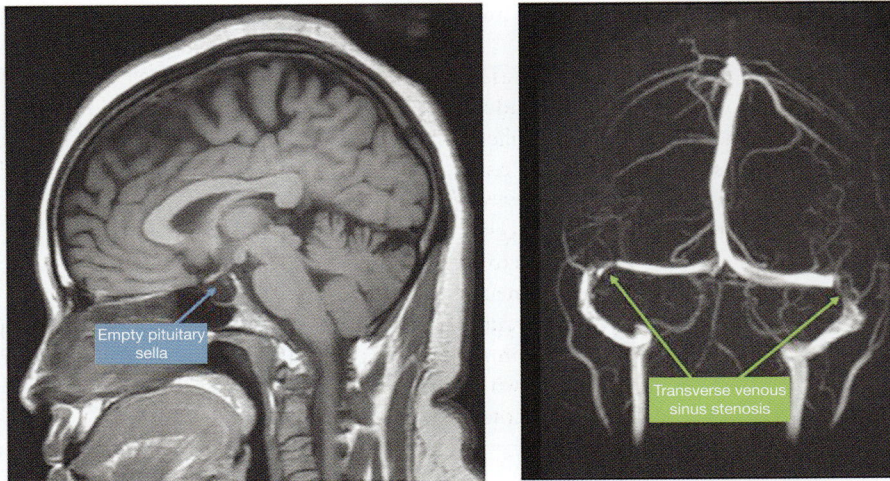

FIGURE 12.8 Imaging findings in idiopathic intracranial hypertension. Common imaging findings seen in patients with idiopathic intracranial hypertension include an "empty" or partially empty pituitary sella, with flattening of the pituitary gland and expansion of the sella turcica, and stenoses of the transverse venous sinuses.

spuriously elevated measurements. Opening pressures between 20 and 25 cm H_2O are in the borderline range, but pressures above 25 cm H_2O are considered abnormally elevated.

Idiopathic intracranial hypertension (pseudotumor cerebri). Idiopathic intracranial hypertension, also referred to as pseudotumor cerebri, causes elevated intracranial pressure without any clear structural cause. This condition is more frequent in women than men, and it is highly associated with weight gain. Retinoid medications (such as those prescribed for acne) and tetracycline antibiotics can cause a similar syndrome. MRI does not show a structural etiology of elevated intracranial pressure, although alterations in venous anatomy may be observed on MRV such as a congenitally hypoplastic or stenotic segment of one of the transverse venous sinuses (Figure 12.8). Weight loss is critical to managing this condition successfully. In addition, to improve the visual deficits and reduce headache, many patients require medical treatment to lower the intracranial pressure. Acetazolamide is the most commonly used medication, but may cause paresthesias and alteration of taste.[2] If visual deficits do not respond to these conservative measures, ventriculoperitoneal shunt, lumboperitoneal shunt, optic nerve sheath fenestration, or stenting of venous sinus stenosis should be considered.

Ischemic Optic Neuropathy

Ischemic optic neuropathy is classified as arteritic (caused by arteritis, ie, blood vessel inflammation) or nonarteritic. Arteritic ischemic optic neuropathy is most commonly caused by giant cell arteritis (GCA). Patients with GCA tend to be older and frequently have other symptoms such as scalp tenderness, jaw claudication, myalgias, and weight loss. However, some patients can present with isolated visual symptoms, requiring a high index of suspicion for the condition. The optic disc in GCA can show pallor and swelling, and areas of ischemia elsewhere in the retina (cotton wool spots) may also be present. Elevation of the erythrocyte sedimentation rate (ESR) or C-reactive protein (CRP) is highly suggestive of this condition, but nonspecific. Urgent ophthalmologic referral should be considered. The diagnosis may be made by temporal artery ultrasound or fluorescein angiography, but definitive confirmation usually requires a temporal artery biopsy. Given the high risk of visual loss in GCA, if there is concern for this condition, empiric high-dose steroid treatment should be initiated immediately while awaiting diagnostic results.

Nonarteritic ischemic optic neuropathy causes painless sudden vision loss in one eye. On funduscopic examination, the optic disc appears swollen without evidence of retinal ischemia. Patients at risk for this condition often have a congenitally crowded optic nerve with a small cup-to-disc ratio, and surgery in the prone position is also considered a risk factor. Patients who develop nonarteritic ischemic optic neuropathy in one eye are at risk for the condition occurring in the other eye. Since nocturnal hypotension is also believed to be a contributing factor, patients with this condition should be advised to avoid nocturnal antihypertensive medications.

Lesions Causing a Visual Field Deficit

Visual inputs coming from each eye travel through the optic nerves and then arrive at the optic chiasm. The visual inputs coming from the nasal half of the retina of each eye (representing the temporal visual field) cross at the optic chiasm to enter the contralateral optic tract. The visual inputs coming from the temporal half of the retina of each eye (representing the nasal visual field) travel through the optic chiasm without crossing to the other side, entering the ipsilateral optic tract. Because of this arrangement, the visual pathways posterior to the optic chiasm (ie, the optic radiations and the visual cortex in the occipital lobe) represent the contralateral visual field as seen by both eyes: The left visual field in both eyes is represented in the right cerebral hemisphere and the right visual field in both eyes is represented by the left cerebral hemisphere. Lesions affecting the visual pathways posterior to the optic chiasm (ie, in the brain) cause a contralateral homonymous visual field deficit in both eyes that respects the vertical midline (eg, hemianopia, quadrantanopia). Patients with a homonymous visual field deficit require brain imaging to identify the underlying etiology, which may be vascular, neoplastic, infectious, or inflammatory.

Patients with a complete homonymous hemianopia have significant functional impairments resulting from their vision loss. When patients turn their head to the affected side, they will see what is there, but when they hold their eyes and head still, they will only see an object once it has crossed the midline in front of them and entered the intact visual field. Most states have legal restrictions that forbid driving with a significant homonymous visual field deficit. Patients with visual field deficits often have reduced reading fluency as they may miss parts of words or sentences.

Bitemporal hemianopia refers to loss of vision in the temporal field of each eye. This deficit localizes to a lesion affecting the optic chiasm where a subset of fibers from each eye cross to reach the opposite optic tract. The most common cause is a pituitary macroadenoma that compresses the optic chiasm inferiorly (Figure 12.9).

The prognosis for visual field recovery depends on the etiology. In general, visual field deficits following ischemic stroke may improve somewhat in the months after a stroke, but recovery following this period is generally minimal, leaving patients with a permanent visual field deficit.

Conditions Affecting Higher Visual Functions

Lesions of some regions of the cerebral cortex can cause visual processing deficits despite preserved visual

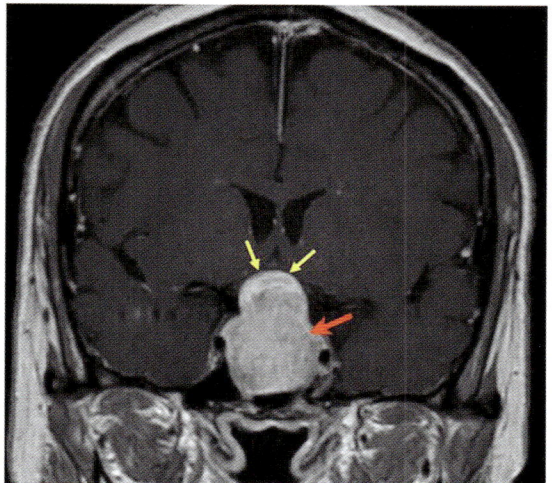

FIGURE 12.9 Pituitary macroadenoma. The large pituitary macroadenoma (red arrow) compresses the optic chiasm (yellow arrows).

acuity. These higher order visual processing deficits can be caused by stroke, metastases and other brain tumors, and neurodegenerative diseases such as dementia with Lewy bodies and Alzheimer disease (see Chapter 18).

Neglect

A lesion affecting the right parietal lobe can cause left hemispatial neglect. The parietal lobes play a key role in shifting spatial attention to different objects in the visual field. With a right parietal lesion, an individual develops a bias for visuospatial attention toward the right, with an impaired ability to shift attention toward the left. If the visual environment is very simple, the individual may be able to attend to some objects on the left, but if the complexity of the environment increases with multiple objects competing for visual attention, items on the left are no longer consciously perceived. For example, if a patient with left-sided neglect is shown a piece of paper with many targets on it and asked to cross them out, they will often cross out only the targets on the right side of the page and miss many of the targets on the left side. Similarly, if they are asked to make a drawing of an object, such as a house or a flower, they will draw the details on the right side of the object but fail to draw details on the left (Figure 12.10). A common etiology of acute left hemispatial neglect syndrome is a right middle cerebral artery (MCA) infarct, although other conditions affecting the right hemisphere can be the cause (eg, neoplasm).

Balint Syndrome

Bilateral parieto-occipital lesions can cause a severe impairment of visuospatial attention known as Balint syndrome. A key feature is simultanagnosia, in which the patient can visually process only one item at a time but cannot disengage visual attention in order to shift it to other portions of the scene to understand how they fit together. For example, when shown the "cookie thief picture" (in which two children are climbing a stool to steal cookies from a jar in a cupboard, while their parent is standing by the sink and the sink is overflowing with water), an individual with bilateral parieto-occipital lesions may only describe the water coming out of the sink but would be unable to shift spatial attention to see the other elements of the picture.

DOUBLE VISION (DIPLOPIA)

When a patient describes double vision (diplopia), the history and examination should determine whether it is monocular (in one eye only) or binocular (present only when both eyes are open). This can be determined by asking the patient to cover each eye separately: Binocular diplopia resolves if either eye is closed, whereas monocular

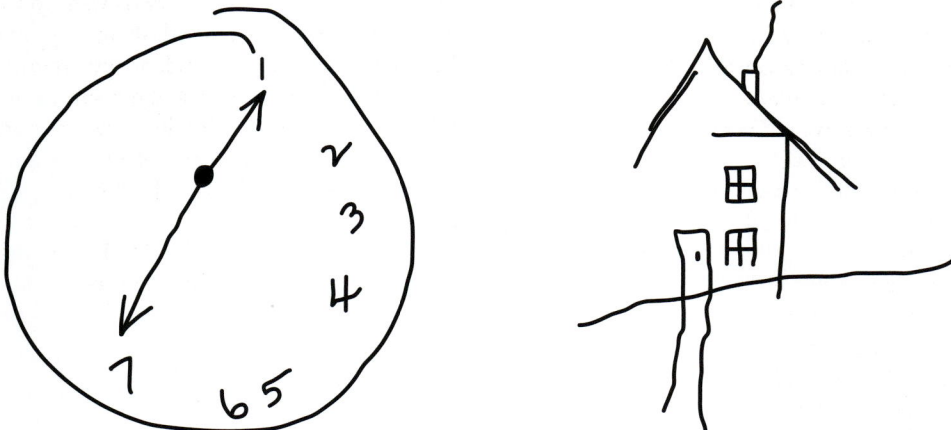

FIGURE 12.10 Left-sided spatial neglect. These drawings made by a patient with left-sided spatial neglect following a right middle cerebral artery stroke demonstrate reduced capacity to shift spatial attention toward the left side.

diplopia persists in one eye when the other eye is closed. Monocular diplopia indicates an ocular cause (eg, an abnormality of the cornea, lens, or retina), and ophthalmologic consultation should be sought.

Binocular diplopia is caused by misalignment of the eyes, which can be secondary to a process affecting the cranial nerves controlling eye movements (cranial nerves 3, 4, and 6), their interconnections in the brainstem (via the medial longitudinal fasciculus), the neuromuscular junction (eg, myasthenia gravis), the extraocular muscles (eg, thyroid eye disease), or an orbital mass restricting eye movement.

Diplopia Due to a Cranial Nerve or Brainstem Lesion

Dysfunction of cranial nerve 3 (the oculomotor nerve) causes limited adduction, elevation, and depression of the eye, as well as ptosis and, in some cases, pupillary dilation with impaired pupillary constriction to light. Dysfunction of cranial nerve 4 (the trochlear nerve) causes impairment of the superior oblique muscle, which causes vertical diplopia that increases when the patient looks away from the side of the lesion (with the affected eye adducted). Dysfunction of cranial nerve 6 (the abducens nerve) causes limited abduction of the eye and produces horizontal binocular diplopia that is worse when the patient looks toward the side of the weak cranial nerve 6 and when the patient looks into the distance. A variety of etiologies can affect these cranial nerves, including compressive lesions (ie, tumor or aneurysm), trauma, infectious and inflammatory conditions, and metastatic cancer. Microvasculopathic cranial nerve palsies occur acutely in patients with diabetes and/or hypertension. These generally have an excellent prognosis for recovery within 3 months. Most cases of binocular diplopia due to cranial neuropathy require MRI of the brain and orbits to evaluate for structural causes.

Dysfunction of the medial longitudinal fasciculus in the dorsal brainstem that connects the nuclei of cranial nerve 6 and cranial nerve 3 causes internuclear ophthalmoplegia: limited adduction of one eye on attempted lateral gaze, often accompanied by nystagmus in the abducting eye. Internuclear ophthalmoplegia is often a sign of demyelinating disease, but it can also be caused by stroke.

Diplopia Due to Neuromuscular Junction Pathology

Myasthenia gravis is an autoimmune disorder in which antibodies block acetylcholine receptors at the synapse between nerve terminals and muscle fibers (see Chapter 25). The primary symptom is fatigable muscle weakness, in which weakness worsens with repetitive use. Binocular diplopia and ptosis are very common features of myasthenia gravis. The examination shows ptosis that worsens with sustained upgaze (as the levator palpebrae muscle fatigues) and improves with rest (eye closure). On examination, the pattern of eye movement abnormalities may mimic one or more specific cranial nerve palsies or internuclear ophthalmoplegia and may vary from one examination to another because of the variable involvement of multiple eye muscles. Pupillary function remains normal in myasthenia gravis because autonomic signaling is preserved.

Diplopia Due to Extraocular Muscle and Orbital Pathology

Thyroid eye disease is the most common condition that directly affects the eye muscles. In thyroid eye disease, one or more extraocular muscles become inflamed and fibrotic due to an autoimmune response to orbital tissues. Patients often have eyelid retraction and proptosis (bulging of the eye) in addition to limited eye movements. CT, MRI, or orbital ultrasound shows enlargement of the eye muscles. Thyroid evaluation should be performed, since patients with thyroid eye disease may be hyperthyroid, hypothyroid, or euthyroid.

Binocular diplopia can also result from a variety of orbital mass lesions that limit eye movements due to mechanical displacement of the eye and the eye muscles. Examples include orbital hemangioma, lymphoma, and metastatic tumors. These are diagnosed by their appearance on CT or MRI of the orbit, often followed by biopsy or resection of the lesion.

Symptomatic Treatment of Binocular Diplopia

In addition to treatment of the underlying etiology (when possible), binocular diplopia can be treated symptomatically. Since binocular diplopia is due to ocular misalignment, occlusion of one eye eliminates double vision. This can be done either with an opaque eye patch or with transparent tape placed over one lens of a pair of eyeglasses. The transparent tape method is successful because it makes one image so blurred that the patient easily ignores it and no longer perceives double vision. In addition, it is more cosmetically appealing than an eye patch, and it can be more comfortable because it allows some light to enter the eye. When the ocular misalignment causing binocular diplopia is relatively stable, a prism can be used to shift the image entering the eye by the right amount so that the patient experiences single instead of double vision. A temporary (Fresnel) prism can be pasted on the glasses, and if this is successful, a permanent prism can be ground into the lenses. Finally, if the patient has longstanding, stable ocular misalignment, eye muscle surgery can be performed to shift the position of the eyes the appropriate amount so that normal ocular alignment is achieved in most directions of gaze.

ANISOCORIA

Anisocoria refers to asymmetry in the size of the pupils. The key to determining whether anisocoria is physiologic or pathologic is to assess the size of the pupils in darkness and in light. With normal physiologic anisocoria, the asymmetry in pupillary size is essentially the same in darkness and in light. However, with pathologic anisocoria, the amount of anisocoria may be greater in darkness or in light.

An asymmetry in pupillary size that is greater in darkness suggests a problem with the dilation of the smaller pupil (ie, Horner syndrome). Other features of Horner syndrome include subtle ptosis (1-2 mm). Horner syndrome is caused by impaired sympathetic innervation of the eye and can result from lesions anywhere along the course of the sympathetic pathway in the brainstem, upper chest, neck (eg, carotid dissection), or cavernous sinus. Diagnostic evaluation for a patient with new Horner syndrome should include imaging of the brain and chest, and vascular imaging of the carotid artery to evaluate for dissection.

Anisocoria that is greater in the light suggests a problem with constriction of the larger pupil. In the case of a third nerve palsy, the anisocoria is usually accompanied by limitation of eye movements and/or ptosis (because the muscles that accomplish those actions are also innervated by the third cranial nerve). Isolated abnormality of pupillary constriction, without other features of a third nerve palsy, may be due to pharmacologic dilatation of the pupil (eg, after accidental exposure to a medication or chemical) or due to tonic pupil (which refers to a presumed postinfectious inflammation of the ciliary ganglion that conveys parasympathetic innervation to the pupillary constrictor). Diagnostic evaluation of a pupil-involving third nerve palsy should include urgent neuroimaging with CT or MRI and CT angiogram or MR angiogram to assess for lesions that can compress the third nerve, such as an aneurysm of the posterior communicating artery. Tonic pupil and a pharmacologically dilated pupil do not require diagnostic evaluation with neuroimaging.

PTOSIS

Ptosis of the eyelid can have various etiologies. With third nerve palsy, there is weakness of the levator palpebrae eye muscle, which can cause significant ptosis leading to complete closure of the lid. With Horner syndrome, there is reduced sympathetic innervation of the Müller muscle, causing only mild ptosis (the lid usually still remains above the pupil). Variable ptosis that increases when the levator palpebrae muscle is fatigued (with sustained upgaze) is a feature of myasthenia gravis. Often, ptosis does not have a neurologic cause but is due to mechanical changes in the position of the eyelid muscle (eg, levator dehiscence).

OSCILLOPSIA

Oscillopsia refers to the illusory perception of motion. There are two main circumstances in which patients can describe oscillopsia: nystagmus and impaired vestibulo-ocular reflex. Nystagmus refers to rhythmic eye movements that disrupt visual fixation. It can result from pathology in either the peripheral or central vestibular system. Examples of peripheral causes of nystagmus include vestibular neuritis, vestibular schwannoma, and Ménière disease. Examples of central causes of nystagmus include stroke or demyelination in the brainstem or cerebellum. These conditions and the clinical distinction between peripheral and central nystagmus are also discussed in Chapters 9 and 22.

The vestibulo-ocular reflex coordinates eye movements with head movements to maintain visual fixation when the head is moving. With impairment of the vestibulo-ocular reflex, these normal eye movements no longer occur when the patient is moving, leading to dizziness and oscillopsia. An impaired vestibulo-ocular reflex can be caused by pathology of the eighth cranial nerve (eg, vestibular schwannoma) or inner ear (eg, gentamicin toxicity).

SUMMARY

Whether the symptom is visual loss or double vision, a key aspect of the history and examination is to determine whether the problem is monocular or binocular. Monocular conditions may be related to either pathology of the eye or the optic nerve. Visual field deficits in both eyes and binocular diplopia are due to lesions in the nervous system that require localization, appropriate diagnostic evaluation, and referral to neurology. Anisocoria can be physiologic, pharmacologic, or due to a structural lesion of cranial nerve 3 or the oculosympathetic pathway (Horner syndrome). Ptosis can be due to cranial nerve 3 palsy (usually accompanied by extraocular muscle weakness and dilated pupil), Horner syndrome, myasthenia gravis, or mechanical changes of the lid. A careful examination can often localize the cause of a patient's visual symptom, determining whether the patient needs brain imaging and whether they should be referred to an ophthalmologist or a neurologist.

EDITORS' KEY POINTS

- Visual loss in only one eye localizes to the eye or optic nerve.
- Visual loss in the same visual field in both eyes (ie, left or right hemianopia or quadrantanopia) localizes to the cerebral hemisphere contralateral to the visual field deficit.
- Bitemporal hemianopia localizes to the optic chiasm and is most commonly caused by lesions of the pituitary gland.

- Optic nerve disease (optic neuropathy) is most commonly inflammatory (optic neuritis) or vascular (ischemic optic neuropathy, which may be due to GCA or vascular risk factors) in etiology, but can rarely be toxic (eg, ethambutol) or inherited (eg, Leber hereditary optic neuropathy).
- Optic neuritis causes unilateral (or less commonly bilateral) visual loss occurring over days, and can be due to primary neurologic conditions (eg, multiple sclerosis, NMOSD, MOG-associated disease), systemic immune-mediated diseases (eg, sarcoidosis), or infections (eg, Lyme disease and syphilis).
- Double vision (diplopia) that resolves when covering either eye is due to ocular misalignment, which can be caused by a cranial nerve palsy (of cranial nerves 3, 4, or 6), a brainstem lesion, a condition of the extraocular muscles (eg, thyroid eye disease or orbital mass), or myasthenia gravis.
- Unequal pupils (anisocoria) can be due to a failure of pupillary constriction (cranial nerve 3 palsy), failure of pupillary dilation (Horner syndrome), or medication affecting one pupil (eg, ipratropium nebulizer).
- Ptosis of the eyelid can be caused by cranial nerve 3 palsy (usually accompanied by a dilated pupil and eye movement abnormalities), Horner syndrome (usually accompanied by a small pupil), myasthenia gravis (usually fatigable with sustained upgaze), or a mechanical problem (eg, levator dehiscence).

REFERENCES

1. Beck RW, Cleary PA, Anderson Jr MM, et al. A randomized, controlled trial of corticosteroids in the treatment of acute optic neuritis. *N Engl J Med*. 1992;326:581-588.
2. NORDIC Idiopathic Intracranial Hypertension Study Group Writing Committee, Wall M, McDermott MP, et al. Effect of acetazolamide on visual function in patients with idiopathic intracranial hypertension and mild visual loss: the idiopathic intracranial hypertension treatment trial. *JAMA*. 2014;311(16):1641-1651.

13

Approach to the Patient With Abnormal Movements

Emily Anne Ferenczi

INTRODUCTION

The term *movement disorder* refers to disruption of movement initiation, speed, rhythm, and/or coordination despite preserved strength and sensation. Movement disorders are broadly classified into three categories: too little movement (the hypokinetic disorder parkinsonism), too much movement (the hyperkinetic disorders: tremor, dystonia, chorea, myoclonus, and tics), and uncoordinated movements (ataxia; Table 13.1). Each movement disorder has a particular differential diagnosis that includes primary neurologic disorders, systemic conditions, and medication toxicity.

Therefore, recognizing the type of abnormal movement based on the examination is key to diagnosis and treatment. Movement disorders arise from pathology of the circuitry involving the basal ganglia or cerebellum.

NEUROANATOMY AND PATHOPHYSIOLOGY

A simplified model of higher-level control of movement consists of a two-layered system. The first layer of motor control is the pyramidal system, which directly activates muscles to execute a movement (see Chapter 11); diseases affecting this pathway lead to weakness. The second layer of motor control is the extrapyramidal system, which is responsible for more complex aspects of motor control, such as movement initiation, speed, rhythm, sequencing, and coordination. The extrapyramidal system includes the basal ganglia, the cerebellum, and their circuits involving the thalamus and cerebral cortex.

The Basal Ganglia: Control of Movement Selection, Initiation, and Sequencing

Located deep within the cerebral hemispheres, the basal ganglia are a collection of nuclei (groups of cell bodies) that participate in a loop circuit (cerebral cortex—basal ganglia—thalamus—cerebral cortex). Through this loop circuit and other connections, the basal ganglia receive input about the environment, internal state, and goal of a movement. The basal ganglia process and integrate this information,

TABLE 13.1   Definitions and Phenomenology of Movement Disorders

Type of movement disorder	Definition	Examples
Hypokinetic		
Parkinsonism	• Slowed movements with decrement in amplitude over time • Rigidity • Resting tremor	• Idiopathic Parkinson disease • Atypical parkinsonian syndromes • Drug-induced parkinsonism
Hyperkinetic		
Tremor	• Rhythmic oscillatory movement about a joint axis	• Drug-induced tremor • Parkinsonian tremor • Essential tremor • Dystonic tremor
Chorea	• Random, irregular nonpurposeful involuntary movements • Flow from one part of the body to another	• Tardive dyskinesia • Drug-induced dyskinesias • Huntington disease • Sydenham chorea
Dystonia	• Involuntary sustained or intermittent co-contraction of muscle groups • Repetitive twisting movements, abnormal postures, or tremor	• Cervical dystonia • Writer's cramp • Musician's dystonia
Myoclonus	• Shock-like, brief, irregular jerking movements	• Myoclonic epilepsy • Drug-induced myoclonus • Postcardiac arrest hypoxic-ischemic injury • Drug-induced myoclonus
Ataxia		
	• Loss of coordination, leading to abnormal rhythm, rate, and force of movement	• Cerebellar pathology

then communicate back to the cerebral cortex by way of the thalamus. This circuit underlies movement selection and sequencing, allowing for the precise type and amount of movement to be performed at each moment. The complex fine-tuning of movements is achieved through competition between two basal ganglia subcircuits: the direct pathway and the indirect pathway. The delicate balance of activity between these two pathways determines the type and degree of movements. Overactivity in the direct pathway relative to the indirect pathway is thought to be the basis of hyperkinetic movement disorders, leading to involuntary movements such as chorea or dystonia, whereas overactivity in the indirect pathway relative to the direct pathway is thought to be the basis of hypokinetic movement disorders, namely, parkinsonism. The basal ganglia are also involved in processing reward and motivation, so nonmotor symptoms such as apathy, impulsivity, anhedonia, or anxiety are frequently seen in basal ganglia disorders.

The Cerebellum: Control of Movement Coordination

Located posterior to the brainstem and inferior to the cerebral hemispheres, the cerebellum is part of another loop circuit (cerebral cortex-cerebellum-thalamus-cerebral cortex) like that of the basal ganglia, but it also receives input about the position of the body (proprioception) and head (vestibular input). While the basal ganglia subserve initiation and selection of movements, the cerebellum provides real-time feedback to coordinate ongoing movement rhythm, rate, and amplitude. The cerebellar hemispheres control the limbs, whereas the midline cerebellum (the vermis) controls the trunk and is essential for posture and balance. Cerebellar pathology leads to loss of coordination (ataxia). Unilateral focal lesions of one cerebellar hemisphere, for example, due to stroke or hemorrhage, cause unilateral (ipsilateral) limb ataxia, whereas lesions of the midline cerebellum cause truncal and gait ataxia. Cerebellar pathology can also lead to repetitive involuntary movements of the eyes (nystagmus) and irregular rhythm and volume of speech (dysarthria). Like the basal ganglia, cerebellar disease can also affect cognition and emotion.

COMMON PRESENTATIONS

Parkinsonism

Parkinsonism refers to the triad of bradykinesia (slowed movement with progressive decrement in speed and amplitude of movement), rigidity (stiffness of movement), and resting tremor (a tremor present when the affected part of the body is inactive but not when the part of the body is active). In clinical practice, the term *parkinsonism* is an umbrella term to describe the presence of bradykinesia in addition to at least one of rigidity or tremor. There are many possible causes of parkinsonism, the most common being idiopathic Parkinson disease. Patients with bradykinesia and/or rigidity may describe feeling slow or stiff but often report the experience of these symptoms as "weakness" despite having full strength. Patients may note difficulty with fine motor movements (eg, tying their shoelaces, flossing their teeth, typing on a smartphone, using a keyboard, or handwriting) and larger movements (eg, trouble turning in bed, getting dressed, buckling a seatbelt). Shoulder and back pain are common. They may notice difficulty walking or falls. If only one half of the body is affected (as occurs early in idiopathic Parkinson disease), patients may report that one leg is lagging or "scuffing," causing them to trip, or a partner or friend might comment that one arm is swinging less than the other.

Tremor

Tremor is an involuntary rhythmic oscillatory movement around a joint, which patients may describe as "shaking" or "trembling." The impact of tremor on an individual depends on when the tremor occurs (at rest or with action), which parts of the body are affected, and the severity of the tremor. Patients with an action tremor (a tremor that occurs when the affected body part is held in an antigravity posture or engaged in a voluntary action, as can be seen in drug-induced tremor and essential tremor) often describe difficulty drinking (spilling liquids, needing to hold a cup tightly with both hands) and eating (food falling off the fork or spoon),

messy handwriting, and difficulty with other fine motor tasks. In contrast, resting tremor, as occurs in parkinsonism, often does not impact action and so may only be noticed by others or by the patient when trying to relax or fall asleep at night.

Dystonia

Dystonia refers to abnormal twisting movements or postures caused by involuntary sustained muscle contraction. Dystonia may be focal (eg, cervical dystonia [torticollis] or writer's cramp) or generalized; generalized dystonia is usually inherited. Patients with dystonia describe muscles "cramping" or "locking," which may be painful. Some types of dystonia may only occur during specific tasks, such as writing or playing a musical instrument. Patients often report ways they have discovered of diminishing the dystonia (called *sensory tricks*), such as a change in position or touching a particular place (eg, wearing a scarf in cervical dystonia).

Chorea, Athetosis, and Ballism

Some involuntary movements may be more apparent to others than to the patient, such as chorea, athetosis, or ballism. Examples include drug-induced dyskinesias (such as tardive dyskinesia), dyskinesias caused by autoimmune disease or stroke, or genetic conditions such as Huntington disease. These involuntary movements can vary in appearance and severity from what may resemble subtle fidgeting to flowing, writhing, or flailing movements.

Myoclonus

Myoclonus is a brief, sudden, brisk involuntary jerking movement. It can be seen in many different conditions, including drug-induced myoclonus, myoclonic epilepsy, or myoclonus due to anoxic brain injury. Patients may describe that one or multiple parts of the body "jump," "jerk," or "twitch" at random times, disrupting ongoing movement.

Tics

Tics are brief, sudden, complex movements that may appear purposeful (eg, shoulder shrug or grimace).

Tics may occur transiently in children and resolve with age, whereas complex and persistent tics can be seen in Tourette syndrome. Patients describe a preceding urge or compulsion to complete the movement and a subsequent sense of release after the movement.

Ataxia

Ataxia is loss of coordination of movement, which causes an abnormal rhythm, rate, and force of movement. Ataxia can be caused by disorders of the cerebellum, which may be acquired (eg, cerebellar stroke, paraneoplastic cerebellar degeneration, alcohol-associated cerebellar ataxia) or genetic (eg, Friedreich ataxia or spinocerebellar ataxia), or may also be caused by diminished proprioception due to peripheral neuropathy or dorsal column disease (called *sensory ataxia*). Patients with cerebellar ataxia may report slurred speech, clumsiness, imbalance, or falls; they may describe observers saying that they sound or look "drunk."

CLINICAL APPROACH

The Movement Disorder History

The history of a patient with a movement disorder should determine the type(s) of abnormal movement, the body parts affected, the time course of symptom onset and evolution, other symptoms that may be related to the patient's chief concern, medical and medication history to look for potential causes of movement disorders, and the impact of the symptoms on the patient's life. During the history, the examiner can often begin to observe the movement disorder and how it may change with the patient's attention and movement while speaking and gesturing.

History of the Presenting Illness

A movement disorder history begins with asking patients to describe the symptom(s) of concern to them and/or their accompanying friends/family in the visit. The tempo of symptom progression is a critical diagnostic clue—slowly progressive symptoms suggest neurodegenerative or genetic causes, subacute progression may suggest an inflammatory (eg, paraneoplastic), infectious, or neoplastic process, and acute onset is more suggestive of a vascular etiology.

Whether symptoms are symmetric or unilateral is also an important element; for example, idiopathic Parkinson disease tends to present unilaterally and progress asymmetrically, whereas atypical parkinsonian disorders (eg, progressive supranuclear palsy, multiple system atrophy) are often more symmetric at presentation. Certain movement disorders may have a predilection for different parts of the body; for example, a tremor only involving the head but not the arms is suggestive of dystonic tremor, whereas a tremor of both hands and the head is more suggestive of essential tremor.

Further diagnostic clues may be provided by the presence of other neurologic symptoms. For example, a change in speech, such as a soft voice (hypophonia), can be seen in parkinsonism, whereas slurred speech (dysarthria) is more characteristic of cerebellar ataxia. For a patient with falls, knowing the nature of the falls can be helpful—for example, in progressive supranuclear palsy, patients often describe falling "like a tree," whereas in cerebellar ataxia, patients stagger or trip.

Nonmotor symptoms may not be the primary presenting feature of movement disorders but may point toward the underlying diagnosis. For example, violent acting out of dreams (rapid eye movement [REM] sleep behavior disorder) is common in idiopathic Parkinson disease, dementia with Lewy bodies, and multiple system atrophy, whereas loss of sense of smell is common in Parkinson disease and dementia with Lewy bodies but not in multiple system atrophy. In rare cases, nonmotor features may be a presenting symptom, such as cognitive impairment in dementia with Lewy bodies or profound dysautonomia in multiple system atrophy.

The history should also assess for systemic symptoms that may point toward a secondary cause for a movement disorder, such as symptoms of malignancy that may suggest a paraneoplastic condition, or symptoms of rheumatologic disease since conditions such as systemic lupus erythematosus (SLE) and antiphospholipid antibody syndrome may be associated with movement disorders such as chorea.

Finally, the history can elicit the impact of symptoms on day-to-day function and quality of life as this will often determine the approach to treatment. Specific tasks to inquire about include fine motor tasks such as writing, typing, texting, tying shoelaces, brushing or flossing teeth, eating, and drinking; gross motor tasks such as putting on clothing, turning in bed, and buckling a seatbelt; and any changes in gait or balance.

Past Medical History

In some patients, movement disorders may be caused by an underlying medical condition—known or unknown to the patient—rather than a primary neurologic disorder. For example, parkinsonism can occur in neuroinvasive infections (eg, West Nile virus encephalitis) or due to overly rapid correction of hyponatremia (extrapontine myelinolysis). Tremor can be caused by hyperthyroidism, whereas dystonia can be caused by hypoparathyroidism. Chorea be seen in hyperglycemic nonketotic states, pregnancy (chorea gravidarum), SLE, polycythemia vera, and after streptococcal infection (Sydenham chorea). Myoclonus can be caused by renal failure, hepatic failure, medications, or hypoxic-ischemic brain injury caused by cardiac arrest. Most systemic causes of movement disorders lead to bilateral abnormal movements, with some exceptions (eg, acute unilateral chorea caused by hyperglycemic nonketotic states). Patients who are immunocompromised have a higher risk for infections that have a predilection for the basal ganglia (eg, toxoplasmosis) and the cerebellar peduncles (eg, JC virus causing progressive multifocal leukoencephalopathy).

Structural brain lesions can also cause movement disorders. For example, in a patient with a history of vascular risk factors, sudden-onset hemiballism/hemichorea can be caused by an acute stroke (ischemic or hemorrhagic) in the subthalamic nucleus or other basal ganglia nuclei. In a patient with a history of malignancy or immunocompromise, subacute onset of hemichorea can be caused by space-occupying lesions in the basal ganglia such as brain metastases or cerebral abscesses (eg, toxoplasmosis). In a patient with multiple sclerosis, ataxia or tremor can result from plaques in the subcortical white matter tracts, where they can disrupt cerebellar-thalamic circuits.

Medication History

Many medications cause movement disorders. Drug-induced parkinsonism can be caused by chronic use of dopamine receptor blocking agents such as antipsychotic drugs, and some antiemetic medications (eg, metoclopramide, prochlorperazine). Action tremor can be caused by psychiatric medications (eg, selective serotonin reuptake inhibitors [SSRIs], serotonin norepinephrine reuptake inhibitors [SNRIs], lithium, neuroleptic agents); antiseizure medications, asthma medications (eg, β-agonists, theophylline), and immunosuppressive agents (eg, cyclosporin and tacrolimus). Drug-induced dyskinesias (choreiform involuntary movements), dystonia, and tic disorders can also result from chronic exposure to dopamine receptor blocking agents (antipsychotic agents are the most common culprits). Myoclonus can be provoked by many different classes of medications, including psychiatric mediations (eg, SSRIs, tricyclic antidepressants, antipsychotics, benzodiazepines), opiates, and cephalosporin antibiotics.

In patients with an established movement disorder (eg, Parkinson disease), the medication history should include a discussion of all current and previous medications tried for the condition, their effectiveness, and any side effects. One helpful approach in patients with Parkinson disease or essential tremor is to ask the patient to "walk through their day," starting with how they feel when they first wake up, the timing and amount of each medication dose, how much and how soon their symptoms change with each dose, whether there is any wearing off of the benefit prior to the next dose, and any side effects that correlate with doses.

Family History

Some movement disorders are familial. Although most cases of Parkinson disease are sporadic, individuals with young-onset Parkinson disease (onset before age 50) are more likely to have a family history of parkinsonism (~25%) compared to individuals with later onset Parkinson disease (older than age 50, and most commonly after age 60). Essential tremor often runs in families, but many patients have no family history of the condition. The onset of generalized dystonia at a young age raises concern for an inherited dystonia. A family history of chorea, especially if accompanied by progressive psychiatric or cognitive symptoms, suggests a history of an inherited neurodegenerative chorea such as Huntington disease.

Social History

The social history should assess for use of alcohol or drugs and occupational exposures. Essential tremor often (but not always) improves with alcohol, although the volume of alcohol required is variable between individuals. Some patients with essential tremor may self-medicate with alcohol, and alcohol use disorder can run in families with essential tremor. Chronic amphetamine use has been associated with the development of parkinsonism, as has the neurotoxin MPTP (1-methyl-4-phenyl-1,2,3,6-tetrahydropyridine), a contaminant of synthetic heroin that caused parkinsonism in the 1970s to 1980s and is now used in research as the basis for animal models of parkinsonism. Cocaine can cause choreoathetosis. Occupational or residential exposure to environmental toxins such as pesticides (eg, through well water exposure in rural areas), heavy metals, or certain solvents has also been linked in epidemiologic studies to Parkinson disease risk.

The social history provides an opportunity to gather background information about the patient's life, values, and priorities including occupation and living circumstances, and the support networks they have in place to navigate their symptoms. The impact of a patient's symptoms will depend on their profession and pastimes. A musician or clockmaker may be impacted by even the mildest of tremors, an avid athlete may be acutely aware of early balance disturbance or slowing of gait, and some patients may find a tremor highly embarrassing, whereas other patients may be less impacted by their symptoms. Since treatment of movement disorders is largely symptomatic, the type and timing of treatment depends on these individual patient factors.

THE MOVEMENT DISORDER EXAMINATION

Observation During the History

The examination begins as the patient walks into the clinic room, at which time the gait can be observed (see "Gait and Posture" section). Throughout the history, the patient's cognition, range of facial expression, speech, and any spontaneous movements can be noted.

Decreased facial expression (hypomimia) and reduced blink rate are common in idiopathic Parkinson disease, whereas an "astonished" expression with vertical wrinkling of the forehead (procerus sign) may be seen in progressive supranuclear palsy. A soft voice that gets progressively quieter during a sentence (hypophonia) is common in Parkinson disease; a tremulous voice may be present in essential tremor, breathy or strained speech can be caused by spasmodic dysphonia (laryngeal dystonia), and irregular rate and volume of speech is a feature of cerebellar dysarthria (called *scanning speech*). Any abnormalities in body movement can also begin to be assessed during the history: Is there a paucity of movement (hypokinesia) or an excess (hyperkinesia)? Do abnormal movements occur at rest, with action, or both? Does the patient appear aware of the movements?

General Examination

The general examination may provide clues about the presence of a systemic illness underlying the patient's movement disorder. Conjunctival pallor may suggest iron deficiency anemia, which can cause restless legs syndrome (leg discomfort relieved by voluntary movements of the legs, usually in the evenings). Proptosis, excessive sweating, and tachycardia may be seen in hyperthyroidism, which can be associated with action tremor. A characteristic malar (butterfly) rash may unveil SLE as the cause of chorea. Kayser-Fleischer rings (golden-green rings around the irises, often only visible on slit-lamp examination) and scleral icterus are clues for Wilson disease (a cause of tremor, chorea, or dystonia in young people). The general examination may also reveal systemic manifestations of primary movement disorders, such as orthostatic hypotension, which is often seen in multiple system atrophy, Parkinson disease, and dementia with Lewy bodies.

Neurologic Examination

In addition to evaluating the movement disorder, a complete neurologic examination should be performed to evaluate for other neurologic features that may provide clues to the underlying disorder and assess for concurrent conditions (such as peripheral sensorimotor neuropathy or spinal disease) that may compound the disability from a movement disorder. Areas of the neurologic examination requiring particular attention in patients with movement disorders include extraocular movements, head and limb movements, tone, coordination, and gait.

Extraocular Movements

Many disorders that affect the movements of the body also affect the movements of the eyes. Nystagmus (involuntary beating of the eyes in one or more directions) can be seen in cerebellar conditions. Square wave jerks (involuntary lateral deviations of gaze from the intended focal point) can be seen in atypical parkinsonian syndromes such as progressive supranuclear palsy and multiple system atrophy, as well as in cerebellar disease. Overshoot or undershoot of the patient's eyes when making saccades (tested by assessing movement of the eyes rapidly from the midline to a target such as the examiner's finger) is a common finding in cerebellar disease. Slowed vertical saccades may be seen in progressive supranuclear palsy. Limited upgaze is common in older individuals, but limited downgaze is a specific finding of progressive supranuclear palsy. Saccadic breakdown of smooth pursuit (interrupted rather than smooth eye movements when tracking the examiner's finger) can be seen in cerebellar and parkinsonian conditions but may also be a normal finding in older individuals.

Head, Facial, and Mouth Movements

The head is tilted or twisted to one side in cervical dystonia (torticollis), which may be accompanied by a jerky and irregular head tremor. A more rhythmic head tremor—forward (called a *yes-yes* tremor) or side-to-side (called a *no-no* tremor)—is seen in essential tremor. A head tremor is uncommon in Parkinson disease, although a tremor of the jaw or chin can be seen in addition to a limb tremor. Facial expression and blink rate are often diminished in Parkinson disease (hypomimia), whereas a surprised expression can be seen in progressive supranuclear palsy. Frequent and sustained bilateral eye blinking is seen in blepharospasm and rapid contractions of muscles on one side of the face occur in hemifacial spasm. Orofacial dyskinesias (involuntary choreiform movements such as tongue protrusion, pursing of the lips, or grimacing) are common in drug-induced tardive dyskinesia caused by antipsychotics and antiemetics.

Tremor in the Limbs

One of the most valuable features of tremor to assess is the circumstance in which it occurs: at rest or with action (including posture and ongoing movement). Rest tremor with resolution on action is characteristic of Parkinson disease. The rest tremor of Parkinson disease may be subtle, involving only a single digit, such as the thumb or index finger. If a rest tremor is not observed during the history or examination, it may be brought out by asking the patient to perform a cognitively demanding task, such as subtracting 7s from 100. Tremor present with action (eg, with antigravity posture or on moving the finger between the nose and examiner's finger) is characteristic of an enhanced physiologic tremor, medication-related tremor, essential tremor, and cerebellar or midbrain disease. Cerebellar tremor leads to increasing inaccuracy as the target (nose or finger) is approached, whereas physiologic, medication-related, and essential tremor are generally consistent throughout the range of movement. Other clinical features used to characterize tremor include amplitude, frequency, anatomic distribution, and improvement of the tremor with position or sensory input (Table 13.2). Patients may report specific circumstances that can bring out a tremor, such as drinking from a cup or holding a phone. It is useful to try to recreate these situations in the clinical evaluation, for example, asking patients to take a sip from a cup, pour water from one cup to another, or use their phone to elicit the tremor. Asking patients to draw an Archimedes spiral provides objective documentation of the degree of tremor (Figure 13.1). The patient's handwriting can be assessed for the progressive decrease in the size of writing (micrographia) seen in Parkinson disease.

Tone

Tone is assessed by passively moving the patient's relaxed limbs. Increased tone can be caused by spasticity or rigidity. Spasticity refers to increased tone with velocity dependence: If a limb is moved quickly, the tone increases suddenly, causing a spastic catch. Spasticity is

TABLE 13.2   Features of Tremor

	Medication-related or enhanced physiologic tremor	Parkinsonian tremor	Essential tremor	Dystonic tremor	Rubral tremor[a]
Activation	On action (posture or kinetic)	At rest (+/– postural/ kinetic tremor)	On action (posture, kinetic); at rest if severe	At rest and/or on action	At rest and on action
Anatomic distribution	Distal upper extremities	Distal upper extremities, lower extremities, and jaw	Upper extremities, head, and voice	Dystonic body part	Proximal upper or lower extremities
Rhythmicity	Regular	Regular	Regular	Irregular	Irregular
Frequency	High frequency (6-12 Hz)	Low frequency (4-6 Hz)	Moderate frequency (4-10 Hz)	Variable frequency	Low frequency (2-5 Hz)
Amplitude	Low	Low to high	Low to high	Low to high	High
Other features	Temporal relationship to medication or dose changes	Asymmetry common in early Parkinson disease	Family history often present, may improve with alcohol	Sensory trick Position-dependence Dystonic head tremor persists on lying down	Associated with structural CNS lesion

CNS, central nervous system.
[a]Tremor caused by structural brain lesions. usually in the midbrain and associated circuits, also known as a Holmes tremor or midbrain tremor.

caused by central nervous system lesions of the pyramidal pathway (ie, the corticospinal tracts in the brain or spinal cord) and is not a feature of most movement disorders. In contrast, rigidity refers to an increase in tone that is present throughout the range of movement and is not velocity dependent.

Rigidity is characteristic of parkinsonism and consists of the following components: lead pipe rigidity (non-velocity-dependent increased tone) and cogwheeling (tremor superimposed on increased tone, resulting in a ratcheting resistance to passive movement). The wrist and elbow joints are sensitive

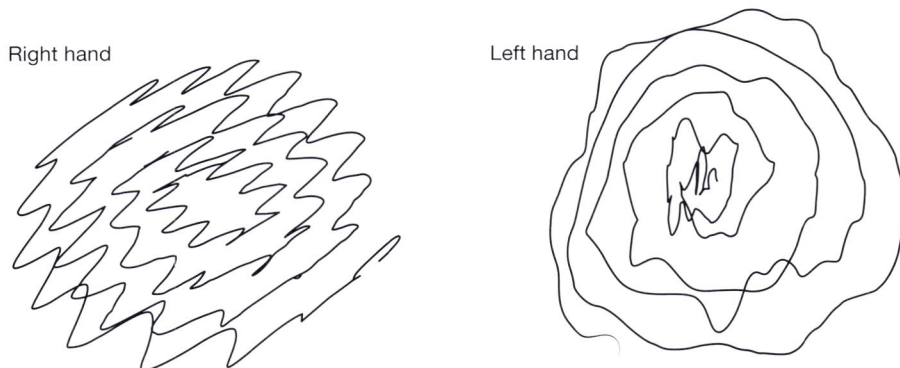

Right hand

Left hand

FIGURE 13.1 Archimedes spiral drawing in a patient with essential tremor. The image shows a rhythmic, high-amplitude tremor that has a consistent axis in the 8 to 2 o'clock direction (which is typical for right-hand spirals, whereas left-hand spirals usually show a 10-4 o'clock axis). This example demonstrates asymmetry between the two hands, with less tremor on the left.

locations to assess for cogwheel rigidity. Tone at the wrist is assessed by supporting the patient's forearm and passively rotating the wrist, and tone at the elbow is assessed by supporting the patient's arm at the elbow and flexing and extending the forearm. Subtle rigidity in a limb may become more perceptible to the examiner if the patient simultaneously performs a voluntary movement with the contralateral limb (the limb that is not being tested), such as drawing a circle in the air or opening and closing the hand. Axial tone can be examined by passively moving the neck and is usually a prominent feature of progressive supranuclear palsy, although pain and stiffness of the neck associated with osteoarthritis can sometimes make axial tone challenging to assess. In contrast, tone may be decreased in cerebellar disease. Cerebellar hypotonia can be demonstrated by asking the patient to hold their arms outstretched firmly, then giving the arms a gentle push downward and releasing; a hypotonic limb will have an exaggerated upward rebound.

Bradykinesia

Bradykinesia is defined as slowed movements with progressive decrement in speed and amplitude of repetitive movements. The progressive decrement is an important characteristic that distinguishes true parkinsonian bradykinesia from slowed movement caused by other conditions, such as psychomotor slowing in depression or a functional neurologic disorder. Bradykinesia can be assessed by rapid tapping of the index finger to the thumb, rapid opening and closing of the fist, rapid pronation and supination of the arm, and rapid tapping of the foot. It is important to ask the patient to make these movements as big and fast as possible and perform the movements on one side of the body at a time to prevent entrainment of one side by the other. In true bradykinesia, the movement will not only be slowed but also demonstrate progressive decrement in speed and/or amplitude over time.

Coordination

Coordination testing such as finger-nose, heel-shin, and rapid alternating movements (as described in Chapter 3) is done to evaluate for signs of cerebellar ataxia.

Gait and Posture

Patients with parkinsonism have reduced arm swing on one or both sides, reduced stride length with small shuffling steps, and require multiple steps to make a turn. They may exhibit sudden stopping (freezing) or sudden speeding up with multiple small steps (called *festination*). Walking may cause the emergence of resting tremor in Parkinson disease, dystonic postures in dystonia, or choreiform movements in patients with dyskinesia or chorea from various etiologies. The gait in patients with cerebellar ataxia is wide-based, and patients are unstable when walking heel to toe (tandem gait), often needing to step to the side to avoid falling.

Postural reflexes may be impaired in parkinsonian disorders and are affected particularly early in progressive supranuclear palsy. Postural reflexes can be assessed by asking the patient to stand from a sitting position with their arms crossed, assessing the speed and stability of the movement. The "pull test" also evaluates postural reflexes by assessing for retropulsion. It is performed by standing behind the patient and asking them to maintain their balance while being briefly pulled backward. The patient should be warned that they will be pulled backward, and the pull from the shoulders should be firm enough to generate at least one step backward. If the patient takes more than one step backward or simply falls backward with no steps, this is retropulsion, an indication of impaired postural reflexes. This test should be performed with a wall behind the examiner for support should the patient begin to fall backward.

DIAGNOSTIC EVALUATION

The type of movement disorder is often determined clinically at the bedside without the need for further diagnostic testing. In some primary neurologic conditions, such as Parkinson disease, the diagnosis is entirely clinical. However, laboratory testing for systemic causes of movement disorders (Table 13.3) and neuroimaging for structural lesions is necessary in some scenarios. In general, neuroimaging should be obtained for acute or subacute unilateral movement disorders to evaluate for a stroke or an other focal process. Advanced imaging (eg, positron emission tomography

TABLE 13.3   Screening Laboratory Tests to Consider for Different Movement Disorders (Targeted to the Individual Patient History and Examination Findings)

Movement disorder	Laboratory test
Hypokinetic	
Parkinsonism	• B_{12}, TSH (to rule out hypothyroidism/vitamin B_{12} deficiency as common, treatable causes of gait and cognitive dysfunction) • If concern for infection—viral serology (eg, HIV, EBV, VZV, and arbovirus) • If subacute onset—autoimmune/paraneoplastic Ab panel • If exposure history—heavy metal screen • If younger than 50 years old—serum ceruloplasmin and 24-h urinary copper
Hyperkinetic	
Tremor	• TSH and complete metabolic panel (including glucose) • If younger than 50 years old—serum ceruloplasmin and 24-h urinary copper
Chorea	• Complete metabolic panel, complete blood count, TSH, ANA, dsDNA Ab, antiphospholipid Ab panel, and autoimmune encephalopathy panel • If concern for infection: HIV and toxoplasma serology (serum/CSF) • In children: antistreptolysin Abs and streptococcus culture
Dystonia	• Complete metabolic panel and parathyroid hormone • If subacute onset: antiphospholipid Ab panel, autoimmune encephalopathy/paraneoplastic Ab panel • If young onset: genetic testing, serum ceruloplasmin, and 24-h urinary copper
Myoclonus	• Complete metabolic panel, liver function tests, HbA_{1c}, TSH, and parathyroid hormone • Antithyroid Ab and paraneoplastic/autoimmune encephalopathy Ab panel • If concern for infection: viral serology (serum/CSF), treponemal Ab, and Lyme serology • If rapidly progressive: CSF RT-QuIC for prion disease
Ataxia	
	• Complete metabolic panel, complete blood count and smear, HbA_{1c}, TSH, SPEP, ACE, vitamin E, vitamin B_{12}, homocysteine, folate, ESR • ANA, antithyroid Ab, celiac Ab, and paraneoplastic anticerebellar Ab (Yo, Ri, Hu, CV2, Tr, Ma1, mGluR1, amphiphysin, and GAD) • If rapidly progressive: CSF RT-QuIC • If concern for infection: HIV, treponemal Ab, Lyme serology, and viral serology • If young onset: genetic testing, serum ceruloplasmin and 24-h urinary copper, lipids, serum amino acids, and lactate/pyruvate • If slowly progressive or family history: genetic testing (repeat expansion panel + whole exome sequencing)

Ab, antibody; ACE, angiotensin-converting enzyme; ANA, antinuclear antibody; CSF, cerebrospinal fluid; dsDNA, double-stranded DNA; EBV, Epstein-Barr virus; ESR, erythrocyte sedimentation rate; GAD, glutamic acid decarboxylase; RT-QuIC, real-time quaking-induced conversion; SPEP, serum protein electrophoresis; TSH, thyroid-stimulating hormone; VZV, varicella zoster virus.

[PET] or single-photon emission computerized tomography [SPECT]) and cerebrospinal fluid (CSF) biomarkers may be considered in diagnostically challenging cases.

Laboratory Tests

Patients with symmetric action tremor should be evaluated for hyperthyroidism by serum TSH. If the patient is on medications that may cause tremor (eg, lithium, antiseizure medications, tacrolimus), drug levels may be informative (although many medications can cause tremor even at standard levels). Patients younger than 50 years old with tremor, dystonia, chorea, and/or parkinsonism should be evaluated for Wilson disease by serum ceruloplasmin, 24-hour urine copper, and liver function tests. Serum copper levels are less informative than levels of urinary copper excretion.

Patients with sudden-onset chorea should be evaluated for a hyperglycemic nonketotic state (serum glucose), stroke (with brain imaging), or intoxication (urine drug testing). Patients with subacute bilateral chorea should be evaluated for immune-mediated causes (SLE lupus, antiphospholipid antibody syndrome, paraneoplastic syndromes such as anti-Hu, anti-CRMP5 [collapsin response mediator protein 5], anti-NMDA [*N*-methyl-D-aspartate], and anti-IGLON5 [immunoglobulin-like cell adhesion molecule 5]) and polycythemia vera. Children who develop chorea should be evaluated with antistreptolysin titers for Sydenham chorea. Patients with unilateral chorea should be evaluated with neuroimaging to assess for stroke.

Myoclonus requires evaluation of renal and hepatic function. If accompanied by rapidly progressive dementia, the patient should be evaluated for Creutzfeldt-Jakob disease with brain magnetic resonance imaging (MRI) and CSF real-time quaking-induced conversion (RT-QuIC) testing.

Patients with cerebellar ataxia not explained by a structural lesion should be evaluated for a paraneoplastic process (with computed tomography [CT] or PET imaging of the chest/abdomen/pelvis), celiac disease, vitamin deficiencies (eg, vitamin B_{12}, vitamin E), and if slowly progressive and/or a family history of ataxia is present, genetic testing with a cerebellar triplet repeat expansion panel or whole exome sequencing.

In patients who develop movement disorders in childhood or young adulthood (eg, dystonia, chorea) or younger than age 50 in the case of parkinsonism and/or have a family history of a similar disorder, genetic counseling and genetic testing should be considered.

Cerebrospinal Fluid Testing

CSF testing is indicated if there is suspicion for an antibody-mediated or paraneoplastic cause of a movement disorder (to look for inflammation and causative antibodies), or in rapidly progressive conditions suggestive of prion disease (for which CSF RT-QuIC is diagnostic).

Structural Neuroimaging

MRI or CT should be considered in patients with unilateral movement disorders to look for a causative structural lesion. An exception is idiopathic Parkinson disease, which is often unilateral at onset, diagnosed clinically, and typically has no associated structural neuroimaging findings. In patients with acute-onset unilateral movement disorders, neuroimaging may reveal ischemic stroke or intracerebral hemorrhage. In patients with subacute progressive movement disorders, imaging may diagnose a neoplasm or features of prion disease. In patients with a history of immunosuppression, imaging may show an infectious lesion (eg, toxoplasmosis of the basal ganglia), and in patients with systemic cancer, imaging may diagnose brain metastasis.

Structural imaging may demonstrate specific findings helpful in the diagnosis of atypical parkinsonian syndromes: midbrain atrophy in progressive supranuclear palsy, pontine or cerebellar atrophy in multiple system atrophy, and asymmetric parietal lobe atrophy in corticobasal syndrome. Prominent periventricular and subcortical microvascular changes may contribute to parkinsonism, predominantly affecting the lower limbs (vascular parkinsonism). If myoclonus involves the trunk or is unilateral and exclusively below the neck, structural imaging of the spine should be considered.

Advanced Brain Imaging and Other Diagnostic Modalities

Dopamine transporter SPECT imaging is a nuclear medicine test that evaluates dopamine binding in the basal ganglia. This test shows reduced dopamine binding in neurodegenerative parkinsonian diseases (eg, idiopathic Parkinson disease, multiple system atrophy, dementia with Lewy bodies, progressive supranuclear palsy, and corticobasal degeneration) but cannot distinguish between them. As these are clinical diagnoses, the test is generally only obtained in clinically ambiguous or challenging scenarios, such as distinguishing drug-induced parkinsonism from idiopathic Parkinson disease, or distinguishing rare cases of asymmetric essential tremor from idiopathic Parkinson disease. New pathologic tests for neurodegenerative parkinsonism using skin biopsy to evaluate for abnormal deposits of the protein α-synuclein are now available.

SUMMARY

Movement disorders may be caused by primary neurologic disease or secondary to systemic illness or medications. The clinical features of a movement disorder help guide the differential diagnosis and treatment and usually fall into three major categories: hypokinetic movements (parkinsonism), hyperkinetic movements (tremor, chorea, dystonia, myoclonus, and tics), and uncoordinated movements (ataxia). The pace of onset and progression, the age at onset, the family history, medications, and any associated neurologic or systemic features on examination provide key information for determining the underlying etiology. A focused set of diagnostic tests may provide additional diagnostic clues, depending on the clinical context. Treatment for most primary movement disorders is often symptomatic, although disease modifying approaches are an active area of research. Chapter 19 explores the diagnosis and treatment of specific movement disorders in more detail.

EDITORS' KEY POINTS

▶ Movement disorders are classified into three categories: too little movement (hypokinetic disorders such as parkinsonism), too much movement (hyperkinetic disorders, such as tremor, dystonia, chorea, myoclonus, and tics), and uncoordinated movements (ie, ataxia).

▶ Parkinsonism consists of the triad of bradykinesia, rigidity, and resting tremor, although in clinical practice, the term can be used to describe the presence of bradykinesia in addition to rigidity or tremor.

▶ Tremor is an involuntary rhythmic oscillatory movement around a joint.

▶ Dystonia consists of abnormal twisting movements/postures caused by involuntary sustained muscle contraction.

▶ Chorea, athetosis, and ballism exist on a continuum and can vary in appearance and severity from subtle fidgeting to flowing, writhing, or flailing movements.

▶ Myoclonus is a brief, sudden, brisk involuntary jerking movement.

▶ Tics are brief, sudden, complex movements that may appear purposeful; patients describe a preceding urge to complete the movement followed by a sense of release after the movement.

▶ Ataxia refers to loss of coordination causing abnormal rhythm, rate, and force of movement.

▶ Characterizing the type of movement disorder, its tempo of onset and evolution, its distribution in the body, and its exacerbating and alleviating factors based on the neurologic history and examination guide the evaluation for etiology and potential initial treatments.

▶ The differential diagnosis of movement disorders includes primary neurologic diseases, medications/drugs, and systemic conditions.

Approach to the Patient With Abnormal Gait

Carrie Katherine Grouse

INTRODUCTION

Gait disorders—and the falls they may lead to—become more common with increasing age. The ability to walk normally relies on many neurologic functions, including balance, strength, proprioception, coordination, and higher-order motor control. Therefore, gait dysfunction can arise from problems anywhere in the nervous system, including motor control systems in the frontal lobes and basal ganglia, coordination circuitry in the cerebellum, proprioception pathways in the spinal cord and peripheral nerves, and motor pathways in the spinal cord, peripheral nerves, neuromuscular junction, and muscle. Difficulty walking may also be caused by pain due to orthopedic conditions of the knees and/or hips. In older patients, gait disorders are most commonly multifactorial, caused by a complex combination of deficits in balance, strength, and sensation due to common conditions, including spinal stenosis and neuropathy, in combination with orthopedic conditions causing pain. A careful history and neurologic examination can generally allow the clinician to identify the likely cause of gait dysfunction and guide appropriate evaluation.

COMMON PRESENTATIONS

Difficulty walking may be described as imbalance, weakness, incoordination, slowness, shuffling, stiffness, or increased fatigue when walking. Some patients with gait disorders may present with falls. Therefore, all patients presenting with falls should have a careful evaluation of their gait before concluding that the fall was mechanical (ie, due to tripping on an obstacle).

NEUROANATOMY AND PATHOPHYSIOLOGY

Higher-order control of movement occurs in the frontal lobes and basal ganglia, which initiate the movements of walking. Coordination of movements involved in gait occurs in the midline cerebellum, which relies on input from the vestibular system (inner ear, cranial nerve 8, and brainstem). The corticospinal tracts span the brain and spinal cord and communicate with peripheral nerves that transmit signals to muscles, providing for strength and speed of movement. Proprioception refers to the awareness of body position in space, and this information is carried by the peripheral nerves and dorsal columns of the spinal cord, which relay this information to the brain.

Due to the numerous functions and systems involved in gait, difficulty walking can be caused by a wide variety of conditions, including frontal lobe disorders (eg, normal pressure hydrocephalus; see Chapter 18), basal ganglia disorders (eg, Parkinson disease; see Chapter 19), cerebellar disorders (eg, stroke, multiple sclerosis, chronic alcohol use, and degenerative conditions; see Chapter 19), spine disorders (most commonly degenerative; see Chapter 23), peripheral neuropathy (eg, due to diabetes or vitamin B_{12} deficiency; see Chapter 24), and diseases affecting the neuromuscular junction or muscle (see Chapter 25). Gait disorders can also be caused by orthopedic conditions that cause pain when walking.

CLINICAL APPROACH

The evaluation of gait begins when observing the patient walking into the examination room. Can they walk independently or do they require support from a caregiver, a cane, a walker, or a wheelchair? Does their gait fit a particular pattern? How do they navigate thresholds, turns, and tight spaces?

History

As with any neurologic symptom, the time course of onset and evolution of the gait disorder should be established. Common causes of gait difficulty, such as peripheral neuropathy, degenerative disease of the cervical and/or lumbar spine, and Parkinson disease, most commonly present over a chronic or subacute time course. Sudden-onset gait disorders should raise concern for stroke or acute nerve root or spinal cord compression. The time course can be established by asking about when the patient began relying on ambulatory aids such as a cane or walker and the timing of falls.

The history can begin the process of localization by asking about symptoms related to the different structures that contribute to gait:

- *Frontal lobes:* Is the patient experiencing any cognitive changes or urinary incontinence?
- *Basal ganglia:* Is the patient experiencing stiffness, slowness, or tremor?

- *Cerebellum:* Is the patient experiencing a loss of coordination in the extremities or slurred speech?
- *Vestibular system:* Is the patient experiencing vertigo or dizziness?
- *Proprioceptive system:* Is the patient experiencing any numbness or paresthesia? Note that patients with loss of proprioception may describe incoordination, requiring detailed examination to distinguish sensory ataxia from cerebellar ataxia (see Chapter 10).
- *Motor system:* Is the patient experiencing any weakness? Is the weakness distal (ie, in the feet) suggesting neuropathy, proximal (ie, in the hips) suggesting myopathy, or fluctuating and fatigable suggesting myasthenia gravis?
- *Spine:* Is there neck pain or back pain? Does the patient describe progressive pain, numbness, or weakness when walking longer distances that resolves with leaning forward (eg, over a shopping cart at the grocery store) or rest, suggesting lumbar canal stenosis (see Chapter 23)?

Examination

All elements of the neurologic examination can provide potential clues as to the etiology of the patient's gait difficulties and should be included in the evaluation. Mental status testing can assess for cognitive, personality, or executive function changes suggestive of a frontal lobe disorder. The cranial nerve examination should focus on visual acuity and eye movements: vertical gaze paresis can indicate a basal ganglia disorder (although diminished upgaze can be normal in older individuals), whereas nystagmus could indicate a cerebellar or vestibular disorder. A detailed motor examination assesses for weakness and determines whether it is symmetric or asymmetric and proximal or distal. The motor examination also evaluates for rigidity and tremor, which may indicate a parkinsonian disorder. The sensory examination assesses vibration and proprioception, which can be impaired in peripheral neuropathy or dorsal column disease. Hyporeflexia or areflexia signifies peripheral neuropathy or polyradiculopathy. Hyperreflexia is seen with conditions of the brain and spinal cord. The coordination examination evaluates cerebellar function. Patients should also be assessed for pain and passive range of motion to evaluate for the contribution of any orthopedic conditions to the patient's walking difficulty.

If the general neurologic examination is normal or reveals only mild abnormalities that would not explain the patient's gait difficulty, observing the patient's gait may still reveal patterns that suggest particular conditions. Walking should ideally be observed in a hallway rather than in the clinic room so that longer distances of walking and turns can be evaluated. The patient's walking should be observed while they are dressed in their normal clothes (ie, rather than a gown) both so that they feel more comfortable and as this usually allows better visualization of their hip and leg movements that are often obscured by the gown.

The following are common patterns of gait abnormality that may be observed.

Gait Disorders Due to Frontal Lobe Dysfunction

Frontal lobe lesions may cause gait apraxia: failure to walk despite normal strength, coordination, and sensation in the legs. The gait may be described as magnetic, in which the patient struggles to lift their feet from the floor (as if their feet are pulled to the ground by magnets). Other signs of a frontal lobe disorder may include difficulty with initiating the first steps of walking, small steps, a shuffling gait, freezing of gait, and a wide-based stance. Patients can generally perform other non-gait coordinated movements normally, such as bicycling the legs in bed, confirming that the apraxia is specific to gait. Frontal lobe lesions can also be accompanied by cognitive dysfunction, abulia (decreased motivation), and urinary incontinence. An example of a frontal gait disorder is the gait seen in patients with normal pressure hydrocephalus (see Chapter 18).

Gait Disorders Due to Basal Ganglia Dysfunction

The most common condition affecting the basal ganglia is parkinsonism, which may be caused by Parkinson disease, or by medications and other neurodegenerative disorders (see Chapter 19). A parkinsonian gait is characterized by stooped posture, short steps, shuffling, en bloc turning (requiring multiple steps to turn), and decreased arm swing (often unilateral or asymmetric in Parkinson disease). Patients may also demonstrate slowness of movement (bradykinesia), cogwheel rigidity, resting tremor, and postural instability (see Chapters 13 and 19).

Gait Disorders Due to Cerebellar Dysfunction

Patients with cerebellar disorders have a wide-based, unsteady gait. However, this pattern can also be seen in patients with severe proprioceptive dysfunction. Subtle cerebellar gait dysfunction may manifest as only difficulty with tandem gait (walking heel to toe on a straight line), although this can sometimes be difficult for healthy older individuals. Cerebellar conditions may also cause additional signs such as nystagmus, dysarthria, and ataxia on finger-nose and heel-shin testing.

Gait Disorders Due to Proprioceptive Dysfunction

Gait difficulty due to proprioceptive dysfunction can look similar to a cerebellar gait disorder: wide-based and unsteady. If the problem is proprioceptive (eg, due to neuropathy or dorsal column dysfunction), patients will have decreased vibration sensation and proprioception, a Romberg sign, and no evidence of cerebellar signs such as nystagmus or dysarthria. If the proprioceptive problem is due to peripheral neuropathy, reflexes will be diminished or absent. Vitamin B_{12} deficiency is a common cause of proprioceptive dysfunction.

Gait Disorders Due to Muscle Weakness

The lower extremity muscles are strong enough to support the entire weight of the body, and subtle weakness may not be detected on standard testing. Proximal muscles can be evaluated by having the patient stand from a chair without using the arms. Proximal weakness can cause a waddling (Trendelenburg) gait, in which the pelvis drops to the affected side with each step. Distal strength can be evaluated by having the patient stand on the toes (plantar flexion) and heels (dorsiflexion). Weak dorsiflexion of the foot can cause a steppage gait in which the patient lifts the affected foot to avoid scraping the toe and slaps it down to the ground. Lesions of the corticospinal tracts in the brain or spinal cord cause a spastic gait in which the leg is fully extended with the foot plantarflexed, and the leg is circumducted (swung outward and around from the hip). After a stroke, this may be present on one side; with spinal cord dysfunction, this can be bilateral, causing a scissoring gait.

Gait Disorders Due to Musculoskeletal Pain

An antalgic gait is one due to pain, often caused by musculoskeletal conditions. The gait does not fit into any of the abovementioned neurologic patterns, patients may report pain in affected joints, and pain may be elicited by various examination maneuvers of the hips or knees.

Gait Disorders Due to Functional Neurologic Disorders

Functional neurologic disorders are conditions in which neurologic symptoms are present despite the absence of a structural lesion or identifiable alternative neurologic or medical condition (in the past, these were attributed to conversion disorder). Functional gait disorders often demonstrate variability in pattern, inconsistency in degree, and/or sudden onset. In some patients, a functional gait disorder is suspected because the abnormality of gait appears profound, and yet the patient maintains balance and does not fall. Functional gait disorders are very challenging to diagnose since movement disorders (eg, chorea or dystonia) or combinations of multiple underlying conditions (eg, multifactorial gait disorder and/or gait disorder due to fear of falling) may be hard to classify as falling under one clear pattern and functional gait disorders may coexist with other gait disorders. Therefore, a careful assessment for each of these underlying disorders is necessary before considering a functional gait disorder.

Multifactorial Gait Disorder

A multifactorial gait disorder describes gait difficulties due to any combination of the abovementioned gait patterns. It is common, for example, to see a combination of sensory ataxia from peripheral neuropathy and antalgic gait due to pain from hip, spine, or knee pathology.

Gait Disorders Due to Fear of Falling

Patients with abnormal gait due to any reason and patients with normal gait who have a mechanical fall may develop severe anxiety due to fear of falling, which can result in them maintaining a very slow and cautious gait pattern that may be the entirety of the gait disorder, or may be superimposed on an underlying cause of gait dysfunction.

Table 14.1 summarizes the major gait disorders, their descriptions, and some typical causes.

DIAGNOSTIC EVALUATION

Diagnostic evaluation of gait disorders depends on what is thought to be the most likely cause based on the history and examination. Neuroimaging may be indicated to evaluate for conditions affecting the brain or spine (see Chapter 23), and laboratory evaluation should be considered to evaluate for common causes of neuropathy if present (see Chapter 24).

MANAGEMENT

All patients with gait difficulty should be referred for physical therapy to assist with improving strength, coordination, and balance. The physical therapist can also evaluate whether the patient would benefit from a cane or walker. A home safety evaluation may be indicated to develop strategies that can minimize fall risk by keeping walking paths in and around the home clear of items that the patient could trip over, installing grab bars in the bathroom, and adding lighting to improve visibility when walking in the home at night.

Discussion of treatment of specific conditions affecting gait is found in other chapters.

SUMMARY

Assessment of the patient presenting with abnormal gait requires consideration of the multiple neurologic processes required to ambulate. This should include a thorough history and systematic neurologic examination, with special attention to close observation of the patient's gait, to localize the cause of the gait dysfunction to appropriately guide diagnostic evaluation and treatment.

TABLE 14.1 **Patterns of Gait Dysfunction, Examination Findings, and Typical Causes**

Gait disorder	Description of gait	Accompanying signs/symptoms	Etiologies
Frontal lobe gait disorder (called an *apractic gait* or *magnetic gait*)	• Wide-based stance • Difficulty initiating steps • Shuffling gait • Freezing of gait	• Cognitive dysfunction • Lack of motivation and spontaneity (*abulia*) • Urinary incontinence	• Normal pressure hydrocephalus • Obstructive hydrocephalus • Frontal lobe tumors • Anterior cerebral artery stroke • Neurodegenerative disease
Parkinsonian gait	• Slowness of movement (*bradykinesia*) • Short-stepped, shuffling gait • Stooped posture • Postural instability (*retropulsion*) • *En bloc* turning • Reduced arm swing	• Resting tremor • Rigidity of the arms and legs • Decreased facial expression (*masked facies*) • Soft speech (*hypophonia*) • Small handwriting (*micrographia*)	• Parkinson disease • Drug-induced parkinsonism • Atypical parkinsonian syndromes (progressive supranuclear palsy, multiple system atrophy, corticobasal syndrome)
Ataxic gait	• Wide-based and unsteady (*truncal ataxia*) • Inability to tandem (heel-to-shin) walk	*Cerebellar ataxic gait:* • Lack of smooth tracking eye movements (*saccadic pursuit*) • Gaze-evoked nystagmus • Difficulty with finger-to-nose and heel-to-shin maneuvers (*appendicular ataxia*) • Falling or deviating to the side of the lesion with lesions lateral to the vermis *Sensory ataxic gait:* • Romberg sign • Diminished vibration sense and diminished proprioception • Diminished reflexes if peripheral neuropathy (reflexes may be increased in dorsal column disease if adjacent corticospinal tracts are affected)	*Cerebellar ataxia:* • Cerebellar stroke • Cerebellar tumor • Acute alcohol intoxication or chronic alcohol-related cerebellar degeneration • Paraneoplastic disease • Neurodegenerative disease (eg, spinocerebellar ataxia) *Sensory ataxia:* • Spinal cord dorsal column dysfunction (eg, vitamin B_{12} deficiency, copper deficiency, syphilis, demyelinating disease, structural spine disease) • Peripheral neuropathies (diabetes, vitamin B_{12} or B_1 deficiency, chronic alcohol use, HIV) • Ganglionopathy/neuronopathy (vitamin B_6 toxicity, paraneoplastic, Sjögren syndrome)
Hemiplegic gait	• Leg dragging and swinging in semicircle when walking (*circumduction*)	• Hyperreflexia • Spasticity • Extensor muscle weakness in the affected leg	• Cerebral hemisphere or brainstem lesion (stroke, tumor) • Spinal cord lesion (demyelinating disease, spinal cord compression)
Spastic gait	• Narrow base with scissoring (knees/thighs pressed together or crossing when walking) • Dragging of both legs	• Weakness of muscles of the legs • Increased muscle tone, increased reflexes • Babinski sign	• Spinal cord disease • Bilateral cerebral hemisphere lesions
Trendelenburg gait	Unilateral weakness: dropping or sagging of pelvis on opposite side of weak gluteus medius/minimus muscles Bilateral weakness: alternating dropping of the pelvis to unsupported side with each step, causing waddling gait	Weakness of proximal arm and leg muscles	• Myopathy (genetic or acquired) • Lumbar radiculopathy • Hip pathology
Steppage gait	Exaggerated elevation of thigh and flexion of the knee with dropped/insufficiently dorsiflexed foot at the ankle	Weakness of ankle dorsiflexion	• L5 nerve root injury • Peripheral neuropathy • Peroneal or sciatic nerve injury • Motor neuron disease
Antalgic gait	• Limping • Pain with bearing weight		Orthopedic or rheumatologic disorders
Functional gait	Gait abnormalities are as follows: • Variable • Distractable • May demonstrate excessive swaying/overcorrection without falling		Etiology unclear
Slow/cautious gait	Slow, cautious gait pattern		Fear of falling
Multifactorial gait	Any combination of the abovementioned patterns		Combination of multiple etiologies

- Gait dysfunction can arise from problems anywhere in the nervous system, including motor control systems in the frontal lobes and basal ganglia, coordination circuitry in the cerebellum, proprioception pathways in the spinal cord and peripheral nerves, and motor pathways in the spinal cord, peripheral nerves, neuromuscular junction, and muscle. The history, examination, and evaluation aim to determine the most likely cause(s) of a patient's gait disorder among these possibilities.

- Frontal lobe lesions dysfunction (eg, normal pressure hydrocephalus) can cause gait apraxia in which the patient has a magnetic gait (struggles to lift their feet from the floor), has difficulty with initiating the first steps of walking, walks with small shuffling steps, and may have freezing of gait. This may sometimes be accompanied by other frontal signs such as abulia (decreased motivation) and urinary incontinence.

- Basal ganglia disorders are associated with a parkinsonian gait characterized by a stooped posture, short shuffling steps, needing multiple steps to turn, and decreased arm swing. A parkinsonian gait is often associated with other signs of parkinsonism such as slowness of movement (bradykinesia), cogwheel rigidity, resting tremor, and postural instability.

- Cerebellar disorders cause a wide-based, unsteady gait; patients have particular difficulty with tandem gait and may have additional signs of cerebellar dysfunction, including nystagmus, dysarthria, and clumsiness on finger-nose and heel-shin testing.

- Proprioceptive dysfunction causes a wide-based gait disorder similar to a cerebellar gait disorder: In addition, patients will have decreased sensation to vibration and proprioception and a Romberg sign (inability to maintain balance with the feet together and eyes closed), and the absence of cerebellar signs such as nystagmus or dysarthria.

- Proximal muscle weakness affecting the gluteal muscles can cause a Trendelenburg gait, in which the pelvis drops to the affected side with each step.

- Distal weakness affecting foot dorsiflexion causes a steppage gait in which the patient lifts the affected foot to avoid scraping the toe and slaps it down to the ground.

- Lesions of the corticospinal tracts cause a spastic gait in which the stiff, extended leg is circum-ducted; when bilateral, the patient may have a scissoring gait.

- Musculoskeletal conditions can cause an antalgic gait, related to pain in the back and/or the affected extremity.

- Multifactorial gait disorders occur due to a combination of factors affecting gait and are increasingly common in older age.

- Patients with gait difficulty should be referred for physical therapy to assist with improving strength, coordination, balance, and safety.

Primary Headache Disorders

Carrie Dougherty and Jessica Ailani

INTRODUCTION

Headache is a common symptom that can be due to an underlying condition (secondary headache disorder [eg, giant cell arteritis and subarachnoid hemorrhage]) or a primary headache disorder (eg, tension-type headache and migraine). Chapter 8 discusses the initial approach to determining whether a patient's headache is most likely to be secondary and require additional evaluation, or whether it represents a primary headache disorder. Here, the diagnosis and treatment of the most common primary headache disorders—migraine and tension headache—are discussed along with less common headache disorders, the trigeminal autonomic cephalalgias. Trigeminal neuralgia is also discussed. Criteria for the diagnosis of primary headache disorders can be found in the International Classification of Headache Disorders.[1]

MIGRAINE

Diagnosis of Migraine

Migraine is characterized by moderate to severe head pain that is usually throbbing or pulsating, unilateral, worse with physical exertion, and associated with photophobia, phonophobia, nausea, and/or vomiting. Migraine typically lasts hours to days. A patient does not need to have all features described to meet the diagnostic criteria of migraine. Some patients report a prodrome of symptoms that may precede migraine headache, including motion and smell sensitivity, dizziness, cognitive fog, fatigue, changes in emotional state, neck stiffness, dizziness, nausea, yawning, and food cravings (particularly for chocolate and carbohydrates).

Up to 30% of people with migraine have an aura that most commonly precedes the headache and lasts 5 to 60 minutes. The most common type of aura is visual, described as flashing lights or zigzag lines followed by loss or blurring of vision. Less common auras include sensory (numbness/tingling often starting in the mouth and traveling to the unilateral arm, sometimes to the leg), motor (hemiplegic attacks), vestibular (vertigo, imbalance), or speech changes (dysarthria or other difficulty with speech). Some patients report more than one type of aura. In patients who have migraine with aura, not all headaches are accompanied by aura, and not all auras are accompanied by headache. If a person has a change in their aura symptoms or they last longer than their usual time frame, this is considered a red flag requiring urgent neuroimaging to evaluate for migrainous infarct.

Migraine is classified into three categories: migraine without aura, migraine with aura, and chronic migraine.

Unlike in other medical disorders, the term "chronic" in chronic migraine does not refer to the duration of illness but instead indicates that the person has more than 15 days of headache per month, with at least eight of those headaches being migraine (with or without aura) and that this occurs for more than 3 months. Nonmodifiable risk factors for the development of chronic migraine include female sex, stressful life events, and low educational status, whereas modifiable risk factors include obesity, ineffective acute treatment, frequent migraine attacks, and overuse of acute treatment. The primary differential diagnosis for chronic migraine is medication-overuse headache caused by excessive use of analgesic agents, defined as more than 15 days per month of a single non-opiate analgesic or more than 10 days per month of multiple analgesics, triptans, or opiate analgesics.

Migraine is a clinical diagnosis based on history. Headache diaries describing symptoms before, during, and after a headache can aid in diagnosis, and headache calendars can help gauge the frequency and severity of migraine to plan treatment and assess treatment response. Patients generally have a normal neurologic examination during and between migraine attacks. While taking a headache history or performing a neurologic examination, there are several "red flags" to look for that are concerning for a secondary headache and warrant further investigation for another cause for headache (see Chapter 8). These include an abnormal neurologic examination (even if the patient is having a migraine attack during the examination) or if the patient describes a prolonged migraine aura (lasting >1 hour), which raises concern for migrainous infarct (requiring urgent bin imaging).

The risk of stroke in patients with migraine is slightly increased, with particular elevation in risk related to migraine with aura, female sex, smoking, and estrogen-containing oral contraceptives. Therefore, patients with migraine should be counseled to abstain from smoking. Historically, it has been suggested to avoid exogenous estrogen in patients with migraine, especially migraine with aura; however, estrogen-containing compounds that contain less than 35 µg of exogenous estrogen are likely safe to use in people with migraine; progesterone-only contraception is another option.[2] Risk and benefit of the use of hormonal contraception in people with migraine should be considered in each individual case.

Treatment of Migraine

Migraine treatment is divided into lifestyle modification, acute treatment for acute attacks, and preventive treatment to reduce the severity and frequency of attacks. Various guidelines for treatment have been published,[3-6] but treatment should be tailored to each individual patient, taking into account migraine frequency, patient comorbidities, and medication side effect profiles.

Lifestyle and Behavioral Management

Lifestyle modifications associated with improvement in migraines include stress reduction/management, regular sleep, healthy and consistent diet, and exercise. While some patients may report dietary triggers (monosodium glutamate, caffeine, and alcohol), these are highly individual and generally only elucidated by a migraine diary kept by the patient.

Acute Treatment

The goal of acute treatment for a migraine attack is rapid, sustained, and consistent freedom from pain and other migraine symptoms (such as photophobia, phonophobia, and nausea) with minimal side effects. Acute abortive treatment must be taken by the patient as early as possible after migraine onset to be most effective. Before considering an abortive treatment ineffective, it should be determined when the patient took the medication in relation to symptom onset and the route of administration; for example, if a patient with nausea and vomiting as part of their migraine vomits an oral abortive treatment, the treatment itself may not be ineffective but rather the route of administration.

Acute treatments include over-the-counter analgesics (eg, ibuprofen and acetaminophen) and migraine-specific treatments such as triptans, ergots, gepants, and ditans (Table 15.1). Migraine-specific treatments should be used in patients with moderate to severe attacks in whom over-the-counter treatments have been unsuccessful. Opioids and butalbital-containing medications should be avoided.

Triptans (5-HT1B/D agonists) are considered first-line acute therapy due to their efficacy, low cost, and various routes of administration, including oral, sublingual, intranasal, and injectable, with the latter three particularly helpful in patients with significant nausea and vomiting during migraine. Two triptans have longer

TABLE 15.1   Acute Treatments for Migraine

Drug class	Mechanism of action	Formulation	Side effects	Contraindications	When to consider use
Triptans	5-HT 1B/D agonist	Oral (sumatriptan, rizatriptan, zolmitriptan, eletriptan, almotriptan, naratriptan, and frovatriptan) Nasal (sumatriptan and zolmitriptan) SQ (sumatriptan)	Chest pain, dizziness, drowsiness/fatigue, flushing, nausea, neck pain, sweating, and paresthesia	Coronary artery disease, history of stroke, peripheral vascular disease, and chronically uncontrolled high blood pressure Caution with concomitant serotonin medication	Generally considered first-line migraine-specific medication unless patient with contraindication Sumatriptan is second line in pregnancy (after acetaminophen)
DHE	5-HT1B/D receptor agonist	Nasal SQ/IM	Dizziness, drowsiness, nausea, vomiting, diarrhea, flushing, sweating, and anxiety	Coronary artery disease, a history of stroke, peripheral vascular disease, and chronically uncontrolled high blood pressure	Prolonged/status migrainosus Menstrual migraine Wake up migraine Later-to-treat migraine Triptan or gepant ineffective
Ditans	5-HT1F agonist	Oral	Dizziness, drowsiness, nausea, and paresthesia Impaired driving for 8 h	Caution with concomitant serotonin medications No driving for 8 h after use	For patients with vascular risk factors who can avoid driving after use Rescue treatment after NSAID or gepant
Gepants	CGRP receptor antagonist	Oral (Ubrogepant, rimegepant) Nasal (zavegepant)	Nausea and somnolence	Consider CYP3A4 interactions	Does not cause medication-overuse headache, so anyone who needs frequent acute treatment, even on prevention For patients with vascular risk factors For patients who do not tolerate triptans
NSAIDs	Inhibition of the enzyme cyclooxygenase	Oral (ibuprofen, naproxen, and diclofenac) Oral solution (celecoxib and diclofenac powder) Nasal (ketorolac) SQ/IM (ketorolac)	Indigestion, peptic ulcer disease, drowsiness, dizziness, and renal dysfunction	Caution with vascular disease Avoid with history of peptic ulcer disease Caution with concomitant use with SNRI due to increased GI bleed risk	Can be first line for most patients with migraine Preference of low side effects and ease of use Can be added on to any above treatment for better efficacy

CGRP, calcitonin gene-related peptide; CYP, cytochrome P450; GI, gastrointestinal; IM, intramuscular; NSAIDs, nonsteroidal anti-inflammatory drugs; SNRI, serotonin norepinephrine reuptake inhibitor; SQ, subcutaneous.

half-lives (naratriptan and frovatriptan) and are therefore useful in patients with longer migraine attacks. Triptans as a class should not be considered ineffective until patients have trialed at least two different triptans with confirmation that they are taking them early in their migraine. Triptan use should be limited to 10 days a month to avoid medication-overuse headache. Triptans cause vasoconstriction and are therefore contraindicated in patients with coronary artery disease. Concomitant use of triptans while on other serotonin agents, such as selective serotonin reuptake inhibitors (SSRIs), may be considered after advising the patient about the potential of serotonin syndrome and monitoring for signs and symptoms of this over time. Sumatriptan may be considered in pregnancy as a second-line acute treatment if the patient does not respond to acetaminophen and/or metoclopramide.[7,8]

In patients in whom triptans are ineffective or contraindicated, gepants or ditans may be considered. Gepants (calcitonin gene-related peptide [CGRP] receptor antagonists) are available in oral (ubrogepant and rimegepant) and nasal (zavegepant) formulations with minimal side effects (eg, nausea and sedation; dysgeusia with zavegepant). Aside from pregnancy, there are no contraindications to gepants, but there may be drug-drug interactions with CYP3A medications, so evaluating for potential interactions should be undertaken before prescribing gepants.

There is currently one available ditan (5-HT1F receptor agonist), lasmiditan, the usage of which is limited by the side effects of dizziness and sedation requiring abstaining from driving for 8 hours after administration. Lasmiditan can also cause serotonin syndrome either on its own or when combined with other serotonin agents, so it would be advisable to monitor patients who are concomitant serotonin agents. Lasmiditan does not cause vasoconstriction, so it can be an option in patients who have vascular disease.

Dihydroergotamine (DHE) is available for patients to use at home as a nasal option in either a spray or as a nasal device. While DHE is rapid in onset for treating a migraine attack, its benefits include the ability to be effective late in an attack as well as having a sustained response. It is often used for longer migraine attacks, especially in status migrainosus (migraine lasting >72 hours), where repeat doses can be helpful to break a patient out of status. DHE has been evaluated and found effective in those who wake up with migraine, have menstrual migraine, have allodynia (pain induced by a nonpainful stimulus, eg, in migraine, touching the scalp), are triptan resistant, have severe migraine, or who treat their migraine up to 8 hours after the start of an attack. DHE is contraindicated in patients with vascular disorders, uncontrolled hypertension, during pregnancy, and is not used concomitantly with triptans and ditans. DHE use should be limited to 10 days per month to avoid medication-overuse headache.

Preventive Treatment

Preventive treatments reduce migraine frequency and severity and should be offered to patients with four or more migraines per month, or any number that significantly interferes with daily activities. Pharmacologic agents for migraine prevention include antihypertensive medications (propranolol, metoprolol, nadolol, and candesartan), anti-seizure medications (topiramate and valproate), antidepressant medications (tricyclic antidepressants and serotonin norepinephrine reuptake inhibitor [SNRIs]), migraine-specific medications (CGRP inhibitors: gepants and anti-CGRP monoclonal antibodies), and botulinum toxin (Table 15.2). Nutraceuticals such as riboflavin, magnesium, and melatonin have shown efficacy as migraine preventives in small trials. Aside from diarrhea with magnesium, these medications are well tolerated and can be considered as an initial choice in patients reluctant to try pharmaceutical agents. Butterbur was previously used, but this is now best avoided as cases of hepatotoxicity have been reported.

Preventive agents have not been compared in head-to-head trials, so the choice of agent is based on patient comorbidities and medication side effect profile. Some patients may require multiple agents. Many preventive agents take several months before an effect is noted. Unless there are intolerable side effects, medications should be trialed for at least 3 months at the appropriate dose before considering treatment failure and moving to another agent. Many patients who report having tried medications in the past that were ineffective had been on an insufficient dose or not trialed on the medication for long enough

TABLE 15.2   Preventive Treatments for Migraine

Drug class	Mechanism of action in migraine	Formulation	Side effects	Contraindications	When to consider use
Gepants	CGRP antagonist	Oral	Nausea, constipation (atogepant), fatigue (atogepant), and weight loss (atogepant)	Consideration of CYP3A4 interactions Avoid in pregnancy	Level A In patients who prefer oral medication and migraine-specific treatment
CGRP monoclonal antibodies	CGRP receptor antagonist (erenumab) CGRP ligand binder (eptinezumab, fremanezumab, and galcanezumab)	SQ monthly (erenumab, galcanezumab, and fremanezumab) SQ quarterly (fremanezumab) IV quarterly (eptinezumab)	Constipation (erenumab) HTN (erenumab) Injection site reaction (erenumab, fremanezumab, and galcanezumab) Hypersensitivity reaction	Avoid in pregnancy	Level A In patients who prefer injectable monthly or quarterly medication and migraine-specific treatment
Anti-seizure medication	Unknown	Oral	Weight loss (topiramate), weight gain (valproate), concentration problems, hair loss, paresthesia (topiramate), kidney stones (topiramate), and liver disease (valproate)	Avoid in pregnancy and women of child-bearing age	Level A Topiramate is often used when patient is considering weight loss Folate should be added in women of child-bearing age Valproate is often avoided due to side effects
β-blocker	Unknown	Oral	Fatigue, weight gain, and shortness of breath	Caution in the first trimester of pregnancy Caution in patients with low blood pressure or low heart rate	Propranolol, metoprolol, and timolol are level A Used with concomitant anxiety or hypertension
ARB	Unknown	Oral	Arm, back, or jaw pain, bleeding gums, chest tightness, cough, hoarseness, fainting, fast or irregular heartbeat, and joint pain	Avoid in pregnancy	Candesartan is level A and the only used ARB in migraine
ACE inhibitor	Unknown	Oral	Blurred vision, body aches, dizziness, cough, fainting, and angioedema	Avoid in pregnancy	Lisinopril is level B and the only ACE inhibitor used in migraine, cough is a limiting factor
SNRI	Unknown	Oral	Mood changes, fatigue, insomnia, nausea, and hypertension		Venlafaxine is level B Considered for patients with comorbid depression/anxiety
Tricyclic antidepressant	Unknown	Oral	Fatigue, sedation, dry mouth, difficulty urinating, weight gain, and increased heart rate		Amitriptyline is level B Considered for patients with comorbid insomnia, neck pain, neuropathy, and irritable bowel syndrome

Medications with level A evidence should be preferentially given to patients over level B evidence.
ACE, angiotensin-converting enzyme; ARB, angiotensin receptor blocker; CGRP, calcitonin gene-related peptide; CYP, cytochrome P450; HTN, hypertension; IV, intravenous; SNRI, serotonin norepinephrine reuptake inhibitor; SQ, subcutaneous.

to assess efficacy. Most migraine-preventive agents, such as topiramate, valproate, candesartan, amitriptyline, CGRP monoclonal antibodies, and gepants, are contraindicated in pregnancy and should therefore be avoided in women of childbearing age unless concurrent effective contraception is used.[7]

Migraine-Specific treatments

Studies have shown that CGRP fluctuations are related to migraine and that suppression of CGRP activity relates to migraine activation. There are currently two classes of CGRP-inhibiting medications: CGRP receptor antagonists (gepants) and CGRP monoclonal antibodies. Often, health systems and insurance plans will only cover these medications if the patient fails to respond to (or does not tolerate) other migraine-preventive treatments.

Gepants are small-molecule CGRP receptor antagonists developed for the treatment of migraine. There are three approved gepants for the acute treatment of migraine and two approved gepants for the preventive treatment of migraine (atogepant and rimegepant). Atogepant is a daily oral tablet that carries adverse effects of constipation, nausea, and weight loss and comes in three doses, which allows for adjustment if needed due to potential drug-drug interactions. Rimegepant is an every-other-day dissolvable tablet and can have the adverse effect of nausea. Atogepant is approved for episodic and chronic migraine, while rimegepant is approved for the prevention of episodic migraine. In female patients of childbearing age, gepants can be stopped shortly prior to pregnancy planning. The differences in side effect profile, type of dosing regimen, and type of approval for episodic migraine and/or chronic migraine are summarized in Table 15.2.

CGRP monoclonal antibodies bind either to the CGRP receptor (erenumab) or the CGRP ligand (eptinezumab, fremanezumab, and galcanezumab). All four CGRP monoclonal antibodies have shown efficacy as migraine-preventive treatment options for both episodic and chronic migraine. Overall, the CGRP monoclonal antibodies are well tolerated, although some treatment-related side effects have been noted since U.S. Food and Drug Administration (FDA) approval. Erenumab, fremanezumab, and galcanezumab all cause injection site reactions, the latter two to a

greater extent. Erenumab causes constipation and can cause hypertension, the latter of which was not seen in clinical trials. Eptinezumab causes nasal congestion and can cause hypersensitivity reactions (at a greater rate than seen in clinical trials). There have been reports of Raynaud phenomenon with both the CGRP monoclonal antibodies and with gepants, and there have been patient reports of alopecia with all CGRP-targeted treatments. CGRP monoclonal antibodies should be stopped 5 months prior to pregnancy and, in case of unanticipated pregnancy, should be stopped immediately, although no maternal or fetal toxicities have been observed in pharmacovigilance databases documenting a small number of accidental exposures during pregnancy.

Once treatment with a CGRP monoclonal antibody is started, migraine reduction may take several months, although it can occur sooner. For patients with chronic migraine, response times can be longer. After 3 months (or two treatment cycles for eptinezumab), a majority of people who will respond to treatment will have shown some treatment response. If a patient is responding to treatment, continuation is generally needed indefinitely since cessation often results in the return of migraines. If a patient does not respond to one CGRP monoclonal antibody, they may respond to another; switching from a ligand to a receptor-binding monoclonal antibody or vice versa should be considered.

Onabotulinumtoxin A

Onabotulinumtoxin A is an approved preventive treatment for chronic migraine, with injections typically administered every 12 weeks. Side effects include neck pain, headache, muscle/injection site pain, and ptosis.

Neuromodulation

There are currently five neuromodulation devices available for the treatment of primary headache disorders: supraorbital transcutaneous neurostimulation (STNS) for acute and preventive treatment of migraine, single-pulse transcranial magnetic stimulation (sTMS) for acute and preventive treatment of migraine, noninvasive vagal nerve stimulator (nVNS) for acute and preventive treatment of migraine and for the acute treatment of cluster headache, remote electrical neuromodulation (REN) for the acute and preventive treatment of migraine, and the external combined occipital and trigeminal nerve stimulator (eCOT-ns) for the acute treatment of migraine. Currently, most devices are not covered by insurance, and data are varied in their efficacy for migraine, although they are generally well tolerated and can be beneficial in some patients refractory to medications, with intolerable side effects from medications, or in whom medications are contraindicated due to medical comorbidities. Neuromodulation devices are contraindicated in patients with epilepsy or with other electrical implantable devices such as a pacemaker.

TENSION-TYPE HEADACHE

Diagnosis of Tension-Type Headache

Tension-type headache is the most common primary headache disorder. It causes a bilateral, dull, pressure-like pain, often described as a "band-like" sensation around the head. Unlike migraine, there is generally no associated nausea, vomiting, or aura, although photophobia may rarely be observed. Also, unlike migraine, tension-type headache often improves with exercise. On examination, patients with tension-type headache may have muscle tenderness on manual palpation of the frontal, temporal, masseter, pterygoid, sternocleidomastoid, splenius, and trapezius muscles, although this is not universally present. The differential diagnosis for tension-type headache includes migraine without aura, medication-overuse headache, and secondary headaches due to obstructive sleep apnea, sinusitis, or intracranial processes such as mass lesions or other causes of elevated intracranial pressure. If the onset of tension-type headache is daily from onset, begins at age 50 or older, or is associated with neurologic or systemic symptoms or signs, neuroimaging and laboratory testing to evaluate for a possible secondary etiology should be pursued.

Tension-type headache is classified by headache frequency into infrequent episodic (<1 day/month), frequent episodic (1-14 days/month for >3 months), and chronic (≥15 days/month for >3 months).[1] In each, the headache may last from minutes to days.

Treatment of Tension-Type Headache

Analgesics such as acetaminophen, aspirin, or nonsteroidal anti-inflammatory drugs (NSAIDs) are used for episodic tension-type headache. Ibuprofen and ketoprofen have more evidence to support their use than combination caffeine-containing analgesics. Topical peppermint oil may also provide acute relief in tension-type headache. Muscle relaxants are not recommended.

In patients with frequent tension-type headache, preventive treatment should be offered. The tricyclic antidepressant amitriptyline is the only preventive medication for tension-type headache with level A evidence. Common side effects include weight gain, dry mouth, constipation, and orthostasis. Amitriptyline is contraindicated in patients with ventricular arrhythmias. Older patients should be monitored with electrocardiogram (ECG) and may be more susceptible to the adverse effects of urinary retention and cognitive impairment. Mirtazapine and venlafaxine are both supported by level B evidence. Third-line options include tizanidine, topiramate, and valproate. If sustained reduction in headache frequency is achieved, preventive medication may be tapered and discontinued to see whether it is still indicated.

Lifestyle modifications such as regular diet, sleep, and exercise as well as complementary therapies such as biofeedback, cognitive behavioral therapy, and relaxation therapy can be helpful in patients with tension-type headache. Patients should be screened for underlying mood disorders, which may co-occur with tension-type headache.

MEDICATION-OVERUSE HEADACHE

Medication-overuse headache occurs when a person with a headache disorder uses acute treatment medications for more than 10 days per month (for triptans, opioids, and multiple analgesics) or more than 15 days per month (for acetaminophen or NSAIDs) for greater than 3 months and develops a headache that occurs more than 15 days per month. Treatment of medication-overuse headache begins with education about the underlying primary headache disorder, about limits and appropriate use of acute treatment, and the benefits of preventive treatment. Withdrawing the overused medication along with initiation of a preventive agent is needed, and patients should be counseled that there may be an initial worsening of headaches due to rebound after withdrawal of analgesics before improvement. Management of underlying anxiety disorder and other mood disorders is important for successful treatment. Avoiding the use of butalbital-containing products and opioids in the treatment of migraine can greatly reduce the risk of developing medication-overuse headache.

TRIGEMINAL AUTONOMIC CEPHALALGIAS

Trigeminal autonomic cephalalgias are a group of primary headache disorders characterized by unilateral head pain with associated autonomic features, including lacrimation, rhinorrhea, conjunctival injection, and ptosis. Trigeminal autonomic cephalalgias are subdivided into four different headache disorders, cluster headache, paroxysmal hemicrania, hemicrania continua, and short-lasting unilateral neuralgiform headache attacks (SUNHA). Although

the trigeminal autonomic cephalalgias share similar clinical features, they vary by headache attack duration, frequency, and treatment (Table 15.3). There is an inverse relationship between attack duration and frequency, which ranges from seconds of pain occurring hundreds of times a day in SUNHA to a single continuous attack that persists for months in hemicrania continua. Paroxysmal hemicrania and hemicrania continua are unique in their response to indomethacin. Trigeminal autonomic cephalalgias may be primary or secondary headache disorders, and all patients should therefore undergo MRI of the brain with particular attention to the pituitary region, as trigeminal autonomic cephalalgias can be associated with pituitary lesions.

Cluster Headache

Cluster headache is the most common trigeminal autonomic cephalalgia. Cluster headache attacks are characterized by unilateral pain, most commonly around or behind the eye, a sense of restless or agitation that drives the patient to rock or pace, and autonomic symptoms (lacrimation, rhinorrhea,

TABLE 15.3   Clinical Features of Trigeminal Autonomic Cephalalgias

	ICHD duration	Typical duration	ICHD frequency	Typical frequency	Triggers	Male vs Female predominance	Preventive treatment	Primary headache differential diagnosis
Hemicrania continua	>3 mo	Continuous	Continuous	Continuous		F	Indomethacin	Chronic migraine New daily persistent headache
Cluster headache	15-180 min	45-90 min	QOD-8 ×/d	1-3 ×/d	EtOH	M	Verapamil Galcanezumab	Migraine Paroxysmal Hemicrania
Paroxysmal hemicrania	2-30 min	26 min	≥5 ×/d	6 ×/d	EtOH Neck movement occipital pressure	F	Indomethacin	Cluster headache Short unilateral neuralgiform headache attacks
Short unilateral neuralgiform headache attacks	1-600 s	1 min	≥20 ×/d	100/d	Tactile	Similar	Lamotrigine	Paroxysmal hemicrania Trigeminal neuralgia

The International Classification of Headache Disorders (ICHD) diagnostic criteria include the extremes of headache duration and frequency (number of headaches per day) allowable to make the diagnosis, but because these can overlap between the various TACs (eg, a headache lasting 2 minutes could meet criteria for both short unilateral neuralgiform headache and paroxysmal hemicrania), the typical presentation is also provided to help aid in clinical recognition. The trigeminal autonomic cephalalgias are uncommon, and, thus, some clinical features, triggers, and gender predominance are unknown.
EtOH, alcohol; ICHD, International Classification of Headache Disorders; TACs, trigeminal autonomic cephalalgias.

conjunctival injection, and ptosis). Cluster attacks typically last 45 to 90 minutes and occur 1 to 3 times each day but can range from 12 to 180 minutes in duration and occur up to 8 times daily. Cluster headaches tend to occur over a 6- to 12-week period (hence the name "cluster" for the clustering of these headaches over a specific time period). Most patients experience cycles about twice yearly, often with season change in the spring and fall. Attacks often occur at the same time each day (often in the predawn hours), and cycles present at the same time of the year. Unlike migraine, which causes a desire to rest, cluster headache causes agitation and restlessness during attacks. Cluster headache is more common in men. A minority of patients experience chronic cluster headache with cycles lasting 9 months or more each year. As with all trigeminal autonomic cephalalgias, brain MRI should be obtained with attention to the pituitary, as pituitary lesions can impinge upon the V1 branch of the trigeminal nerve, causing secondary cluster headache.

Treatment of cluster headache involves three types of intervention, acute medication for pain relief, preventive treatment with daily or long-acting medication to reduce the frequency of cluster headache attacks and hasten the end of a cycle, and transitional or bridge therapy, which can temporarily suppress cluster headache attacks during the titration of preventive intervention.

Acute treatment includes high-flow oxygen or triptans in intranasal or injectable formulation since oral triptans are not sufficiently fast acting to alleviate cluster headache. Preventive treatment should be initiated promptly at the onset of a cluster headache cycle. First-line options include galcanezumab and verapamil; second-line options include lithium and topiramate. Since doses of verapamil are often higher than those used for cardiovascular indications, patients should be followed up with ECG at initiation and 1 to 2 weeks after each dose escalation. Noninvasive vagal nerve stimulation can be considered in refractory cases. Transitional/bridge interventions that can temporarily suppress cluster headache attacks include an oral steroid taper (eg, over 10-12 days) or greater occipital nerve block ipsilateral to the side of cluster headache attacks. Due to the risk of osteonecrosis, steroid treatment should be limited to 2 to 3 times per year.

Paroxysmal Hemicrania

Paroxysmal hemicrania attacks are shorter in duration than cluster headaches (ranging from 2 to 30 minutes) but occur more frequently (typically 5-6 times daily). They can occur throughout the year and do not cluster in a particular schedule, as do cluster headaches. As in other trigeminal autonomic cephalalgias, pain is unilateral, periorbital, or temporal and has a sharp, stabbing, or throbbing quality. Patients do not have the same sense of agitation as in cluster headache. Between attacks, patients may have mild facial pain and migrainous features.

The diagnosis of paroxysmal hemicrania is confirmed by a complete and dramatic cessation of attacks with indomethacin treatment. Initial treatment is typically with 25 mg 3 times daily and then increased to 50 mg 3 times daily, and finally up to a maximum of 75 mg 3 times if symptoms do not improve at lower doses. Patients whose headaches stop with indomethacin treatment can often maintain benefit at lower doses. Eventually, indomethacin can be discontinued, and patients may remain in remission.

Indomethacin can be difficult to tolerate due to gastrointestinal irritation and should be avoided in patients with a history of bleeding, impaired kidney function, or cardiovascular disease. All patients should receive concomitant treatment with a histamine receptor 2 blocker or proton pump inhibitor while taking indomethacin. Common adverse effects include nausea, heartburn, diarrhea, dizziness, and, paradoxically, headache. Patients who cannot tolerate indomethacin may respond to other cyclooxygenase inhibitors, melatonin, topiramate, verapamil, or noninvasive vagal nerve stimulation.

Hemicrania Continua

Hemicrania continua is characterized by continuous side-locked unilateral, frontal or temporal, sharp or throbbing pain that may vary with intensity and is associated with autonomic symptoms (tearing, conjunctival injection, and ptosis) and migrainous features (photophobia, phonophobia, and nausea). Many patients also describe a foreign body or gritty sensation in the eye. The principal differential diagnosis is chronic migraine.

Like paroxysmal hemicrania, hemicrania continua is an indomethacin-responsive headache, and the diagnosis is confirmed by elimination of symptoms with indomethacin. If indomethacin is intolerable or contraindicated, the alternative treatment options listed with paroxysmal hemicrania may be effective as well as peripheral nerve blocks. If indomethacin does not provide complete relief of presumed hemicrania continua, alternative diagnoses, such as chronic migraine, should be considered.

Short-Lasting Unilateral Neuralgiform Headache Attacks

SUNHA encompasses two similar headache disorders, short-lasting unilateral neuralgiform headache attacks with conjunctival injection and tearing (SUNCT) and short-lasting unilateral neuralgiform headache attacks with cranial autonomic symptoms (SUNA). SUNCT has more autonomic features, including both conjunctival injection and tearing; SUNA has only one or neither.

SUNHA attacks last seconds and can occur hundreds of times a day. Pain is typically described as sharp, stabbing, or like an electric shock, and individual attacks can be isolated or superimposed on baseline pain. Similar to trigeminal neuralgia, attacks can have physical triggers, including talking, chewing, touching the face, and brushing teeth. The presence of cranial autonomic symptoms distinguishes SUNHA from trigeminal neuralgia. Prominent pain between episodes can mimic paroxysmal hemicrania or cluster headache, but these conditions lack the brief episodes occurring with high frequency in a day.

First-line preventive treatment for SUNHA is lamotrigine; topiramate, gabapentin, carbamazepine, oxcarbazepine, or duloxetine may also be effective. In refractory cases, intravenous lidocaine can be considered with appropriate cardiovascular monitoring.

TRIGEMINAL NEURALGIA

Trigeminal neuralgia is characterized by severe unilateral paroxysmal lancinating pain in the distribution of the V2 and V3 branches of the trigeminal nerve (ie, over the maxilla or mandible). The pain is typically shock-like, stabbing, or sharp; occurs in brief paroxysms for seconds to minutes; and may be provoked by physical triggers, including chewing, touching the face, brushing teeth, eating, talking, or cold wind, but may also occur spontaneously. The pain can be so severe that patients may avoid eating or drinking out of fear of triggering paroxysms of pain, resulting in anorexia and dehydration. Many patients describe a dull persistent baseline pain that persists for hours or days in between acute attacks.

The neurologic examination in idiopathic trigeminal neuralgia is usually normal. In classical trigeminal neuralgia (with a normal neurologic examination), an MRI should be obtained and may reveal contact between the trigeminal nerve and an adjacent blood vessel. If sensory loss is found over the distribution of the trigeminal nerve, this increases concern for an underlying cause other than a vascular loop, such as multiple sclerosis or neoplasm.

First-line preventive medications for trigeminal neuralgia are carbamazepine and oxcarbazepine. Laboratory work, including complete blood count and comprehensive metabolic panel, and ECG should be performed at initiation, with any dose adjustment, and periodically with long-term use. The most common side effects of these agents include fatigue, dizziness, ataxia, nausea, hyponatremia, and leukopenia. If these agents are ineffective or have intolerable side effects, alternatives include lamotrigine, gabapentin, pregabalin, or phenytoin. Some patients may require multiple agents.

Long-term use of carbamazepine, oxcarbazepine, lamotrigine, and phenytoin can be associated with low bone mineral density, so vitamin D and calcium supplementation should be provided with chronic use. Both carbamazepine and oxcarbazepine are enzyme inducers and can lower the concentrations of other medications, such as warfarin or oral contraceptives. In patients who are refractory to medications, botulinum toxin, microvascular decompression, or trigeminal ganglion ablation (radiofrequency, thermocoagulation, and gamma knife) can be considered, and neurologic consultation is indicated to discuss these options.

SUMMARY

There are a wide variety of primary headache disorders with unique clinical features. Understanding these features allows clinicians to make the correct diagnosis and prescribe appropriate acute and preventive therapies tailored to the headache syndrome, patient preferences and comorbidities, and side effect profile.

EDITORS' KEY POINTS

▶ Migraine is characterized by severe, throbbing, often unilateral headache lasting hours to days accompanied by photophobia, phonophobia, nausea, and/or vomiting. About a third of patients have an accompanying aura, most commonly visual.

▶ Treatment for migraine includes both abortive therapies (taken acutely during a migraine) and preventive therapies (taken regularly to reduce migraine severity and frequency).

▶ Preventive treatment of migraine is generally offered to patients with four or more migraines per month or any frequency of migraine that interferes with the patient's daily activities.

▶ Tension-type headache is characterized by mild to moderate, bilateral, and dull headache lasting 30 minutes to days.

▶ Treatment for tension-type headache includes analgesics for acute headache (acetaminophen or NSAIDs) and, in patients with frequent disabling tension-type headaches, preventive treatment with tricyclic antidepressants.

▶ Patients who use analgesics for headache should be counseled on limiting use to severe headaches to avoid medication-overuse headache.

▶ The trigeminal autonomic cephalalgias are rare headache disorders causing severe unilateral pain accompanied by lacrimation, rhinorrhea, conjunctival injection, and/or ptosis. The most common (although still rare) trigeminal autonomic cephalalgia is cluster headache.

▶ Trigeminal neuralgia is characterized by brief episodes of severe unilateral lancinating shock-like pain over the maxilla and/or mandible. Patients should be evaluated for an underlying structural cause with MRI. First-line treatment is with carbamazepine.

REFERENCES

1. Headache Classification Committee of the International Headache Society (IHS) the international classification of headache disorders, 3rd edition. *Cephalalgia*. 2018;38(1):1-211.
2. Sheikh HU, Pavlovic J, Loder E, Burch R. Risk of stroke associated with use of estrogen containing contraceptives in women with migraine: a systematic review. *Headache*. 2018;58(1):5-21.
3. Marmura MJ, Silberstein SD, Schwedt TJ. The acute treatment of migraine in adults: the American headache society evidence assessment of migraine pharmacotherapies. *Headache*. 2015;55(1):3-20.
4. American Headache Society. The American headache society position statement on integrating new migraine treatments into clinical practice. *Headache*. 2019;59(1):1-18.
5. Ailani J, Burch RC, Robbins MS; Board of Directors of the American Headache Society. The American headache society consensus statement: update on integrating new migraine treatments into clinical practice. *Headache*. 2021;61(7):1021-1039.
6. Sacco S, Amin FM, Ashina M, et al. European Headache Federation guideline on the use of monoclonal antibodies targeting the calcitonin gene related peptide pathway for migraine prevention—2022 update. *J Headache Pain*. 2022;23(1):67.
7. American College of Obstetricians and Gynecologists. Headaches in pregnancy and postpartum: ACOG clinical practice guideline no. 3. *Obstet Gynecol*. 2022;139(5):944-972.
8. Marchenko A, Etwel F, Olutunfese O, Nickel C, Koren G, Nulman I. Pregnancy outcome following prenatal exposure to triptan medications: a meta-analysis. *Headache*. 2015;55(4):490-501.

CHAPTER 16

Cerebrovascular Disease

Nicholas A. Morris, Shadi Yaghi, and Seemant Chaturvedi

INTRODUCTION

Cerebrovascular disease is a leading cause of death and disability worldwide. Stroke can be classified into ischemic stroke or hemorrhagic stroke, with hemorrhagic stroke further divided into intracerebral hemorrhage (ICH) and subarachnoid hemorrhage (SAH). The majority of strokes are ischemic (70%-90% depending on world region), followed in incidence by ICH; SAH is the least common. Both ischemic stroke and ICH present with sudden-onset focal neurologic deficits (eg, unilateral weakness, ataxia, numbness, or visual loss; difficulty speaking; vertigo and imbalance). In contrast, SAH typically presents with a sudden, severe headache that may rapidly progress to coma. Since ischemic stroke and ICH present similarly, computed tomography (CT) of the head is critical for diagnosis and acute treatment. Ischemic changes on head CT may be absent in the first hours after stroke, but ICH (and most SAH) is evident on CT at presentation. Once CT has determined the type of stroke, acute treatment and further diagnostic evaluation for the cause of stroke proceed accordingly.

ISCHEMIC STROKE

Ischemic stroke presents with focal neurologic symptoms and signs such as unilateral weakness, speech difficulty, visual loss, or gait difficulty. The majority of strokes will occur in the territory of the internal carotid artery (ICA). The two major branches of the ICA are the middle cerebral artery (MCA) and anterior cerebral artery (ACA). About 20% of strokes occur in the posterior circulation, encompassing the two vertebral arteries, the basilar artery, and their respective arterial branches that supply the brainstem and cerebellum, as well as the posterior cerebral arteries (PCA).

Classic ischemic stroke syndromes include left MCA syndrome (aphasia with right-sided weakness and sensory loss) and right MCA syndrome (left-sided weakness, sensory loss, and neglect). In the acute stage of an MCA stroke, there may be gaze deviation toward the side of the lesion (and away from the side of weakness), due to involvement of the frontal eye fields. PCA strokes cause contralateral visual field deficits. Strokes in the posterior circulation can cause a variety of symptoms and signs involving the cranial nerves and cerebellum including dizziness/vertigo, dysarthria, diplopia, and weakness and/or sensory loss in one side of the face and the opposite side of the body.

Transient ischemic attacks (TIAs) are temporary episodes of neurovascular dysfunction, typically lasting less than 1 hour. They can represent a harbinger of future stroke, especially for patients with large vessel atherosclerotic lesions. Implementing early treatment for stroke prevention, as detailed further, is important for patients with a TIA.[1]

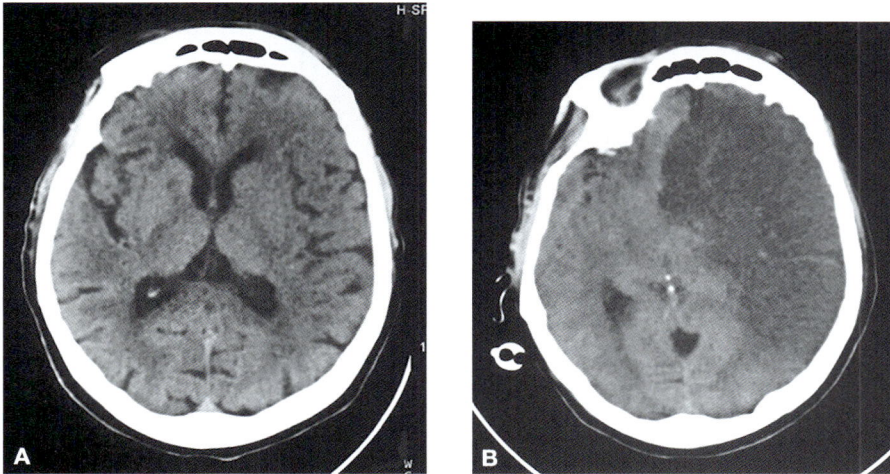

FIGURE 16.1 A. Early hypodensity in the left middle cerebral artery territory at 4 hours after stroke onset. B. Large area of hypodensity with edema in the left middle cerebral artery territory.

Initial head CT in acute ischemic stroke may be normal; over time, the infarcted area becomes increasingly hypodense (Figure 16.1). In the acute stage, the occluded vessel may appear hyperdense before hypodensity develops in the brain parenchyma. Diffusion-weighted magnetic resonance imaging (MRI) sequences can detect stroke with very high sensitivity; the ischemic area appears hyperintense on diffusion-weighted imaging (DWI) and hypointense on corresponding apparent diffusion coefficient (ADC) sequences[2,3] (Figure 16.2).

Acute Treatment of Ischemic Stroke

When a patient presents with ischemic stroke, the most immediate priorities are determining the time the patient was last seen normal to assess whether they are within the window for time-sensitive acute interventions (thrombolysis and thrombectomy), obtaining head CT to evaluate for intracranial hemorrhage, and determining whether there are any contraindications to intravenous (IV) thrombolysis.

IV thrombolysis (with alteplase [also known as recombinant tissue plasminogen activator (r-tPA)] or with tenecteplase) has been shown to improve outcomes of eligible patients with acute ischemic stroke when treated within 4.5 hours from the time

they were last seen normal. Obtaining information on the last known well time from family members or onlookers is therefore critical. For patients without a clear time of onset (eg, patients who wake up with stroke symptoms), comparison of certain

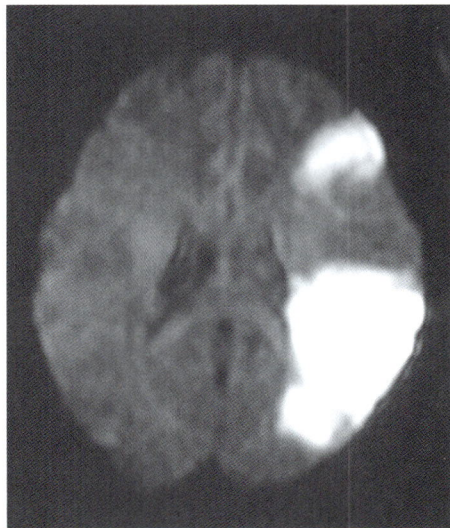

FIGURE 16.2 Two separate areas of increased signal on diffusion-weighted imaging on the left, representing acute infarction.

MRI sequences may be able to determine the approximate age of the stroke to identify potential thrombolysis candidates.[4] For patients being considered for thrombolysis, absolute contraindications include presence of hemorrhage on head CT, recent ingestion of direct oral anticoagulants (within the previous 48 hours), and recent gastrointestinal or genitourinary bleeding (within the previous 3 weeks). Recent surgery (within the previous 2 weeks) is considered a relative contraindication and requires balancing risks (and compressibility of the surgical site should bleeding occur) and potential benefits based on stroke severity.

In patients with proximal occlusion of a large artery (such as the proximal MCA), catheter-based procedures such as mechanical thrombectomy significantly improve outcome in select patients up to 24 hours from the time they were last seen normal. For patients who can be treated within 6 hours, only head CT and CT angiography (CTA) are required to choose appropriate candidates for this procedure; between 6 and 24 hours advanced imaging (eg, CT perfusion) is often utilized to select treatment candidates based on radiologic evidence of salvageable brain tissue.

In patients who are not candidates for thrombolysis or thrombectomy, antiplatelets are administered. All patients should receive aspirin, and patients with a small stroke may receive dual antiplatelet therapy with aspirin and clopidogrel for 21 days (see "Secondary Prevention of Ischemic Stroke" section). For patients who receive thrombolysis, aspirin and other antithrombotic medications are typically not administered until 24 hours after thrombolytic initiation.

Treatment of blood pressure in patients with acute stroke varies according to whether the patient received thrombolysis or thrombectomy. If the patient receives thrombolysis, the systolic blood pressure should subsequently be maintained less than 180 mm Hg for the first 24 hours.[5] If the patient undergoes thrombectomy, there are no clear guidelines as to optimal blood pressure goals, but a common practice is to keep the systolic blood pressure less than 160 mm Hg for the first 24 hours.[6] For patients who do not receive thrombolysis or thrombectomy, permissive hypertension for the first 24 to 48 hours after ischemic stroke is recommended, allowing the patient's blood pressure to autoregulate in the range of 160 to 220 mm Hg systolic. Lowering of blood pressure should be avoided in the first 24 hours, but blood pressure may be progressively lowered following this period.

Diagnostic Evaluation for Etiology of Ischemic Stroke

Etiology of stroke can be broadly classified into one of the following categories: (1) large vessel atherosclerosis; (2) cardioembolism; (3) small vessel occlusion (also known as lacunar); (4) stroke of other determined cause; (5) stroke of undetermined cause (cryptogenic stroke).[7] Large artery atherosclerosis is typically divided into extracranial stenosis (such as ICA stenosis) and intracranial stenosis (such as MCA or basilar artery stenosis). Embolic sources are divided into major, high-risk sources (eg, atrial fibrillation [AF], mechanical valve, and endocarditis) and minor, lower-risk sources (eg, reduced cardiac ejection fraction and patent foramen ovale [PFO]). Small vessel occlusion refers to involvement of the small penetrating arteries leading to lacunar infarction in deep brain structures (eg, internal capsule, thalamus). Within the category of stroke of other determined cause, etiologies include arterial dissection, sympathomimetic drug use, and hypercoagulable states.

Determining the etiology of ischemic stroke guides appropriate secondary prevention to reduce the risk of recurrent ischemic stroke. Stroke appearance on brain imaging provides some initial clues to etiology. For example, multiple infarcts in more than one vascular territory suggests a proximal embolic source (eg, cardiac or aortic), whereas multiple unilateral infarcts in one vascular territory may suggest ipsilateral large artery atherosclerosis (eg, carotid stenosis). A cortical, wedge-shaped infarct is suggestive of an embolic stroke[7]; if an embolic source is not determined after a thorough evaluation for an embolic-appearing stroke, the term "embolic stroke of undetermined source (ESUS)" is used to describe these infarcts.

The initial evaluation for stroke etiology includes cerebrovascular imaging to evaluate the cervical and intracranial arteries (magnetic resonance angiography [MRA] or CTA; ultrasound can also be used to evaluate the carotid arteries), cardiac evaluation (echocardiogram and cardiac monitoring), laboratory evaluation for vascular risk factors (serum lipid panel to screen for hyperlipidemia and glycosylated hemoglobin to screen for diabetes). If no etiology is found with these tests, further evaluation is guided by presumed stroke mechanism (based on neuroimaging) and patient context. For example, if the stroke is cryptogenic, especially in individuals over age 60, prolonged cardiac monitoring to look for intermittent AF is useful. Cardiac monitoring should be for a minimum of 2 weeks but longer duration can be considered when this is normal and suspicion for embolism is high. Transesophageal echocardiogram (TEE) can be considered in cryptogenic stroke to evaluate for left atrial appendage thrombus, valvular vegetations, or PFO and atrial septal aneurysm.[8] Hypercoagulable testing is recommended in younger adults (less than age 50 years) or if there is a prior history of venous or arterial clots.[1] Hypercoagulability evaluation should include antiphospholipid antibody panel, homocysteine level, D-dimer, and consideration of cancer screening.

Secondary Prevention of Ischemic Stroke

A key priority after ischemic stroke is secondary prevention, which includes risk factor modification (hypertension, diabetes, hyperlipidemia, smoking) and antithrombotic therapy in all patients, and additional treatments in select patients.

In patients with stroke due to AF, anticoagulation is indicated for secondary prevention (using a direct oral anticoagulant or warfarin). In the absence of AF or another indication for anticoagulation (eg, antiphospholipid antibody syndrome or other hypercoagulable state, mechanical heart valve), antiplatelet

TABLE 16.1 Elements of Intensive Medical Therapy for Secondary Prevention of Ischemic Stroke

Condition	Treatment
Antithrombotic therapy	Aspirin (and in some cases clopidogrel for 21-90 d; see text)
Lipids	High-potency statins (and/or ezetimibe, PCSK9 inhibitors)
Blood pressure	Systolic blood pressure <130 mm Hg
Diabetes	Pharmacologic treatments that reduce cardiovascular risk, hemoglobin A1c target of <7
Smoking cessation	Counseling and adjunctive pharmacologic treatments
Physical activity	Regular physical activity (3-5 sessions of aerobic exercise per week)

therapy is the treatment of choice for secondary prevention in the majority of patients after ischemic stroke.[1] In most patients, aspirin is used. Dual antiplatelet therapy (aspirin plus clopidogrel or ticagrelor with a loading dose) for 21 days (then returning to a single antiplatelet agent) after minor ischemic stroke or high-risk TIA was shown to be beneficial in two large trials.[9,10] Dual antiplatelet therapy is also often utilized (for 90 days) after ischemic stroke due to intracranial atherosclerosis. There is otherwise no indication for dual antiplatelet therapy for secondary prevention of ischemic stroke (although there is generally no contraindication if dual antiplatelet therapy is indicated for cardiac reasons).

Risk factor modification goals are currently systolic blood pressure less than 130 mm Hg and low-density lipoprotein (LDL) less than 70 mg/dL, but readers should consult current guidelines as recommendations change over time.[11] An overview of risk factor modification is provided in Table 16.1.

Atherosclerotic Disease

Patients with stroke due to atherosclerosis can have extracranial or intracranial stenosis. Common sites of extracranial stenosis include the origin of the ICA and the origin of the vertebral artery. Common locations for intracranial atherosclerotic disease include the cavernous segment of the ICA, proximal MCA, distal vertebral artery, and proximal or mid-basilar artery.

Carotid stenosis

ICA stenosis due to atherosclerotic disease can lead to ipsilateral stroke caused by artery-to-artery embolism. Risk factors for carotid stenosis include age, hypertension, diabetes mellitus, hyperlipidemia, smoking, and male sex.[12]

Carotid stenosis is most commonly diagnosed by duplex ultrasonography, CTA of the neck, or MRA of the neck. The degree of stenosis can be classified as severe (70%-99%), moderate (50%-69%), or mild (<50%). Some patients may have complete occlusion of the ICA.

Carotid stenosis is considered symptomatic if the patient has had an ipsilateral TIA or ischemic stroke in the territory of the stenotic vessel (ie, MCA or ACA) within the past 6 months.[13] Carotid stenosis is considered asymptomatic if the patient has not had an ipsilateral TIA or stroke in the territory of the affected ICA (eg, incidentally discovered carotid stenosis after a bruit is heard on exam) or has had a referable stroke, but more than 6 months ago. Revascularization with carotid endarterectomy or carotid artery stenting is recommended in select patients. Guideline recommendations are based on randomized trials that occurred before the advent of modern cardiovascular risk factor reduction strategies (eg, statins, aggressive blood pressure control).[13] While there is general consensus that patients with symptomatic severe (70%-99%) ICA stenosis should undergo intervention, prior recommendations for intervention in patients with symptomatic moderate (50%-69%) stenosis and asymptomatic severe stenosis are now controversial and decisions are made on a case-by-case basis considering the factors outlined in Table 16.2.

Carotid artery stenting has a higher perioperative stroke risk compared to carotid endarterectomy but may be considered in patients in whom the operative risk of endarterectomy is prohibitive. Endarterectomy is generally the procedure of choice in patients older than 70 years unless there are significant medical comorbidities.[14]

TABLE 16.2	Factors in Consideration of Carotid Revascularization	
	Favors medical therapy	**Favors revascularization**
Type of ischemic symptom	Retinal	Hemispheric
Patient sex	Female	Male
Timing of most recent ischemic symptom	Greater than 2 wk	Less than 2 wk
Severe comorbidity	Present	Absent
Well-established collaterals	Present	Absent

Intracranial atherosclerosis

Patients with intracranial atherosclerosis (identified on CTA or MRA of the head) as the etiology of an ischemic stroke can be treated with dual antiplatelet therapy (aspirin and clopidogrel) for 90 days based on data from the SAMMPRIS trial.[15] Patients with intracranial atherosclerosis should also be treated with intensive medical therapy to address risk factors (Table 16.1).

Patent Foramen Ovale

A PFO is present in about 25% to 30% of the population and is rarely associated with ischemic stroke, which can be due to in situ thrombosis or paradoxical embolism. A PFO may be visualized by transthoracic echocardiogram with bubble study, though transcranial Doppler ultrasound with bubble study and TEE are more sensitive if suspicion is high and transthoracic echocardiogram does not reveal a PFO.

Due to the high incidence of PFO in the general population, it is often unclear whether a PFO found in a patient with ischemic stroke is causative or incidental.[16] A PFO is more likely to be the presumed cause of the stroke if the patient has few or no vascular risk factors, is under age 60, the stroke appears embolic on neuroimaging, and the PFO is large and/or associated with an atrial septal aneurysm. Scores incorporating these elements (Risk of Paradoxical Embolism [RoPE] and PFO-Associated Stroke Causal Likelihood [PASCAL]) can guide clinicians in determining the likelihood that a stroke was due to a PFO and aid in selecting patients for endovascular PFO closure.[16,17] PFO closure reduces the risk of recurrent ischemic stroke in select patients but carries the risk of transient AF following the procedure.

In a patient with PFO and ischemic stroke with no indication for anticoagulation (eg, AF, hypercoagulable state), antiplatelet therapy is used for secondary prevention whether or not the patient undergoes PFO closure.[1]

Cryptogenic Stroke/Embolic Stroke of Undetermined Source

About a third of strokes are cryptogenic, meaning that no etiology is determined after evaluation for large artery atherosclerosis, cardiac source of embolism, and vascular risk factors as described earlier. If cryptogenic strokes are embolic-appearing on neuroimaging, they are referred to as ESUS.[18] In such patients, additional evaluation could include TEE, prolonged cardiac monitoring, or hypercoagulability testing, depending on the patient's history and age.[19,20] In patients with ESUS, several randomized trials have shown equivalence of aspirin and direct oral anticoagulants for secondary prevention.[21,22]

Prognosis

Ischemic stroke outcomes have improved with the availability of thrombolysis and thrombectomy. Current 90-day outcomes are complete recovery or mild deficits in about 30% of patients, moderate to severe residual deficits in about 60% of patients, and mortality of about 10%. Multidisciplinary rehabilitation therapies are recommended to maximize recovery.

INTRACEREBRAL HEMORRHAGE

Spontaneous ICH refers to bleeding within the brain parenchyma that does not result from traumatic injury. Patients with ICH present with focal neurologic deficits similarly to those with acute ischemic stroke, though headache and depressed level of consciousness are more common at presentation with ICH. Noncontrast CT is required to differentiate between acute ischemic stroke and ICH. Whereas the noncontrast head CT is most often normal or shows subtle hypodensity in acute ischemic stroke, ICH is apparent at presentation as a region of hyperdensity on CT.

Causes of Intracerebral Hemorrhage

The most common causes of ICH are hypertension and cerebral amyloid angiopathy.[23] Hypertensive ICH, resulting from chronic hypertensive stress on small blood vessels, most commonly occurs in the basal ganglia, thalamus, pons, or cerebellum. Cerebral amyloid angiopathy–associated ICH, caused by the pathologic deposition of β-amyloid in small vessels, tends to occur in the cerebral hemispheres closer to the cortex (called *lobar hemorrhage* as it affects a particular lobe of the brain, eg, the occipital lobe). Aside from hypertension and older age, additional risk factors for spontaneous ICH include coagulopathy (intrinsic or due to anticoagulation), sympathomimetic drug use, and high alcohol intake. Additional causes of spontaneous ICH include rupture of intracranial vascular malformations (eg, arteriovenous malformation, arteriovenous fistula, cavernous malformation, and aneurysm), hemorrhagic conversion of an ischemic stroke, cerebral venous sinus thrombosis, and hemorrhage into a brain tumor (more common with brain metastases than primary brain tumors).

Diagnostic Evaluation for Cause of Intracerebral Hemorrhage

In younger patients with ICH (less than 45 years old, or less than 70 years old without a history of hypertension or coagulopathy), evaluation for cerebral vascular malformations should be performed with CTA or MRA, and, if these are normal, catheter angiography (Figure 16.3G, H). The secondary ICH score uses imaging characteristics, age, and risk factors for ICH to predict the likelihood of an underlying vascular lesion to determine which patients warrant this additional evaluation (Table 16.3).[24] CT venogram (CTV) or MR venogram (MRV) should be considered to evaluate for venous sinus

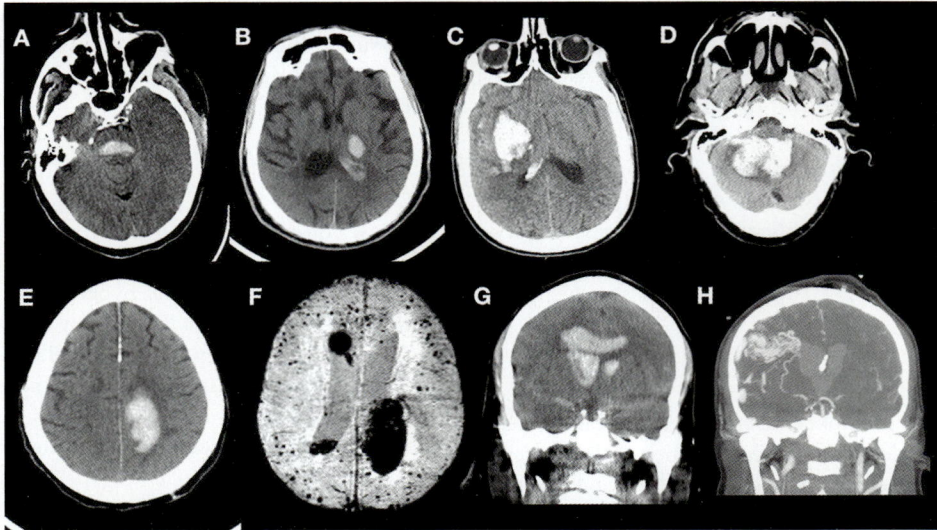

FIGURE 16.3 Diagnosis of intracerebral hemorrhage. Primary intracerebral hemorrhage due to hypertension tends to occur in the pons (A), thalamus (B), basal ganglia (C), or cerebellum (D). Primary intracerebral hemorrhage due to cerebral amyloid angiopathy is usually lobar (E) and associated with microhemorrhages on susceptibility-weighted MRI (F) that give a "Swiss cheese" appearance. In younger patients especially, arteriovenous malformations are an important cause of intracerebral hemorrhage that can be visualized on a CT angiogram (G, H).

TABLE 16.3	Secondary Intracerebral Hemorrhage (ICH) Score	
Parameter		**Points**
• Noncontrast CT categorization[a]		
○ High probability		2
○ Indeterminate		1
○ Low probability		0
• Age group		
○ 18-45 y		2
○ 46-70 y		1
○ ≥71 y		0
• Sex		
○ Female		1
○ Male		0
• Neither known HTN nor impaired coagulation		
○ Yes		1
○ No		0

CT, computed tomography; HTN, hypertension.
Percentage of patients with macrovascular cause of ICH by score: 1 point: <1%, 2 points: <2%, 3 points: 5%-16%, 4 points: 39%-42%, 5 points: 85%, 6 points: 75%-100%. (Derived from van Asch CJ, Velthuis VK, Greving JP, et al. External validation of the secondary intracerebral hemorrhage score in the Netherlands. *Stroke*. 2013;44:2904-2906.)
[a] High probability: enlarged vessels or calcifications along the margins of ICH or hyper-attenuation within a dural venous sinus or cortical vein along venous drainage path. Low probability: no high-risk features, located in basal ganglia, thalamus, brainstem.

thrombosis when hemorrhage occurs adjacent to venous sinuses. MRI with gadolinium to evaluate for an underlying mass can be considered if the cause remains uncertain, although acute blood may obscure an underlying lesion, which may require repeat imaging after several months.

Treatment of Intracerebral Hemorrhage

Immediate priorities of acute treatment of ICH are medically stabilizing the patient, reducing blood pressure, and reversing coagulopathy to reduce the risk of hematoma expansion.[23] Depressed level of consciousness in patients with ICH may require intubation and mechanical ventilation. Current guidelines recommend lowering systolic blood pressure below 140 mm Hg, or below 180 mm Hg in patients with systolic blood pressure higher than 220 mm Hg at presentation.[25,26] Reversal of coagulopathy depends on the anticoagulant (see Table 16.4).[23] Platelet transfusion is not recommended for patients with ICH on aspirin unless they are undergoing surgical evacuation of the hemorrhage.[27]

TABLE 16.4 Acute Treatment of Intracerebral Hemorrhage

Airway	• Intubate all patients unable to protect their airway or with rapidly deteriorating exam.
Blood pressure	• In patients with SBP <220 mm Hg, acutely lower the SBP to 130-150 mm Hg. • In patients with SBP >220, acutely lower the SBP to 160-180 mm Hg. • Intravenous calcium channel blockers such as nicardipine or clevidipine are preferred agents to rapidly achieve blood pressure control while limiting blood pressure variability.
Coagulopathy	• In patients taking warfarin, 4-factor prothrombin complex AND intravenous vitamin K concentrate should be administered (as opposed to fresh frozen plasma) for INR reversal. • In patients taking direct factor Xa inhibitors, andexanet alfa OR 4-factor prothrombin complex concentrate should be administered for reversal. • In patients taking dabigatran, idarucizumab should be administered for reversal. 4-factor prothrombin complex concentrate may be a reasonable alternative. • Activated charcoal should be administered for recent ingestions of direct factor Xa inhibitors and dabigatran: apixaban <6 h, edoxaban <2 h, rivaroxaban <6 h, dabigatran <2 h • In patients on heparin (unfractionated or low molecular weight), protamine should be administered for reversal. • In patients taking antiplatelet agents, platelet transfusion is not recommended for patients that do not require neurosurgical intervention. • In patients taking antiplatelet agents or with significant uremia, desmopressin can be considered to improve hemostasis.

Mass effect	• Medical treatment
	  ○ In patients with mass effect contributing to decreased consciousness, hyperosmolar therapy with either hypertonic saline or mannitol can reduce intracranial pressure.
	  ○ Data do not support the use of early prophylactic hyperosmolar (including elevated serum sodium goals) therapy for improving outcomes.
	  ○ Corticosteroids should generally not be administered.
	• Surgical treatment
	  ○ Craniotomy for hematoma evacuation or decompressive craniectomy can be considered to reduce mortality in severe supratentorial ICH with midline shift or herniation.
	  ○ Minimally invasive surgical approaches can be considered for moderate size (volume >20-30 mL) ICH with mass effect.
	  ○ Suboccipital craniotomy/craniectomy for hematoma evacuation is recommended for cerebellar ICH causing hydrocephalus or brainstem, and generally for ICH volume ≥15 mL.

Hydrocephalus	• For supratentorial ICH or primary IVH causing symptomatic hydrocephalus, an external ventricular drain should be placed for CSF diversion. • For cerebellar ICH causing hydrocephalus, an external ventricular drain should be placed and suboccipital decompressive surgery is recommended. • In patients with significant IVH and stable hemorrhage without a secondary cause, intrathecal thrombolytic therapy is safe and may improve outcomes if >85% of the IVH volume is removed.

Seizure	• Monitoring
	  ○ Unresponsive patients, patients with fluctuating exams, and patients with neurologic deficits out of proportion to their ICH should be monitored for nonconvulsive seizures with continuous EEG.
	• Treatment
	  ○ Patients with seizures should be started on antiseizure medications.
	  ○ Patients without seizures should not be placed on prophylactic antiseizure medications.

Goals of care	• The ICH score should not be used to prognosticate in individual patients or limit life-sustaining therapy. • A trial of aggressive care is reasonable in patients without preexisting goals of care limitations. • A shared decision-making model should be utilized between patients or their surrogates and physicians to align goals of care.
Triage	• Patients should be cared for in dedicated intensive care or stroke units.
DVT prophylaxis	• Chemoprophylaxis should be started as early as 24-48 h after presentation if the hemorrhage is stable.

CSF, cerebrospinal fluid; DVT, deep vein thrombosis; EEG, electroencephalogram; ICH, intracerebral hemorrhage; INR, international normalized ratio; IVH, intraventricular hemorrhage; SBP, systolic blood pressure.

Neurosurgical intervention is only generally considered in patients with large hemorrhages in the posterior fossa causing hydrocephalus or rapidly expanding hemispheric hemorrhages causing life-threatening mass effect. Emerging minimally invasive techniques may lead to an increasing role for surgery in patients with ICH in the future.[28] When hematoma causes mass effect or hydrocephalus in patients who are not surgical candidates, hyperosmolar agents (mannitol, hypertonic saline) and cerebrospinal fluid (CSF) drainage via external ventricular drain should be considered.

Seizures should be treated if they occur, but prophylactic antiseizure medication is not recommended by guidelines.[23,29,30]

Given that the highest risk period for hematoma expansion is within the first 24 hours, patients are generally monitored closely in an intensive care unit (ICU) during this period, and a repeat CT scan is generally obtained at 6 hours and again at 24 hours to assess for stability of the ICH.

Following the acute period, care is supportive with physical therapy, occupational therapy, and deep vein thrombosis prophylaxis (which can be safely started 24-48 hours after presentation if the ICH is stable on 24-hour CT scan).

Outcome

ICH outcomes depend on features of the hemorrhage (eg, size, location, and whether there is accompanying intraventricular hemorrhage), patient factors (age, premorbid functional status), and neurologic examination at presentation. The ICH score, which incorporates many of these variables, was developed as a clinical severity score to improve communication and guide treatment selection (Table 16.5).[31] Clinicians should not use the ICH score to prognosticate in individual patients as it was not meant to do so, performs less reliably than clinician estimates, and overestimates mortality in patients who receive early, aggressive care.[32] Thus, clinicians should not use the score to justify limiting life-sustaining treatment in patients with ICH. Survivors of ICH are at high risk for cognitive impairment, depression, and epilepsy.

TABLE 16.5	Intracerebral Hemorrhage (ICH) Score
Parameter	**Points**
• Glasgow Coma Scale	
○ 3-4	2
○ 5-12	1
○ 13-15	0
• Age	
○ ≥80 y	1
○ <80 y	0
• ICH volume	
○ ≥30 mL	1
○ <30 mL	0
• Intraventricular hemorrhage	
○ Yes	1
○ No	0
• Infratentorial origin of hemorrhage	
○ Yes	1
○ No	0

30-Day mortality predicted by score if early Do-Not-Resuscitate orders are avoided in the first 5 days after intracerebral hemorrhage: 0 points: <1%, 1 point: 5%, 2 points: 10%, 3 points: 20%, 4+ points: ~50%. (Derived from Morgenstern LB, Zahuranec DB, Sánchez BN, et al. Full medical support for intracerebral hemorrhage. *Neurology.* 2015;84(17):1739-1744.)

SUBARACHNOID HEMORRHAGE

SAH refers to bleeding between the arachnoid and the pia (the innermost layers of the meninges). The most common cause of SAH is rupture of a saccular (berry) aneurysm, though SAH can also be caused by trauma, cortical vein thrombosis, arteriovenous malformation, reversible cerebral vasoconstriction syndrome (RCVS), cerebral amyloid angiopathy, and intracranial arterial dissection. Aneurysmal SAH is far less common than ischemic stroke and ICH and affects younger patients (median age of onset of 50-55 years). Risk factors for aneurysmal SAH include female sex, smoking, hypertension, polycystic kidney disease, connective tissue disease, and a family history of aneurysm. The risk of SAH from an unruptured aneurysm is higher in larger aneurysms (greater than 7 mm) and higher for posterior circulation aneurysms (arteries derived from the vertebrobasilar artery supply).[33]

SAH due to aneurysmal rupture most commonly presents with headache that is sudden in onset and maximal intensity at onset (thunderclap headache). The headache is often described as the worst headache of the patient's life and is most commonly unprovoked, though it may be precipitated by physical exertion, emotional stress, or Valsalva maneuver. Associated symptoms include nausea/vomiting, photophobia, and neck pain/stiffness from meningeal irritation. Brief loss of consciousness at onset occurs in 40% of patients and is thought to represent transient cerebral circulatory arrest as the intracranial pressure matches the mean arterial pressure at the time of aneurysmal rupture; this is a poor prognostic sign.[34] Alterations in mental status are common at presentation, ranging from confusion to coma. Seizure occurs in some patients and is associated with a worse prognosis.[35] On examination, patients may have focal deficits such as cranial nerve palsies (eg, cranial nerve 3 palsy with ptosis, dilated pupil, and downward and outward deviation of the eye), hemiparesis, or aphasia, depending on the location of the SAH. Aneurysmal SAH may also cause cardiac arrest and sudden death,[36] and up to one in every four patients with aneurysmal SAH dies before reaching the hospital.

Diagnostic Evaluation of Subarachnoid Hemorrhage

Clinicians should suspect SAH in any patient who presents with sudden-onset severe headache or a severe headache that is unrelenting and qualitatively different from the patient's prior history of headaches. Some patients describe the headache as peaking over 1 hour (as opposed to maximum intensity at onset), others' headaches actually resolve, and many patients do not have meningismus. Because not all patients present "classically" and headache is a very common diagnosis in the emergency rooms, approximately one-quarter of patients with SAH are not diagnosed at first presentation.[37] Misdiagnosis occurs due to failure to recognize red flags (eg, sudden onset, qualitative difference from prior headaches, new neurologic symptoms/signs, onset during exertion), an overreliance on classical symptoms/signs, and underutilization or misinterpretation of diagnostic tests.

If aneurysmal SAH is suspected, a noncontrast head CT should be performed immediately to evaluate for SAH.[38] Unlike subdural hematoma that occurs between the outer layers of dura, SAH occurs within the basal cisterns and tracks into the sulci (Figure 16.4). Head CT is considered nearly 100% sensitive for SAH when performed within 6 hours after symptom onset and read by an expert neuroradiologist, although anemia (which attenuates the density of SAH) and motion artifact may lead to decreased sensitivity. In patients presenting more than 6 hours after onset or in whom suspicion for SAH remains high despite a negative head CT, lumbar puncture should be performed to evaluate for blood. SAH is distinguished from traumatic lumbar puncture by the presence of xanthochromia, a yellow-tinged color of the CSF when analyzed by spectrophotometry after centrifugation indicating red blood cell breakdown. A high CSF red blood cell count that does not clear from tube 1 to tube 4 is a suggestive but unreliable marker of SAH, since the red blood cell count can occasionally decrease from tube 1 to tube 4 after SAH. MRI is most useful in delayed presentations (~3-7 days following rupture) as fluid-attenuated inversion recovery (FLAIR) and susceptibility-weighted imaging (SWI) MRI sequences have better sensitivity than CT for detection of blood in this period.

The location of SAH on neuroimaging correlates with the etiology. SAH within the basal cisterns extending into the major fissures is most likely due to aneurysm rupture (Figure 16.4A and B). SAH in the cerebral sulci (called *convexal SAH*) can occur due to head trauma, RCVS (Figure 16.4C and D), amyloid angiopathy, or cortical vein thrombosis. SAH confined to the anterior basal cisterns (prepontine, interpeduncular, or suprasellar) without extension into the Sylvian or interhemispheric fissures and in the absence of intraparenchymal/intraventricular blood is referred to as *perimesencephalic SAH* and is associated with a very low rate of aneurysm detection and a more benign clinical course.

If CT suggests aneurysmal SAH, a CTA or catheter digital subtraction angiogram (DSA) is required to search for an aneurysm. The sensitivity of CTA for the detection of ruptured aneurysms compared to DSA

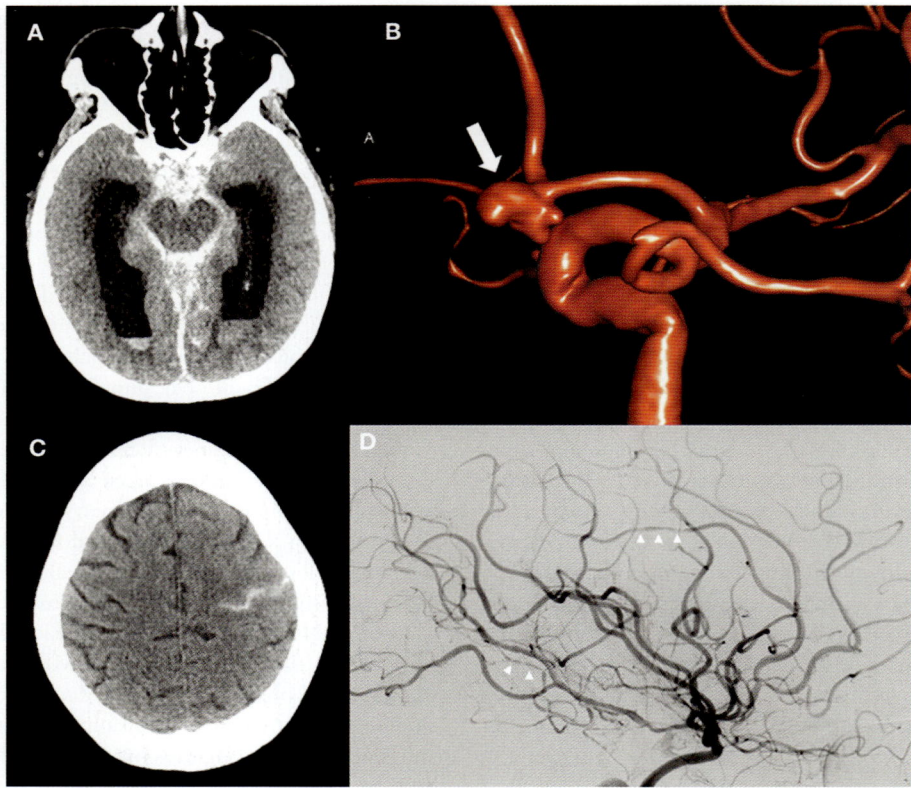

FIGURE 16.4 Diagnosis of subarachnoid hemorrhage. Aneurysmal subarachnoid hemorrhage occurs within the basal cisterns and can cause hydrocephalus (A). A three-dimensional reconstruction of the digital subtraction angiogram shows a multilobed aneurysm of the anterior communicating artery (arrow, B). Convexity subarachnoid hemorrhage occurs within the sulci (C) and in the setting of sudden-onset worst headache of life is suspicious for reversible cerebral vasoconstriction syndrome, which can be demonstrated by segmental narrowing/dilation on the digital subtraction angiogram (arrow heads, D).

is high but not 100%. In aneurysmal-pattern SAH, neither a negative CTA nor a negative DSA rules out the presence of an aneurysm, which may escape detection since a temporary platelet plug may block intraluminal contrast into the aneurysm. In cases in which clinical and radiologic suspicion is high and DSA is unrevealing, DSA should be repeated after 7 days to allow time for thrombus resolution.

Treatment of Subarachnoid Hemorrhage

The initial management of aneurysmal SAH focuses on reducing the risk of rebleeding, ameliorating symptoms, and monitoring for and treating early complications. Rebleeding occurs in 5% to 10% of patients in the first 24 hours after aneurysmal SAH and substantially increases mortality.[39] Aneurysms should be secured by endovascular coiling or open surgical clipping at a high-volume center as soon as possible for definitive management.[40,41] To reduce the risk of rebleeding while awaiting intervention, systolic blood pressure should be reduced to less than 160 mm Hg, any significant coagulopathy should be corrected, and antiseizure prophylaxis should be initiated to prevent seizures. If surgical securing of the aneurysm will be delayed, antifibrinolytic treatment (with tranexamic acid or aminocaproic acid) can be considered. Pain, nausea, and vomiting should be

TABLE 16.6   Subarachnoid Hemorrhage Severity Scores

Severity	Hunt and Hess scale	World Federation of Neurological Surgeons scale	Hospital mortality (%)
Grade 1	Asymptomatic or mild headache only	Glasgow Coma Scale 15	~2
Grade 2	Moderate to severe headache, no focal neurologic deficits other than cranial nerve palsy	Glasgow Coma Scale 13-14 without major motor deficit	~5
Grade 3	Drowsiness, confusion, or lethargy or mild focal deficit other than cranial nerve palsy	Glasgow Coma Scale 13-14 with major motor deficit	~10
Grade 4	Stupor, moderate to severe focal deficit (hemiparesis)	Glasgow Coma Scale 7-12	~25
Grade 5	Coma, extensor posturing	Glasgow Coma Scale 3-6	~70

treated aggressively both to decrease suffering and because they may increase the risk of aneurysmal rerupture due to blood pressure elevation and increased intracranial pressure.

The most common cause of early neurologic decline following aneurysmal SAH is hydrocephalus, presenting as somnolence that may rapidly evolve to coma. In patients with aneurysmal SAH who develop acute hydrocephalus, an external ventricular drain should be placed by a neurosurgeon.

The catecholamine surge caused by SAH can cause systemic complications such as neurogenic pulmonary edema, neurogenic stress cardiomyopathy (known as *takotsubo cardiomyopathy*), and cardiac arrhythmias. Patients must therefore be carefully monitored in an ICU setting, and cardiac enzymes, electrocardiogram (ECG), and echocardiogram should be performed. Patients who develop neurogenic stress (takotsubo) cardiomyopathy may require diuresis, inotropic support, and/or mechanical ventilation to maintain oxygenation and perfusion.

In the 4 to 14 days following aneurysm rupture, patients are at risk for delayed cerebral ischemia due to vasospasm, altered cerebrovascular autoregulation, and other factors. Clinicians often use transcranial Doppler to monitor for the development of vasospasm. Delayed cerebral ischemia can cause new focal neurologic deficits or altered mental status (typically measured by a 2-point decrease in the Glasgow Coma Scale). The calcium channel blocker nimodipine has been shown to improve outcomes after SAH when used prophylactically, although the mechanism is uncertain. Hemodynamic augmentation and endovascular administration of vasodilators or balloon angioplasty are considered when patients develop new focal neurologic deficits or altered mental status due to vasospasm.

Outcome After Subarachnoid Hemorrhage

Though mortality from aneurysmal SAH has decreased over the last several decades, it remains high at 30%.[42-44] Clinical severity correlates with early mortality; the Hunt-Hess and World Federation of Neurological Surgeons scores can be used to estimate mortality (Table 16.6). Survivors often have residual neuropsychiatric symptoms including cognitive impairment, depression, headache, fatigue, and sleep disturbances.

SUMMARY

Ischemic stroke, ICH, and SAH account for substantial morbidity and mortality. Whereas ischemic stroke and ICH both present with sudden-onset focal deficits and cannot be distinguished on clinical grounds alone, SAH most often presents differently with sudden-onset, severe headache. Treatment differs for each, focusing on early reperfusion for ischemic stroke, blood pressure reduction and coagulopathy reversal for ICH, and securing the aneurysm and treating acute complications in SAH. Recent advances in the acute treatment and secondary prevention of ischemic stroke have improved patient outcomes, while much progress remains to be made in hemorrhagic stroke treatment.

► Stroke refers to the sudden onset of neurologic deficits due to a vascular etiology and includes ischemic stroke, ICH, and SAH.

► Ischemic stroke and ICH both commonly present with sudden-onset focal neurologic deficits such as unilateral weakness or sensory loss of the face and/or extremities, visual field defect, aphasia, or ataxia. ICH is more commonly associated with headache and depressed level of consciousness.

► Ischemic stroke and ICH are distinguished on CT: ischemic stroke is hypodense (and may not be apparent very early in acute ischemic stroke) and ICH is hyperdense.

► Patients presenting with stroke symptoms should rapidly undergo CT and CTA since early treatment of ischemic stroke with thrombolysis and/or thrombectomy improves outcomes.

► In acute ischemic stroke, blood pressure should be allowed to autoregulate, whereas in acute ICH, blood pressure should be reduced.

► The etiology of ischemic stroke should be sought with serum lipids and hemoglobin A1c, echocardiogram, cardiac monitoring, and angiographic imaging of the neck vessels (with CTA, MRA, or, for the carotid arteries, ultrasound).

► Secondary prevention of ischemic stroke involves lifestyle modifications, treatment of hyperlipidemia and diabetes, and antithrombotic therapy (aspirin in most cases; anticoagulation in AF-associated ischemic stroke). In patients with a stroke ipsilateral to severe carotid stenosis, surgical or endovascular intervention should be considered.

► Aneurysmal rupture causing SAH should be considered in patients presenting with a sudden severe headache. CT and CTA should be obtained; if normal and suspicion is high, lumbar puncture to look for xanthochromia should be performed.

► Management of aneurysmal SAH focuses on reducing the risk of rebleeding with surgical clipping or endovascular coiling and monitoring for and treating early complications such as hydrocephalus, cerebral vasospasm, and systemic complications.

REFERENCES

1. Kleindorfer DO, Towfighi A, Chaturvedi S, et al. 2021 guideline for the prevention of stroke in patients with stroke and transient ischemic attack: a guideline from the American Heart Association/American Stroke Association. *Stroke*. 2021; 52:e364-e467.
2. Chalela JA, Kidwell CS, Nentwich LM, et al. Magnetic resonance imaging and computed tomography in emergency assessment of patients with suspected acute stroke: a prospective comparison. *Lancet*. 2007;369:293-298.
3. Kang DW, Chalela JA, Ezzeddine MA, Warach S. Association of ischemic lesion patterns on early diffusion-weighted imaging with toast stroke subtypes. *Arch Neurol*. 2003;60: 1730-1734.
4. Thomalla G, Simonsen CZ, Boutitie F, et al. MRI-guided thrombolysis for stroke with unknown time of onset. *N Engl J Med*. 2018;379:611-622.
5. Powers WJ, Rabinstein AA, Ackerson T, et al. Guidelines for the early management of patients with acute ischemic stroke: 2019 update to the 2018 guidelines for the early management of acute ischemic stroke: a guideline for healthcare professionals from the American Heart Association/American Stroke Association. *Stroke*. 2019;50:e344-e418.
6. Morris NA, Jindal G, Chaturvedi S. Intensive blood pressure control after mechanical thrombectomy for acute ischemic stroke. *Stroke*. 2023;54:1457-1461.
7. Yaghi S, Elkind MS. Cryptogenic stroke: a diagnostic challenge. *Neurol Clin Pract*. 2014;4:386-393.
8. de Bruijn SF, Agema WR, Lammers GJ, et al. Transesophageal echocardiography is superior to transthoracic echocardiography in management of patients of any age with transient ischemic attack or stroke. *Stroke*. 2006;37:2531-2534.
9. Wang Y, Wang Y, Zhao X, et al. Clopidogrel with aspirin in acute minor stroke or transient ischemic attack. *N Engl J Med*. 2013;369:11-19.
10. Johnston SC, Easton DJ, Farrant M, et al. Clopidogrel and aspirin in acute ischemic stroke and high-risk TIA. *N Engl J Med*. 2018;379:215-225.
11. Visseren FLJ, Mach F, Smulders YM, et al. 2021 ESC guidelines on cardiovascular disease prevention in clinical practice. *Eur Heart J*. 2021;42:3227-3337.
12. de Weerd M, Greving JP, Hedblad B, et al. Prevalence of asymptomatic carotid artery stenosis in the general population: an individual participant data meta-analysis. *Stroke*. 2010; 41:1294-1297.
13. Chaturvedi S, Sacco RL. How recent data have impacted the treatment of internal carotid artery stenosis. *J Am Coll Cardiol*. 2015;65:1134-1143.
14. Howard G, Roubin GS, Jansen O, et al. Association between age and risk of stroke or death from carotid endarterectomy and carotid stenting: a meta-analysis of pooled patient data from four randomized trials. *Lancet*. 2016;387: 1305-1311.

15. Chimowitz MI, Lynn MJ, Derdeyn CP, et al. Stenting versus aggressive medical therapy for intracranial arterial stenosis. *N Engl J Med.* 2011;365(11):993-1003.

16. Kent DM, Saver JL, Kasner SE, et al. Heterogeneity of treatment effects in an analysis of pooled individual patient data from randomized trials of device closure of patent foramen ovale after stroke. *JAMA.* 2021;326:2277-2286.

17. Kent DM, Ruthazer R, Weimar C, et al. An index to identify stroke-related vs incidental patent foramen ovale in cryptogenic stroke. *Neurology.* 2013;81:619-625.

18. Hart RG, Diener HC, Coutts SB, et al. Embolic strokes of undetermined source: the case for a new clinical construct. *Lancet Neurol.* 2014;13:429-438.

19. Sanna T, Diener HC, Passman RS, et al. Cryptogenic stroke and underlying atrial fibrillation. *N Engl J Med.* 2014;370:2478-2486.

20. Sposato L, Cipriano LE, Saposnik G, et al. Diagnosis of atrial fibrillation after stroke and transient ischemic attack: a systematic review and meta-analysis. *Lancet Neurol.* 2015;14:377-387.

21. Hart RG, Sharma M, Mundl H, et al. Rivaroxaban for stroke prevention after embolic stroke of undetermined source. *N Eng J Med.* 2018;378:2191-2201.

22. Diener HC, Sacco RL, Easton JD, et al. Dabigatran for prevention of stroke after embolic stroke of undetermined source. *N Engl J Med.* 2019;380:1906-1917.

23. Greenberg SM, Ziai WC, Cordonnier C, et al. 2022 guideline for the management of patients with spontaneous intracerebral hemorrhage: a guideline from the American Heart Association/American Stroke Association. *Stroke.* 2022;53(7):e282-e361. doi:10.1161/STR.0000000000000407

24. Van Asch CJJ, Velthuis BK, Greving JP, et al. External validation of the secondary intracerebral hemorrhage score in the Netherlands. *Stroke.* 2013;44:2904-2906.

25. Moullaali TJ, Wang X, Martin RH, et al. Blood pressure control and clinical outcomes in acute intracerebral haemorrhage: a preplanned pooled analysis of individual participant data. *Lancet Neurol.* 2019;18(9):857-864. doi:10.1016/S1474-4422(19)30196-6

26. Qureshi AI, Huang W, Lobanova I, et al. Outcomes of intensive systolic blood pressure reduction in patients with intracerebral hemorrhage and excessively high initial systolic blood pressure: post hoc analysis of a randomized clinical trial. *JAMA Neurol.* 2020;77(11):1355-1365. doi:10.1001/jamaneurol.2020.3075

27. Baharoglu MI, Cordonnier C, Salman RA, et al. Platelet transfusion versus standard care after acute stroke due to spontaneous cerebral haemorrhage associated with antiplatelet therapy (PATCH): a randomised, open-label, phase 3 trial. *Lancet.* 2016;387(10038):2605-2613. doi:10.1016/S0140-6736(16)30392-0

28. Sondag L, Schreuder FHBM, Boogaarts HD, et al. Neurosurgical intervention for supratentorial intracerebral hemorrhage. *Ann Neurol.* 2020;88(2):239-250. doi:10.1002/ana.25732

29. Peter-Derex L, Philippeau F, Garnier P, et al. Safety and efficacy of prophylactic levetiracetam for prevention of epileptic seizures in the acute phase of intracerebral haemorrhage (PEACH): a randomised, double-blind, placebo-controlled, phase 3 trial. *Lancet Neurol.* 2022;21(9):781-791. doi:10.1016/S1474-4422(22)00235-6

30. Naidech AM, Beaumont J, Muldoon K, et al. Prophylactic seizure medication and health-related quality of life after intracerebral hemorrhage. *Crit Care Med.* 2018;46(9):1480-1485. doi:10.1097/CCM.0000000000003272

31. Hemphill JC, Bonovich DC, Besmertis L, Manley GT, Johnston SC. The ICH score: a simple, reliable grading scale for intracerebral hemorrhage. *Stroke.* 2001;32(4):891-897. doi:10.1161/01.str.32.4.891

32. Morgenstern LB, Zahuranec DB, Sánchez BN, et al. Full medical support for intracerebral hemorrhage. *Neurology.* 2015;84(17):1739-1744. doi:10.1212/WNL.0000000000001525

33. Wiebers DO, Whisnant JP, Huston J, et al. Unruptured intracranial aneurysms: natural history, clinical outcome, and risks of surgical and endovascular treatment. *Lancet.* 2003;362(9378):103-110. doi:10.1016/s0140-6736(03)13860-3

34. Suwatcharangkoon S, Meyers E, Falo C, et al. Loss of consciousness at onset of subarachnoid hemorrhage as an important marker of early brain injury. *JAMA Neurol.* 2016;73(1):28-35. doi:10.1001/jamaneurol.2015.3188

35. Butzkueven H, Evans AH, Pitman A, et al. Onset seizures independently predict poor outcome after subarachnoid hemorrhage. *Neurology.* 2000;55(9):1315-1320. doi:10.1212/wnl.55.9.1315

36. Arnaout M, Mongardon N, Deye N, et al. Out-of-hospital cardiac arrest from brain cause: epidemiology, clinical features, and outcome in a multicenter cohort. *Crit Care Med.* 2015;43(2):453-460. doi:10.1097/ccm.0000000000000722

37. Ois A, Vivas E, Figueras-Aguirre G, et al. Misdiagnosis worsens prognosis in subarachnoid hemorrhage with good Hunt and Hess score. *Stroke.* 2019;50(11):3072-3076. doi:10.1161/STROKEAHA.119.025520

38. Connolly ES, Rabinstein AA, Carhuapoma JR, et al. Guidelines for the management of aneurysmal subarachnoid hemorrhage: a guideline for healthcare professionals from the American Heart Association/American Stroke Association. *Stroke.* 2012;43(6):1711-1737. doi:10.1161/STR.0b013e3182587839

39. van Lieshout JH, Mijderwijk HJ, Nieboer D, et al. Development and internal validation of the ARISE prediction models for rebleeding after aneurysmal subarachnoid hemorrhage. *Neurosurgery.* 2022;91(3):450-458. doi:10.1227/neu.0000000000002045

40. Post R, Germans MR, Tjerkstra MA, et al. Ultra-early tranexamic acid after subarachnoid haemorrhage (ULTRA): a randomised controlled trial. *Lancet.* 2021;397(10269):112-118. doi:10.1016/S0140-6736(20)32518-6

41. Molyneux A, Kerr R, Stratton I, et al. International Subarachnoid Aneurysm Trial (ISAT) of neurosurgical clipping versus endovascular coiling in 2143 patients with ruptured intracranial

aneurysms: a randomised trial. *Lancet*. 2002;360(9342):1267-1274. doi:10.1016/s0140-6736(02)11314-6

42. Molyneux AJ, Birks J, Clarke A, Sneade M, Kerr RS. The durability of endovascular coiling versus neurosurgical clipping of ruptured cerebral aneurysms: 18 year follow-up of the UK cohort of the International Subarachnoid Aneurysm Trial (ISAT). *Lancet*. 2015;385(9969):691-697. doi:10.1016/S0140-6736(14)60975-2

43. Foreman B. The pathophysiology of delayed cerebral ischemia. *J Clin Neurophysiol*. 2016;33(3):174-182. doi:10.1097/WNP.0000000000000273

44. Mackey J, Khoury JC, Alwell K, et al. Stable incidence but declining case-fatality rates of subarachnoid hemorrhage in a population. *Neurology*. 2016;87(21):2192-2197. doi:10.1212/WNL.0000000000003353

Seizures and Epilepsy

Lara Jehi

INTRODUCTION

About 1 in 10 individuals will have a seizure during their lifetime, and epilepsy affects about 50 million people worldwide and is associated with significant morbidity and mortality. This chapter reviews the diagnosis and treatment of seizures and epilepsy, including the approach to patients with a first seizure, the approach to patients with epilepsy, the approach to treatment of status epilepticus, and considerations in selection and titration of anti-seizure medications in various patient populations.

An epileptic seizure is a transient neurologic symptom or sign caused by excessive brain activity in one or more cortical regions. Seizures are classified as unprovoked (when no clear trigger is identified) or provoked (when triggered by a reversible factor such as sleep deprivation, alcohol withdrawal, electrolyte imbalance, severe hypoglycemia, medications, or drugs). Epilepsy refers to the condition of recurrent unprovoked seizures.

Seizures are further classified as focal or generalized. Focal seizures begin in a specific area in the brain and cause focal manifestations (eg, unilateral movements, sensations, or visual phenomena); they are usually caused by focal brain lesions (eg, prior trauma or stroke, tumor, and cortical malformation). Generalized seizures result from diffuse or multifocal cortical dysfunction and therefore cause bilateral motor manifestations and altered level of consciousness. Examples of generalized seizures include generalized tonic-clonic seizures (grand mal seizures) and absence seizures (petit mal seizures). An epilepsy syndrome refers to a genetic epilepsy with specific age at onset, type(s) of seizure, and electroencephalogram (EEG) findings.

Most seizures are brief, resolving spontaneously within less than 3 minutes. Status epilepticus is defined as a seizure lasting longer than 5 minutes, or as more than 1 seizure occurring within a 5-minute period without return of consciousness between episodes. This is a medical emergency that can lead to brain damage or death.

Psychogenic nonepileptic seizures (PNES) are transient alterations in neurologic function that are not epileptic on EEG. Features that distinguish PNES from epileptic seizures are discussed subsequently. The diagnosis can be challenging to make, and patients may have both epileptic seizures and PNES. PNES may require EEG monitoring during spells to determine whether the events are epileptic or not. PNES are treated with cognitive behavioral therapy rather than anti-seizure medications.

DIAGNOSIS OF SEIZURES AND EPILEPSY

The first step in evaluating a patient who presents after a possible seizure is determining whether the event was truly a seizure as opposed to another type of transient spell such as syncope or PNES. The history should be obtained from both the patient and a witness since patients may have no recollection of the event(s).

Distinguishing Seizures From Syncope and Psychogenic Nonepileptic Seizures

Stereotyped, sudden, brief events should raise concern for a possible seizure. Seizures may be triggered by fever, dehydration, sleep deprivation, hypoglycemia, severe electrolyte disturbances, or drugs, but may also be unprovoked. An episode that occurs during sleep is usually epileptic. Some seizures are preceded by auras (eg, déjà vu or foul odor) that tend to be specific (stereotyped) in each patient because they arise from activity in a specific epileptic focus in the brain. Patients may report feeling "jittery," "jerky," "confused," or "foggy" preceding a convulsion. Generalized tonic-clonic seizures cause generalized body stiffening (often causing the patient to collapse), followed by rhythmic bilateral jerking movements. Frothing at the mouth, tongue bite (often on the side of the tongue) leading to bloody saliva, ictal cry, grunting, color changes to pale or dusky, and incontinence are common. The duration of a seizure is usually less than 3 minutes. In absence seizures (more common in children), staring with unresponsiveness occurs, which may be accompanied by lip smacking or nonpurposeful hand movements. Following a generalized seizure, the patient often experiences a postictal state in which they may be agitated, confused, or have a depressed level of consciousness; this can last for hours depending on the length of the seizure.

Syncope may be triggered by dehydration, pain, hot weather, standing for too long, or rapid changes in body position (standing up too quickly from a sitting or horizontal position) or vasovagal triggers (eg, urination or straining in the bathroom,

particularly in older patients who are also on medications to lower blood pressure). Syncope may be preceded by lightheadedness, dizziness, sweatiness, palpitations, or vision changes (graying or darkening of vision). During the event, the patient loses consciousness and falls, typically without body stiffening. Loss of consciousness is typically only 10 to 30 seconds. There may be brief tremulousness or jerking and, rarely, urinary incontinence may occur. Patients typically return rapidly to consciousness after syncope with no or only very brief confusion.

PNES may be triggered by an emotional situation, although this is not always the case. A history of physical, emotional, or sexual trauma is common but not universal in these patients. Patients with PNES may describe preceding speech changes, confusion, or numbness, or spells may occur without warning; preceding features may be variable compared to the stereotyped auras preceding epileptic seizures. Clues that a spell may be PNES include retained awareness and eye closure during the spell, nonsynchronous asymmetric movements (compared to the rhythmic symmetric movements of epileptic seizures), gradual onset and offset, long duration (several minutes to an hour or longer), and lack of self-injury or incontinence. Patients are typically responsive after an event (and may be responsive during the event). However, features of PNES may be difficult to differentiate from epileptic events based on clinical features alone, and even experienced epilepsy subspecialists may find the diagnosis challenging. That is why a diagnostic video-EEG evaluation is often necessary to determine whether the events of concern are epileptic (in which case epileptiform changes are expected on the EEG during the captured spell) or not (in which case the EEG shows no epileptic changes during the event).

Additional Key Questions to Ask

Once established that the event is a seizure and any potential provoking factors are elicited, key questions to ask include determining whether it was the first event or whether events have occurred in the past, if the patient has any history of a prior neurologic condition (eg, stroke, head trauma, and meningitis), if they have been on anti-seizure medications in the past, and whether there is any family history of seizures or epilepsy.

DIAGNOSIS AND TREATMENT OF A FIRST SEIZURE

Diagnosis

Patients who have had a first seizure should be evaluated for a provoking trigger by testing serum glucose, complete metabolic panel, complete blood cell count, renal and liver function tests, urinalysis and urine toxicology screen, and brain imaging to evaluate for a causative lesion (eg, hemorrhage, tumor, and infection). A high serum lactate level within the first 2 hours of onset of the event suggests the cause was a generalized seizure rather than syncope or a psychogenic nonepileptic seizure. Creatine kinase, serum prolactin, cortisol, white blood cell count, and lactate dehydrogenase can be abnormal after a generalized tonic-clonic seizure, but these are nonspecific and can be elevated due to other conditions.

If no etiology is found on basic laboratory testing or computed tomography (CT), brain magnetic resonance imaging (MRI) should be obtained to evaluate for lesions that may be missed on CT such as stroke, tumor, sequelae of prior brain injury, mesial temporal sclerosis, cortical dysplasia (a congenital brain malformation that often causes epilepsy), or venous sinus thrombosis. The absence of a lesion does not mean the patient did not have a seizure, since more than half of the patients with known epilepsy have normal neuroimaging studies.[1] It is also important to note that subtle abnormalities that may cause epilepsy may require specialized MRI sequences to visualize them.

Lumbar puncture should be considered if there is clinical concern for meningitis or encephalitis. It is important to note that a convulsive seizure itself can cause an elevation in cerebrospinal fluid white count (usually no more than 10-50 cells/mm^3), despite the absence of infection or inflammation.

EEG should be obtained following a first seizure. Of note, a normal EEG does not rule out a diagnosis of seizures or epilepsy since sensitivity is only about 50% for detection of interictal epileptic abnormalities (ie, epileptiform discharges occurring between seizures). If the patient has recovered to their baseline after a seizure, EEG can be performed nonurgently in the outpatient setting. However, continuous inpatient EEG monitoring should be performed urgently if ongoing seizure activity (status epilepticus) is suspected; for example, if a patient fails to return to their neurologic baseline within 30 to 60 minutes of a convulsion, demonstrates waxing and waning mental status, or has a persistent focal neurologic deficit following a seizure that is not explained by neuroimaging.

If it is unclear whether the event was epileptic or syncopal, evaluation for seizure etiology and possible cardiac etiology may be performed in parallel. Cardiac evaluation generally includes electrocardiogram (ECG), outpatient cardiac monitoring, and echocardiogram.

Management of a First Seizure

If a patient's seizure is found to be provoked by an acute condition (eg, alcohol withdrawal and electrolyte imbalance), the underlying etiology should be treated and anti-seizure medication is generally not indicated. If a patient is found to have a structural lesion on neuroimaging (eg, tumor, prior stroke, or sequelae of prior head trauma), long-term anti-seizure medication is indicated given the ongoing risk of seizures related to the lesion. If a patient has an unprovoked seizure and no lesion on neuroimaging, the risk of a future seizure is guided by EEG, number of prior seizures, and whether there is a history of neurologic disability. If the EEG is abnormal, more than one seizure has occurred prior to presentation, or there is a history of neurologic disability, the risk of recurrence is considered high enough to recommend long-term anti-seizure medication. If none of these factors is present (ie, normal EEG, no seizures prior to the presenting seizure, and no history of a neurologic condition), a joint decision can be made with the patient regarding the risks and benefits of initiating anti-seizure medication.[2] Of the three factors driving this decision, the one where most diagnostic errors typically occur is the determination of whether a patient indeed had seizures prior to the one that triggered the first presentation. Often, the presenting seizure is a generalized tonic-clonic seizure with striking motor manifestations and loss of consciousness, which is obvious to any witness or health care provider. Prior seizures may be more subtle (eg, recurrent panic episodes falsely attributed to an anxiety disorder, abdominal discomfort falsely attributed to gastroesophageal reflux, or recurrent staring spells with momentary unresponsiveness falsely attributed to attention deficit disorder). Thoroughly probing for any history of recurrent stereotyped spells of any nature is essential before dismissing a seizure as "the first and only."

An important part of a patient's care after a seizure includes educating the patient's family about first aid for seizures. It should be explained that most seizures resolve spontaneously within 3 to 5 minutes; emergency services should therefore be contacted if a seizure lasts longer than 5 minutes, the person has another seizure soon after the first one, or there are obvious signs or risk of seizure-related injury (eg, difficulty breathing, not waking up, or injury during the seizure). If the patient has a generalized tonic-clonic seizure, appropriate first aid includes easing the person to the floor and turning them on their side to avoid aspiration, loosening anything tight the person may have around their neck (eg, tie or scarf), removing eyeglasses, and moving them away from anything with sharp or hard edges to avoid injury. Although patients and their families may have heard that something should be put in the mouth of the patient to avoid tongue biting, this should not be done since objects placed in the mouth can lead to choking (and tongue bites are painful but never deadly).

DIAGNOSIS OF EPILEPSY

Making the Diagnosis

Epilepsy is the condition of recurrent unprovoked seizures. This may be due to a structural lesion (eg, brain tumor, prior stroke, or prior head trauma) or a genetic condition. The diagnosis of epilepsy is based on two or more unprovoked seizures, or a single seizure with a high risk of recurrence based on a structural brain lesion on neuroimaging or epileptic discharges on EEG. Some children may be diagnosed with an epilepsy syndrome based on seizure type(s) and EEG findings. Several common pediatric epilepsy syndromes are listed in Table 17.1.

TABLE 17.1   Most Common Pediatric Epilepsy Syndromes

Syndrome	Onset	Main clinical features	EEG findings	Prognosis
Benign childhood epilepsy with centrotemporal spikes	Onset: 3-13 y	Nocturnal seizures with perioral tingling followed by convulsion. Often positive family history	Bilateral asynchronous high-amplitude, sharp and slow wave complexes involving centro-temporal brain regions	Remission by adolescence
Juvenile myoclonic epilepsy	Onset: 13-15 y	Myoclonic jerks in the morning, generalized tonic-clonic seizures, triggered by sleep deprivation; often photosensitive	3-5.5 Hz generalized spike wave or generalized polyspikes	Typically, well controlled with anti-seizure medication (valproic acid, lamotrigine, levetiracetam, topiramate, zonisamide)
Childhood absence epilepsy	Onset: 4-10 y	Multiple brief (few seconds) staring episodes; sometimes with eye fluttering	Generalized 3 Hz spike and wave complexes	Around 40% develop generalized tonic-clonic seizures; 80% remit by adulthood.

Discussing the Diagnosis With the Patient and Family

Delivering the diagnosis of epilepsy requires explaining the condition, discussing seizure first aid (see preceding text), developing a treatment plan and discussing the importance of adherence with medication to avoid breakthrough seizures, and explaining that with appropriate treatment, patients can live a normal life. Until seizures are controlled, the patient needs to abide by certain safety precautions to avoid seizure-related injuries. These safety precautions include no driving, no swimming unsupervised, no using of sharp or moving objects (eg, lawn mowers), no use of heavy machinery, and no heights (eg, ladders). The duration required for these seizure restrictions varies by state within the United States for driving, but, in general, is in the range of 3 to 6 months starting from the date of the last seizure. It should be emphasized to the patient that these restrictions are usually not permanent, but only until seizures are well controlled for a sustained period with medication. Additional factors that are important to discuss include avoiding potential seizure triggers such as sleep deprivation, alcohol, and drugs.

Epilepsy is associated with a 2- to 3-fold risk of premature mortality and reduced life expectancy compared to the general population. While this increased mortality is multifactorial, most premature deaths are directly related to seizures, including drowning and other seizure-triggered lethal accidents, status epilepticus, and sudden unexpected death in epilepsy (SUDEP). SUDEP affects about 0.1% of people with epilepsy each year, most commonly younger individuals. SUDEP risk is increased in patients with uncontrolled generalized tonic-clonic seizures, in patients who are living alone, in patients who are nonadherent with their medications, and in patients with substance and alcohol use disorders. Patients should be educated about SUDEP, its risk factors, and the importance of anti-seizure medication adherence to reduce its risk.

TREATMENT OF EPILEPSY

The goal of epilepsy treatment is to eliminate seizures with minimal side effects. Even rare seizures carry a risk of SUDEP and other seizure-related injuries and prevent patients from driving, thus limiting independence. An evaluation by a neurologist or an epilepsy subspecialist ensures accurate diagnosis of epilepsy and guidance on optimal treatment.

Medical Therapy

Anti-seizure medications are the cornerstone of epilepsy therapy, controlling seizures in up to 75% of patients with epilepsy. Approximately half of patients with newly diagnosed epilepsy become seizure-free with the first anti-seizure medication, around 15% become seizure-free with the second agent, less than 5% with the third, and 2% with subsequent medication trials.[3] Given the relatively comparable effectiveness of anti-seizure medications, choosing which agent to start in an individual patient depends on the patient's medical comorbidities and current medications, and the anti-seizure medication side effect profile and possible benefits beyond seizure control (Table 17.2). For example, levetiracetam is typically avoided in patients with significant depression and anxiety as it could have significant behavioral side effects, but is favored in patients with complex medical comorbidities on multiple medications as it has minimal drug-drug interactions; topiramate is an excellent choice in patients with comorbid migraines as it can also serve as a migraine prophylactic but should be avoided in women of childbearing age due to an elevated risk of cleft palate; and lamotrigine is the drug of choice in women of childbearing age due to its low teratogenicity risk (see "Epilepsy and Pregnancy" section).

To initiate treatment with an anti-seizure medication, a single medication is started and uptitrated until the seizures are controlled. If side effects occur, a new medication should be trialed and the initial medication should be titrated off rather than stopped abruptly. Since anti-seizure medications reduce the risk of seizures through decreased neuronal excitability, common side effects of anti-seizure medications include fatigue, dizziness, word finding difficulties, and memory changes. Starting the anti-seizure medication at a low dose and increasing it gradually, typically over several weeks, is necessary to allow the brain to adapt and minimize these side effects. Explaining this to patients reassures them that side effects with

TABLE 17.2   Commonly Used Anti-Seizure Medications, Their Most Frequent Side Effects, and Practical Considerations That May Favor Their Selection

Drug	Side effects and other disadvantages	Advantages
Levetiracetam (B)	Irritability and mood lability	No drug-drug interactions. Safer in pregnancy Minimal cognitive side effects Exists in intravenous form, so easy to deliver in case of emergency
Lamotrigine (B)	Rash Slow titration	Safer in pregnancy Mood stabilizer
Oxcarbazepine and car-bamazepine (F)	Hyponatremia Osteoporosis Drug-drug interactions	Rapid titration Mood stabilizer
Topiramate (B)	Weight loss Nephrolithiasis Cognitive slowing Slow titration Cleft palate risk	Weight loss Migraine prophylaxis
Valproic acid (B)	Weight gain Rash Osteoporosis Hirsutism Drug-drug interactions Highest teratogenic risk	Most effective treatment for juvenile myoclonic epilepsy Migraine prophylaxis Mood stabilizer
Lacosamide (B)	Significant dizziness when used with some other seizure medications (sodium channel blockers such as la-motrigine or oxcarbazepine) PR prolongation	Excellent effectiveness when combined with levetiracetam Exists in intravenous form
Phenytoin (B)	Osteoporosis Hepatotoxicity Significant drug-drug interactions Gum hyperplasia	Easy to load intravenously in case of emergency
Zonisamide (B)	Nephrolithiasis Depresses mood	Weight loss Migraine prophylaxis Relatively rapid titration (faster than lamotrigine or topiramate, which are often considered in same clinical scenarios of generalized epilepsy)

B, represents appropriate for both focal and generalized epilepsy; F, is used only in focal epilepsy.

a new medication are expected to be transient and encourages adherence. It should be communicated to patients that an anti-seizure medication does not cure epilepsy but can prevent seizures if taken regularly and therefore requires strict adherence to the prescribed dosing schedule to maintain seizure control.

Psychiatric comorbidities are common in epilepsy, with a significant proportion of patients with epilepsy developing anxiety or depression. Therefore, patients with epilepsy should be screened for anxiety and depression and treated appropriately with counseling and/or medication therapy. Bupropion should be avoided since it can lower the seizure threshold, but other commonly used agents used to treat anxiety and depression are safe in epilepsy. In 2008, the U.S. Food and Drug Administration issued a warning that all anti-seizure medications might increase the risk of suicidal ideation, suicide attempt, and completed suicide. Multiple studies since then have questioned this conclusion. Epilepsy itself increases suicidality risk, as one manifestation of commonly associated mood disorders. It is therefore imperative to screen for suicidality in patients with chronic epilepsy, and to avoid using anti-seizure medications that could trigger or worsen anxiety and depression (eg, levetiracetam, topiramate, and zonisamide) in patients with an active mood disorder or at risk for one.

Surgical Therapy

Up to 30% of patients have drug-resistant epilepsy, which is defined as a failure of adequate trials of two medications (as monotherapy or in combination) to achieve seizure freedom. To be characterized as drug-resistant epilepsy, the two medications must have been well tolerated, appropriately dosed, and appropriately chosen for the patient's seizure type(s). This definition reflects the data cited earlier regarding the low probability of seizure freedom after failure of two medications, and the high risk of mortality (eg, SUDEP) in this population.

Patients with drug-resistant epilepsy should be referred to a comprehensive epilepsy center to confirm the diagnosis and for consideration of epilepsy surgery.[4] Patients with focal epilepsy are the best candidates for resection or ablation of a clearly delineated epileptic focus. Resective surgery achieves long-term (>9 years) seizure freedom in more than half of cases, with 1-year (or longer) remission periods observed in more than 90% of cases, and a mean reduction of seizure frequency by more than 75%.[5] These results underscore the importance of referring patients with drug-resistant epilepsy for consideration of surgery as early as possible.

Epilepsy that is not clearly localized to a specific brain region may benefit from nonresective, nonablative procedures that use neuromodulation, such as vagus nerve stimulation, deep brain stimulation, or responsive neurostimulation, all modalities that rely on modulating the brain's epileptic networks, analogous to a sort of "pacemaker" for the brain. Nine-year outcomes following responsive neurostimulation showed a mean seizure-frequency reduction of 75% and 1 year (or greater) seizure freedom in 18% of cases, making it an excellent option in patients who do not qualify for the resective or ablative approach.[6] Overall life expectancy, quality of life, and mood improve after surgery. Individualized outcome prediction tools regarding epilepsy surgery are now available at www.riskcalc.org Evaluating patients for epilepsy surgery requires detailed testing in specialized epilepsy programs (locations available on the Epilepsy Foundation and National Association of Epilepsy Centers' websites listed in Table 17.4).

STATUS EPILEPTICUS

Status epilepticus is defined as more than 5 minutes of continuous seizure activity or two or more sequential seizures without full recovery of consciousness between seizures.[7] Status epilepticus is a medical and neurologic emergency requiring monitoring and stabilization of the ABCs, rapid initiation of anti-seizure medication, and determination and treatment of the underlying etiology with finger-stick blood glucose, laboratory testing (electrolytes, toxicology screening; anti-seizure medication levels in patients on anti-seizure medications), and neuroimaging. First-line treatment for status epilepticus is a benzodiazepine (intravenous [IV] lorazepam or diazepam; or intramuscular [IM] midazolam). If seizures persist after 10 minutes, an IV anti-seizure medication should be administered (fosphenytoin, valproic acid, and levetiracetam are the best studied). If seizures persist after effective loading of IV seizure medication, pharmacologically induced coma (pentobarbital or propofol) and intubation and mechanical ventilation should be pursued. If the patient does not awaken and it is unclear whether the patient is still seizing, continuous EEG monitoring should be initiated to guide treatment. Treatment of status epilepticus is well summarized in a pocket card recently published by Fesler et al.[8] Common etiologies of status epilepticus include fever and infection in children, and stroke, infectious or autoimmune encephalitis, and alcohol withdrawal or intoxication in adults. Nonadherance to seizure medications is a common trigger status epilepticus both in adults and children.

EPILEPSY IN WOMEN

The interaction between seizures and the hormonal milieu in women is complex and affects women with epilepsy throughout their lifetime. Certain epilepsies tend to worsen around the menstrual cycle (called *catamenial epilepsy*). A detailed cataloging of the timing of breakthrough seizures relative to the timing of the menstrual cycle should be maintained by the patient, and patterns could offer opportunities for a predictable "just-in-time" use of benzodiazepines. Standard longitudinal anti-seizure medication therapy still needs to be maintained but could be augmented with acetazolamide or hormonal therapy.

Oral contraceptives can be affected by anti-seizure medications. Hepatic enzyme-inducing anti-seizure medications increase the metabolism of both estrogen and progesterone and reduce the effectiveness of oral contraceptive pills. Women with epilepsy taking strongly enzyme-inducing anti-seizure medications (eg, carbamazepine, oxcarbazepine, phenobarbital, phenytoin, and primidone) need to be warned about this interaction and encouraged to seek other methods of contraception (eg, barrier methods and intrauterine device [IUD]). Weak enzyme inducers such as eslicarbazepine, felbamate, lamotrigine, perampanel, rufinamide, and topiramate may also reduce the effectiveness of contraceptive agents when used at high doses.

Epilepsy and Pregnancy

More than 95% of pregnancies in women with epilepsy result in a healthy baby. Women with epilepsy should not be dissuaded from pregnancy and breast feeding; however, pregnancy should ideally be planned to coordinate any necessary medication changes.

First, seizures must be controlled for at least 6 months on a stable medication regimen before pregnancy is attempted. This will optimize the odds of epilepsy stability prior to introducing the variable of pregnancy.

Second, folic acid (1-2 mg/day) should be started simultaneously with initiation of any anti-seizure medication in a woman of childbearing age to reduce the risk of neural tube defects in case of future pregnancy.

Third, one should strive to achieve seizure control with the lowest number of anti-seizure medications, and preferably anti-seizure medications with the lowest teratogenic potential, if possible (Table 17.3).[9] Levetiracetam and lamotrigine have the lowest teratogenic potential, but lamotrigine has a more favorable mood profile, which is important to consider in pregnancy and during the postpartum period. If the patient is not on these medications and has not tried them previously, cross-titration prior to conception should be considered. However, if the patient's seizures only respond to other agents that have higher teratogenic potential, seizure control should be prioritized as maternal seizures carry high risk for both the mother and fetus. Once the most effective anti-seizure medication regimen is defined, it should be maintained throughout pregnancy to ensure ongoing seizure control and prevent seizure-related injuries in the mother and baby.

Fourth, concentrations of some anti-seizure medications, particularly levetiracetam, lamotrigine, and oxcarbazepine, can decrease during pregnancy due to an increase in the volume of distribution, as well as changes in hepatic metabolism, renal clearance, and protein binding. Blood levels of these

TABLE 17.3	Rates of Major Congenital Malformations With Commonly Prescribed Anti-Seizure Medications[9]	
Anti-seizure medication	Rate of MCM (%)	Notes
Valproic acid	6.7-10.3	Risk of MCM is dose dependent: 5% at <600 mg/d, increasing to 10.4% if >1,000 mg/d
Phenytoin	2.9-6.4	
Topiramate	3.9-4.8	
Carbamazepine	2.6-5.5	
Oxcarbazepine	2.2-3	
Lamotrigine	1.9-2.9	Risk of MCM is dose dependent: 2.5% at ≤325 mg/d, increasing to 4.3% if >325 mg/d
Levetiracetam	0.7-2.8	

MCM, major congenital malformations.

Reprinted from Tomson T, Battino D, Bonizzoni E, et al. Comparative risk of major congenital malformations with eight different antiepileptic drugs: a prospective cohort study of the EURAP registry. *Lancet Neurol.* 2018;17:530-538, with permission from Elsevier.

TABLE 17.4	**Useful Resources**
https://www.cdc.gov/epilepsy/index.html	Centers for Disease Control and Prevention site with excellent information about seizure first aid, and information about Managing Epilepsy Well (MEW) Network self-management programs
https://www.epilepsy.com/	Epilepsy Foundation site addressing frequently asked questions about the basics of epilepsy, tools to track seizures, and other patient-targeted resources. In addition, it includes resources for health care providers (seizure first aid training and certification, and medication resources) and driving restriction laws by state
https://www.aan.com/tools-and-resources/	American Academy of Neurology educational material and resources tailored to health care audiences of various levels of expertise
https://www.naec-epilepsy.org/for-patients/patient-resources/	National Association of Epilepsy Centers site providing a nice compilation of patient resources, including links to consumer, governmental, health professional, and advocacy organizations working to improve care for and advocate for people with epilepsy and their caregivers

anti-seizure medications should be monitored regularly (monthly) during pregnancy. The dose of the medication is often increased during pregnancy to maintain the target blood level, usually defined as the blood level maintained during the period of stable seizure control before pregnancy. The medication dose needs to be reduced back to its prepregnancy level within the first week of delivery to avoid postpartum toxicity. Breastfeeding should be encouraged; sedating effects on the infant may occur with barbiturates, but other agents are considered to have minimal effect.

SUMMARY

Epilepsy is a chronic disease with significant risks and complications, but pharmacologic (and, in some cases, surgical) therapy can be lifesaving and improve quality of life substantially. Patients with epilepsy should ideally be evaluated thoroughly by a neurologist or an epilepsy subspecialist to ensure accurate diagnosis and optimal treatment. Table 17.4 summarizes resources that may be useful to patients, their caregivers, and treating physicians.

EDITORS' KEY POINTS

▶ Seizures are transient neurologic symptoms/signs caused by abnormal electrical activity in the cerebral cortex, and can be classified as focal (causing focal symptoms/signs, eg, unilateral shaking movements) or generalized (causing

bilateral manifestations and altered level of consciousness).

▶ Seizure must be distinguished from syncope and PNES. Prolonged tonic-clonic movements, bowel/bladder incontinence, lateral tongue bite, bodily injury, and postictal confusion are all suggestive of epileptic seizure but distinguishing these on history alone can be challenging.

▶ Seizures may be provoked by an acute reversible etiology (eg, by metabolic disturbances, fever, medications, or drug/alcohol intoxication or withdrawal) or unprovoked due to a fixed structural lesion (eg, prior stroke, prior trauma, prior neurosurgery, brain tumor, arteriovenous malformation) or genetic epilepsy syndrome. Therefore, the initial evaluation of an adult with a first seizure should include a comprehensive metabolic panel, blood glucose, toxicology screen, and neuroimaging to evaluate for a provoking cause or structural lesion.

▶ If a patient has a first unprovoked seizure, normal neurologic examination, normal neuroimaging, and normal EEG, a joint decision can be made with the patient about whether to initiate an anti-seizure medication. If a patient has more than one unprovoked seizure, an abnormal neurologic examination, abnormal neuroimaging, or an abnormal EEG, treatment with an anti-seizure medication is recommended.

▶ Patients with seizures should be counseled on safety: no driving until seizures are under complete control for several months (number of months varies by state law), no activities where seizure could lead to injury or death (eg, swimming alone and working at heights).

▶ Anti-seizure medication should be chosen based on side effect profile and patient medical history. A single agent should be chosen and its dosage increased slowly before adding a second agent if there is inadequate seizure control with the first agent.

▶ If a patient does not respond to adequate trials of two anti-seizure medications (alone or in combination), the patient should be referred to a comprehensive epilepsy center for evaluation of surgical treatment options.

▶ Status epilepticus is defined as more than 5 minutes of continuous seizure activity or two or more sequential seizures without full recovery of consciousness between seizures. First-line treatment is benzodiazepines; second-line treatment (if status epilepticus is not controlled by benzodiazepines) is an IV loading dose of an anti-seizure medication; third-line treatment for status epilepticus refractory to benzodiazepines and anti-seizure medications is induced coma.

▶ The safest anti-seizure medications in pregnancy are lamotrigine and levetiracetam. Drug levels must be monitored carefully and medications titrated accordingly during the course of pregnancy and the postpartum period.

REFERENCES

1. Hakami T, McIntosh A, Todaro M, et al. MRI-identified pathology in adults with new-onset seizures. *Neurology*. 2013;81(10):920-927.
2. Marson A, Jacoby A, Johnson A, et al. Immediate versus deferred antiepileptic drug treatment for early epilepsy and single seizures: a randomised controlled trial. *Lancet*. 2005; 365(9476):2007-2013.
3. Kwan P, Brodie MJ. Early identification of refractory epilepsy. *N Engl J Med*. 2000;342(5):314-319.
4. Jehi L, Jette N, Kwon CS, et al. Timing of referral to evaluate for epilepsy surgery: expert consensus recommendations from the surgical therapies commission of the international league against epilepsy. *Epilepsia*. 2022;64(10):2491-2506.
5. Hsieh JK, Pucci FG, Sundar SJ, et al. Beyond seizure freedom: dissecting long-term seizure control after surgical resection for drug-resistant epilepsy. *Epilepsia*. 2023;64(1):103-113.
6. Nair DR, Laxer KD, Weber PB, et al. RNS System LTT Study. Nine-year prospective efficacy and safety of brain-responsive neurostimulation for focal epilepsy. *Neurology*. 2020;95(9):e1244-e1256.
7. Glauser TA. Designing practical evidence-based treatment plans for children with prolonged seizures and status epilepticus. *J Child Neurol*. 2007;22(suppl 5):38S-46S.
8. Fesler JR, Belcher AE, Moosa AN, et al. The efficacy and use of a pocket card algorithm in status epilepticus treatment. *Neurol Clin Pract*. 2021;11(5):406-412.
9. Tomson T, Battino D, Bonizzoni E, et al. Comparative risk of major congenital malformations with eight different antiepileptic drugs: a prospective cohort study of the EURAP registry. *Lancet Neurol*. 2018;17(5):530-538.

Dementia

Vijay K. Ramanan

INTRODUCTION

Cognitive impairment indicates the presence of decreased mental function compared to expectations for age and educational background. Cognitive impairment exists along a continuum, with mild cognitive impairment (MCI) referring to cognitive changes not severe enough to impact activities of daily living (ADLs) and dementia referring to progressive changes severe enough to affect ADLs. Both MCI and dementia can have a variety of underlying etiologies (Table 18.1). Annually, approximately 10% to 15% of patients diagnosed clinically with MCI will progress to dementia, highlighting the importance of identifying the cause of an individual's cognitive syndrome to guide management and prognosis.

Progressive neurodegenerative diseases such as Alzheimer disease (AD), dementia with Lewy bodies (DLB), and frontotemporal dementia represent common etiologies for progressive dementia syndromes. Neurodegenerative dementias are characterized by particular cognitive deficits associated with particular patterns of neuropathology (which have associated laboratory and neuroimaging findings), but there is wide clinical and pathologic heterogeneity across patients with these diagnoses.

This chapter discusses the diagnosis and treatment of common neurodegenerative diseases and other neurologic conditions that can cause dementia (vascular dementia, normal pressure hydrocephalus [NPH], chronic traumatic encephalopathy, and Creutzfeldt-Jakob disease [CJD]).

DIFFERENTIAL DIAGNOSIS AND BASIC EVALUATION FOR MILD COGNITIVE IMPAIRMENT/DEMENTIA

A priority in the evaluation of cognitive impairment involves assessment and treatment of potentially reversible causes. Examples include hypothyroidism, vitamin B_{12} deficiency (with neurologic symptoms, a vitamin B_{12} level of less than 400 warrants supplementation), sleep disorders, primary psychiatric disease (eg, depression and anxiety), structural intracranial lesions (eg, neoplasm and subdural hematoma), and polypharmacy with medications affecting the central nervous system (see Chapter 5). However, factors warranting treatment should not necessarily preclude additional investigations or follow-up to evaluate for an underlying neurodegenerative disease.

TABLE 18.1 Causes of Dementia

Psychiatric
Depression
Anxiety
Attention deficit disorder
Bipolar disorder
Schizophrenia

Endocrine/metabolic
Vitamin B_{12} deficiency
Thiamine deficiency
Hypothyroidism
Hepatic encephalopathy and other metabolic encephalopathies

Toxic
Side effects/polypharmacy with central nervous system active
   medications
Chronic pain
Sleep disorders (eg, chronic insomnia and obstructive sleep apnea)

Infectious
HIV-associated cognitive impairment
Neurosyphilis

Neurodegenerative
Alzheimer disease
Dementia with Lewy bodies
Frontotemporal degenerative diseases
Creutzfeldt-Jakob disease

Structural
Neoplasm
Normal pressure hydrocephalus

Cerebrovascular
Large territory ischemic stroke
Focal/strategically placed ischemic stroke
Intracerebral hemorrhage
Vascular dementia

Immune Mediated
Autoimmune encephalitis
Paraneoplastic encephalitis

Other
Adult-onset leukodystrophies

ALZHEIMER DISEASE

Background

AD is the most common neurodegenerative cause of dementia, affecting approximately 10% of the population older than 65 years in the United States. Pathologically, AD is characterized by the accumulation of extracellular plaques composed of amyloid-β (a breakdown product from a larger protein known as amyloid precursor protein) and intracellular neurofibrillary tangles made up of tau (a protein that stabilizes components of neurons) that has been hyperphosphorylated (p-tau). Most cases of AD are sporadic, thought to be caused by a combination of genetic predisposition (the ε4 variant of the *APOE* gene imparts the greatest known risk, although it does not solely cause the disease), lifestyle (eg, hypertension and diabetes), and environmental factors, all of which are areas of active study. Rarely (<1%-2% of cases), AD can be familial, caused by single-gene mutations in genes such as *PSEN1*, *PSEN2*, and *APP*, or through chromosomal duplications including these genes (eg, trisomy 21 for *APP*).

Clinical Features

AD most commonly presents after age 70, with slowly progressive cognitive decline predominantly affecting short-term memory as the earliest symptom. Patients or their caregivers may note repetitive questions or stories, forgetting recent events, misplacing objects, or duplicating meals or medication doses. As the disease progresses, other cognitive domains become involved, including visuospatial dysfunction (which may lead to getting lost in familiar environments), executive dysfunction (which may lead to difficulties with multitasking or utilizing appliances or devices), and language dysfunction (which may lead to word finding or comprehension difficulties).

Rarely, patients may present at a younger age (called *early-onset AD*, typically defined by symptom onset before 60-65 years of age). Such patients may not have early memory deficits, but rather other syndromes including dysexecutive AD (causing difficulties with multitasking, organization, sequencing, or device usage); behavioral variant AD (causing personality changes such as disinhibition, apathy, dietary changes, or compulsivity); a language variant known as logopenic primary progressive aphasia (causing naming and word finding difficulties and impaired sentence repetition with other cognitive functions relatively preserved); a visual variant known as posterior cortical atrophy due to atrophy of posterior regions in the occipital lobe involved in vision (causing difficulties with reading, judging distances, and recognizing objects within a field of view); or a motor variant known as corticobasal syndrome (causing unilateral or asymmetric movement disorders such as limb apraxia, dystonia, parkinsonism, myoclonus; cortical sensory loss; and/or oculomotor abnormalities).

The course of AD is typically slowly but inexorably progressive, usually leading to complete dependence within 6 to 8 years of diagnosis. However, symptoms and trajectories vary between patients.

Diagnostic Testing

Structural brain imaging (computed tomography [CT] or magnetic resonance imaging [MRI]) in AD often reveals atrophy that preferentially affects the parietal and medial temporal regions (Figure 18.1). Nuclear imaging studies such as positron emission tomography (PET) and single-photon emission computed

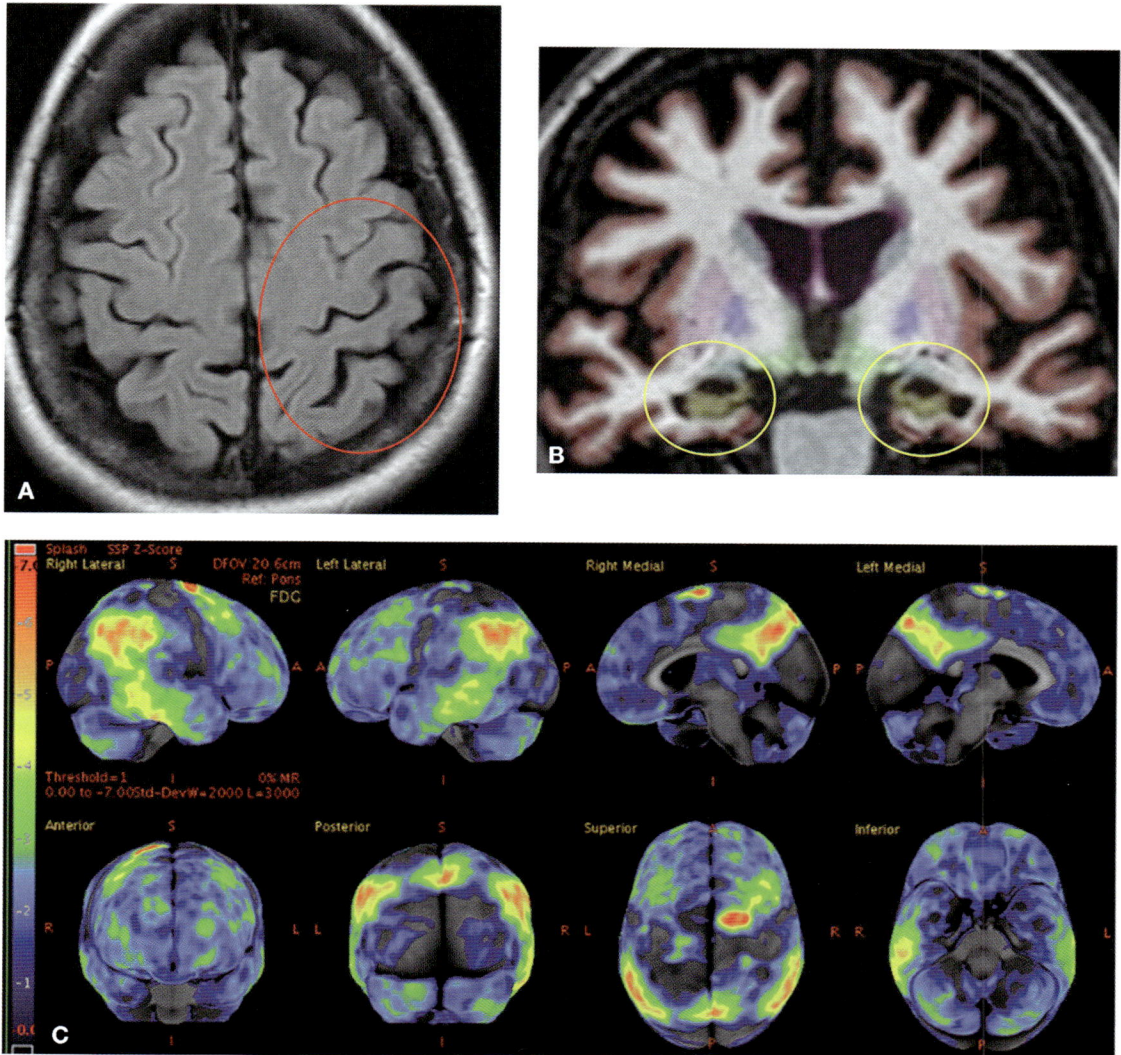

FIGURE 18.1 Neuroimaging in Alzheimer disease. A. Axial fluid-attenuated inversion recovery (FLAIR) magnetic resonance imaging (MRI) demonstrating left parietal atrophy (red circle). B. Coronal MRI demonstrating diffuse atrophy including bilateral hippocampi (yellow circles). C. FDG-PET images showing parietotemporal-frontal hypometabolism; hypometabolism ranging from blue (lowest degree of hypometabolism) to red (highest degree of hypometabolism) on the appended scale.

tomography (SPECT) show hypometabolism in temporoparietal regions, which may be present before atrophy becomes apparent on CT/MRI (Figure 18.1). PET tracers that detect amyloid-β and p-tau are used mostly in specialized centers for research and in challenging clinical cases but may soon come into wider use to ensure precise diagnosis in patients who may qualify for emerging disease-modifying treatments.

Cerebrospinal fluid (CSF) measurement of amyloid-β and p-tau can aid in diagnosis. In AD, CSF amyloid-β levels are low (thought to reflect increased brain parenchymal amyloid deposition) and CSF p-tau levels are high (thought to reflect neurofibrillary tangle pathology). As CSF protein concentrations can be influenced by several factors (eg, collection conditions and coexistent disorders of CSF dynamics), ratios of these protein biomarkers generally have greater specificity than absolute levels (eg, p-tau/amyloid-$β_{42}$). Blood-based biomarkers may soon be available for the purposes of early screening and treatment monitoring.

Treatment

Treatment of AD can be divided into symptomatic and disease-modifying therapy. Symptomatic medications that provide a modest benefit on cognitive functioning include cholinesterase inhibitors (donepezil, rivastigmine, and galantamine) and the *N*-methyl D-aspartate (NMDA) receptor antagonist memantine. In most cases of AD, treatment with these medications is not expected to manifest as an observable improvement in cognitive function. A cholinesterase inhibitor is generally initiated in mild symptomatic stages (ie, MCI or mild dementia due to AD), and memantine is added in moderate to severe AD. Cholinesterase inhibitors can cause bradycardia and should therefore be avoided in patients with preexisting bradycardia or heart block. Oral cholinesterase inhibitors (eg, donepezil and galantamine) can also cause gastrointestinal side effects (eg, nausea/vomiting and diarrhea) that may be mitigated by taking the medication with food or switching to transdermal formulations (ie, rivastigmine patch). Morning dosing of cholinesterase inhibitors is favored to avoid sleep-related side effects (eg, vivid dreams). Memantine has a very favorable side effect profile, although symptoms such as dizziness and headache have been reported. If these medications are tolerated, not contraindicated, and not cumbersome to administer, they should be utilized. If side effects occur or pill burden reduction is needed, these medications can be discontinued, given that they provide only modest benefit.

Other symptoms that should be screened for and treated in patients with AD include mood symptoms and psychosis. Medications that may contribute to cognitive dysfunction should be discontinued if feasible (eg, benzodiazepines, anticholinergic medications, and narcotic pain medications).

Emerging disease-modifying medications for biomarker-confirmed AD use monoclonal antibody infusions targeting the removal of amyloid-β plaques from the brain (eg, lecanemab and donanemab). Preliminary evidence suggests that these agents may slow progression of cognitive decline in some cases of biomarker-confirmed MCI or mild dementia due to AD but carry the risk of cerebral edema and/or bleeding (known as amyloid-related imaging abnormalities [ARIA]) that requires careful patient selection and frequent MRI monitoring. These risks and the significant financial and logistical costs to patients and health systems are current barriers to more widespread use of these medications.

DEMENTIA WITH LEWY BODIES
Background

DLB is the second most common neurodegenerative cause of dementia, affecting over 1 million people in the United States. DLB is characterized by the accumulation of Lewy bodies (which contain α-synuclein protein) in cortical and subcortical neurons. Of note, similar Lewy body inclusions containing α-synuclein are found in a smaller subset of brain regions in Parkinson disease; current frameworks posit that DLB and Parkinson disease exist on a continuum, with the time of onset of cognitive versus motor symptoms distinguishing between these clinical diagnoses (cognitive symptoms concurrent with or preceding motor symptoms in DLB; motor symptoms preceding cognitive symptoms in Parkinson disease).

Clinical Features

Most individuals with DLB have onset of cognitive symptoms around 65 to 70 years of age. Core clinical features include cognitive impairment, prominent fluctuations in attention/alertness, well-formed visual hallucinations, parkinsonism, and rapid eye movement (REM) sleep behavior disorder.

Cognitive dysfunction at onset is characterized by inattention (eg, focus/concentration difficulties), executive dysfunction (eg, difficulties with multitasking or appliance/device usage), and visuospatial deficits (eg, bumping into corners). Fluctuations can manifest as periods of pronounced confusion or abrupt episodes of deep somnolence, at times lasting many hours prior to recovery. Visual hallucinations in DLB are typically recurrent, well formed (eg, of people or animals being in the room), and not frightening. Parkinsonism includes features of bradykinesia, tremor, and/or rigidity (see Chapter 19), and can, at times, be more bilateral or subtle as compared to idiopathic Parkinson disease. Tremor may be predominantly postural as opposed to the resting tremor of Parkinson disease. REM sleep behavior disorder is characterized by dream enactment behavior, which may manifest as running, fighting, or loud screaming during sleep; this may precede the other neurologic symptoms by years or even decades (see Chapter 30).

Other symptoms suggestive of DLB include motor symptoms (eg, postural instability/falls), neuropsychiatric symptoms (eg, presence hallucinations [the feeling that someone is nearby], systematized delusions [false beliefs organized into a coherent theme, such as that of being surveilled]), sleep-related symptoms (eg, daytime hypersomnia and spells of unresponsiveness), autonomic symptoms (eg, orthostatic hypotension, constipation, and erectile dysfunction), and medication-related symptoms (eg, severe sensitivity to neuroleptic medications such as haloperidol).

Diagnostic Testing

Structural brain imaging (CT or MRI) in patients with DLB usually does not show any specific pattern of atrophy; neuroimaging may be normal or show a nonspecific pattern of global atrophy. Nuclear imaging in DLB typically shows hypometabolism on PET imaging and hypoperfusion on SPECT imaging in the occipital, temporal, and parietal cortices (Figure 18.2). Dopamine transporter SPECT in DLB demonstrates reduced dopamine transporter uptake in the basal ganglia. However, this pattern is not specific to this diagnosis and can be seen in other parkinsonian conditions (eg, Parkinson disease, multiple system atrophy; see Chapter 19). Direct detection of α-synuclein in the CSF or skin is being used in research settings and may be available to clinicians in the future.

Treatment

The same cholinesterase inhibitors (donepezil, galantamine, and rivastigmine) used for symptomatic treatment of AD have been shown to be beneficial in DLB,

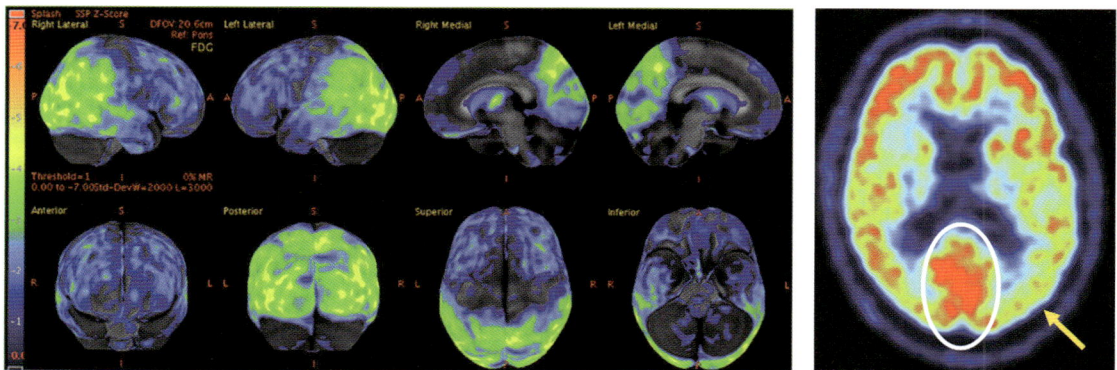

FIGURE 18.2 Neuroimaging in dementia with Lewy bodies. Left panel: FDG PET demonstrating hypometabolism relative to age-matched controls in the occipital, posterior parietal, and inferior temporal regions. Right panel: FDG PET demonstrating preservation of metabolism in the posterior cingulate cortex (white circle) relative to the adjacent precuneus(orange arrow), known as the posterior cingulate island sign and present in patients with dementia with Lewy bodies but not in patients with Alzheimer disease.

particularly in reducing hallucinations and delusions. Some providers have noted a greater impact on cognitive symptoms in patients with DLB compared to patients with AD. REM sleep behavior disorder can be treated with melatonin or clonazepam at bedtime. Psychosis can be treated with quetiapine, olanzapine, or pimavanserin; typical antipsychotics (eg, haloperidol) should be avoided due to the risk of worsening parkinsonian symptoms. Patients should be counseled that antipsychotic medications have been associated with an increased risk of all-cause mortality, a risk that must be balanced with potential symptomatic benefits in individual patients. Depression and anxiety are common and should be screened for and treated. There are currently no disease-modifying treatments available for DLB, but research is ongoing.

FRONTOTEMPORAL DEGENERATIVE DISEASES

Background

Frontotemporal degenerative diseases represent the third most common neurodegenerative cause of dementia overall but are nearly as common as AD in individuals younger than age 65. Common syndromes of frontotemporal degenerative diseases include behavioral variant frontotemporal dementia and several variants of primary progressive aphasia. Pathologically, these conditions are most commonly associated with the accumulation of p-tau (in a different form than seen in AD) or TDP-43 (transactive response DNA-binding protein 43; a protein involved in RNA processing). Similar pathologic findings can be seen in progressive supranuclear palsy and corticobasal syndrome (see Chapter 19). In comparison to AD, a relatively higher proportion (up to 10%-20%) of sporadic cases of frontotemporal degenerative diseases are found to be due to a genetic mutation.

Clinical Features

Most cases of frontotemporal degenerative disease have an onset between 50 and 60 years of age. In behavioral variant frontotemporal dementia, the main symptoms include changes in behavior and personality, including compulsivity, apathy, reduced empathy, disinhibition,

and dietary changes. Patients with behavioral variant frontotemporal dementia may be observed to make inappropriate comments, develop cravings for sweets, engage in repetitive activities (eg, cleaning), or display insensitivity to others' feelings.

Primary progressive aphasia refers to a group of neurodegenerative disease syndromes that predominantly affect language function. Two variants (semantic and nonfluent/agrammatic variants) of this condition are associated with frontotemporal degenerative disease pathology and one (logopenic variant) with AD pathology. Semantic variant primary progressive aphasia (also known as semantic dementia) presents with profound object naming and word meaning deficits, which may manifest with difficulty understanding single words (eg, difficulty retrieving a utensil on command despite being able to utilize it). Nonfluent/agrammatic aphasia is characterized by effortful and halting speech and/or loss of grammar, which may manifest as reduced spontaneous verbal output, loss of sentence connectors (eg, "the"), yes/no reversals, or improper order of words within phrases or sentences.

Diagnostic Testing

Structural neuroimaging (CT or MRI) in frontotemporal degenerative diseases typically demonstrates frontal and/or temporal atrophy and nuclear imaging demonstrates hypometabolism in frontotemporal regions (Figure 18.3). In some cases, amnestic-predominant clinical syndromes resembling AD can have frontal and/or temporal-predominant neuroimaging changes; in these cases, CSF biomarker testing can assess for evidence of AD in order to precisely target symptomatic and disease-modifying treatments. In primary progressive aphasia, detailed language evaluation by a speech-language pathologist can characterize the language disorder more precisely in order to determine the most likely etiologic diagnosis and tailor speech therapy.

Treatment

Unlike AD and DLB, cholinesterase inhibitors are not indicated in frontotemporal dementia. Mood stabilizers such as selective serotonin reuptake

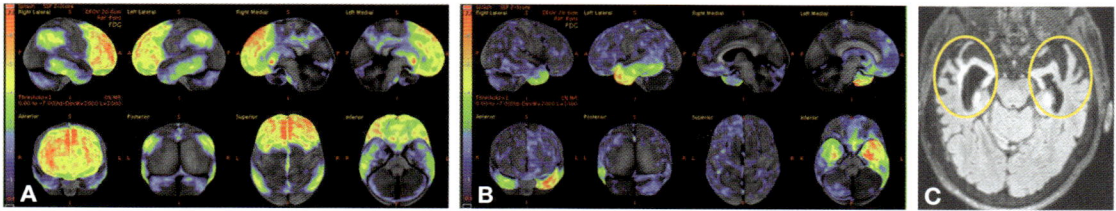

FIGURE 18.3 Neuroimaging in frontotemporal degenerative disease. A and B. FDG-PET demonstrating hypometabolism (indicated by colors spanning light blue to red on the appended scale) of frontal and temporal regions. Hypometabolism ranging from blue (lowest degree of hypometabolism) to red (highest degree of hypometabolism) on the appended scale. C. Axial fluid-attenuated inversion recovery (FLAIR) magnetic resonance imaging (MRI) demonstrating bilateral frontal and temporal atrophy (yellow circles).

inhibitors, lamotrigine, and valproate can be considered for symptomatic treatment of agitation, disinhibition, and behavioral dysregulation.

VASCULAR DEMENTIA

Cerebrovascular disease can cause cognitive dysfunction through a variety of mechanisms, such as a large or strategically placed ischemic stroke or intracerebral hemorrhage, multiple strokes over time, or chronic development of subcortical microvascular disease. The former two etiologies may present with a stepwise decline in cognition, whereas the latter typically presents as a more insidious development of cognitive impairment particularly affecting executive dysfunction and processing speed. Neuroimaging demonstrates diffuse bilateral T2 hyperintensities on MRI or hypodensities on CT in the periventricular and deep subcortical white matter representing chronic small vessel ischemic changes; superimposed areas of encephalomalacia denoting prior infarcts may also be seen. Chronic small vessel ischemic changes are commonly observed in older individuals, however, so these should not be assumed to account for cognitive symptomatology without a thorough evaluation for alternative etiologies.

In the absence of concomitant AD pathology, the likelihood of benefit from cholinesterase inhibitor or memantine therapy in vascular dementia is considered low. However, given the high frequency of dual pathology and generally favorable drug side effect profiles, it is reasonable to consider initiating these medications in the setting of progressive cognitive decline presumed due to cerebrovascular disease.

NORMAL PRESSURE HYDROCEPHALUS

NPH is a condition in which ventricular enlargement causes gait dysfunction, urinary urgency or incontinence, and/or cognitive impairment. Patients with this condition who develop cognitive symptoms often have a preceding gait disorder and/or urinary symptoms before developing cognitive changes. The cerebral ventricles can enlarge asymptomatically with age, so the diagnosis of NPH should only be considered when specific radiologic signs are present (eg, decreased callosal angle, enlarged Sylvian fissures, crowding of gyri at the cerebral convexity) in the appropriate clinical scenario. Gait improvement over the hours to days following large-volume lumbar puncture (removal of 30-40 mL of CSF) predicts a positive response to ventriculoperitoneal shunt placement. Shunt placement often improves gait dysfunction more than cognition.

CHRONIC TRAUMATIC ENCEPHALOPATHY

Dementia can result from repetitive concussive and subconcussive head injuries accumulated through high-level contact sports or repetitive blast exposure. Neuroimaging may show sequelae of prior injury (eg, gliosis or encephalomalacia in an area of prior significant trauma; cavum septum pellucidum [anterior-posterior division of the septum separating the lateral ventricles at the midline]) or may be normal. Diagnosis is confirmed at autopsy, based on pathologic findings of aggregated p-tau distributed irregularly around small blood vessels at the depths of cortical sulci. There are no specific in vivo biomarkers of chronic traumatic encephalopathy, although research is ongoing. Treatment is symptomatic, often targeted to pharmacologic (eg, selective serotonin reuptake inhibitors) and lifestyle therapies for mood and behavioral changes.

CREUTZFELDT-JAKOB DISEASE

CJD is a rare disorder caused by prion accumulation in the brain that can occur sporadically, as an inherited condition, or rarely due to contaminated surgical instruments, transplanted organs, or consumption of infected animal products. Prion proteins are found naturally in the brain and are typically harmless. In CJD, misfolded prion proteins trigger other prion proteins to misfold, ultimately leading to the death of neurons and spread of misfolded protein to other cells. Unlike most neurodegenerative dementias, CJD presents as a rapidly progressive dementia evolving over months and fatal within 1 to 2 years. Dementia in this condition is often accompanied by myoclonus (rapid, lightening-like jerks most commonly seen in the limbs), although this finding is not universally present and has a broad differential diagnosis (see Chapter 13). MRI demonstrates diffusion restriction in the cortex and deep gray matter on diffusion-weighted imaging (DWI)/apparent diffusion coefficient (ADC) sequences, and the diagnosis is confirmed by CSF real-time quaking-induced conversion (RT-QuIC), which detects the abnormal form of prion protein in the nervous system. The disease is irreversible and incurable. Other causes of rapidly progressive dementia to consider in the differential diagnosis of CJD include autoimmune encephalitis (primary or paraneoplastic), toxic/metabolic disorders, central nervous system (CNS) malignancy, and atypically rapid presentations of neurodegenerative diseases.

COUNSELING AND SUPPORTIVE CARE FOR PATIENTS WITH DEMENTIA

Dementia of any cause is a life-altering diagnosis for patients and their family members. Counseling should involve pharmacologic and nonpharmacologic management options, prognosis, advance directive and end-of-life planning, and safety. Strategies to promote brain health should be encouraged, including consistent physical, social, and mental engagement.

Multidisciplinary teams, including social workers, support groups, and other community-based resources can help optimize day-to-day quality of life. Patients or their family members commonly ask about driving, and if the ability to drive (or lack thereof) is not clear clinically, patients should undergo a formal driving safety evaluation.

SUMMARY

Neurodegenerative diseases such as AD represent common causes of MCI/dementia, particularly in older individuals. Recognition of typical clinical syndromes and diagnostic test findings associated with these disorders can help achieve accurate diagnoses, which will be particularly important as disease-modifying treatment options emerge. In all patients presenting with cognitive impairment, a thorough evaluation for reversible causes should be performed (see Chapter 5).

EDITORS' KEY POINTS

▶ MCI refers to cognitive changes not severe enough to impact ADLs, whereas dementia refers to progressive changes severe enough to affect ADLs. MCI carries a 10% to 15% annual risk of progression to dementia.

▶ Evaluation of patients with dementia includes brain MRI, laboratory tests to evaluate for reversible causes of cognitive decline (vitamin B_{12} level, thyroid-stimulating hormone (TSH), HIV, and RPR), and, in some patients, lumbar puncture or nuclear imaging tests (eg, PET).

▶ AD most commonly presents with slowly progressive cognitive decline, initially affecting short-term memory and progressing to affect other cognitive domains. Most patients present after age 70, although patients may rarely present at a younger age. Treatment includes supportive care and symptomatic therapies (eg, cholinesterase inhibitor or NMDA receptor antagonist) that may provide a modest benefit on cognitive functioning; emerging potential disease-modifying medications for biomarker-confirmed AD are monoclonal antibodies targeting the removal of amyloid-β plaques require careful monitoring due to the risk of cerebral edema and bleeding.

- DLB is characterized by cognitive decline, fluctuations in attention/alertness, well-formed visual hallucinations, and parkinsonism. Treatment includes supportive care and symptomatic treatment with cholinesterase inhibitors.
- Vascular dementia refers to cognitive dysfunction due to cerebrovascular disease, including large or strategically placed ischemic stroke or intracerebral hemorrhage, multiple strokes over time, or chronic development of subcortical microvascular disease. Patients typically present with insidious development of cognitive impairment primarily affecting executive dysfunction and processing speed but can also present with stepwise decline in cognition due to accumulation of strokes.
- Frontotemporal neurodegenerative diseases include behavioral variant frontotemporal dementia and variants of primary progressive aphasia. Behavioral variant frontotemporal dementia causes progressive changes in behavior and personality. Primary progressive aphasia causes progressive changes in language function.
- NPH causes gait dysfunction, urinary urgency or incontinence, and cognitive impairment. The gait disorder and/or urinary symptoms typically precede cognitive changes. Neuroimaging demonstrates enlarged ventricles, and gait improvement following large-volume lumbar puncture predicts response to ventriculoperitoneal shunt placement. This condition is rare, and enlarged ventricles are commonly seen in neuroimaging studies in older individuals due to age-related brain atrophy rather than NPH.
- Chronic traumatic encephalopathy is a dementia syndrome resulting from repetitive head injuries accumulated through contact sports or repetitive blast exposures. Diagnosis is confirmed by specific pathologic findings at autopsy.
- CJD is a rare condition causing rapidly progressive dementia evolving over months, often accompanied by myoclonus. DWI brain MRI demonstrates hyperintensity in the cortical ribbon, and the diagnosis is confirmed by CSF RT-QUIC testing. Other causes of rapidly progressive dementia include autoimmune encephalitis (primary or paraneoplastic), toxic/metabolic disorders, CNS malignancy, and atypically rapid presentations of neurodegenerative diseases.

Movement Disorders

Emily Anne Ferenczi

INTRODUCTION

Movement disorders can be broadly classified as those causing too little movement (hypokinetic disorders) and those causing too much movement (hyperkinetic disorders). Hypokinetic disorders fall under the umbrella of parkinsonism, which can be caused either by primary neurodegenerative disease (eg, Parkinson disease [PD] and atypical parkinsonian disorders such as dementia with Lewy bodies [DLB], multiple system atrophy [MSA], progressive supranuclear palsy [PSP], and corticobasal syndrome [CBS]) or occur secondary to medications or structural lesions. Hyperkinetic disorders include tremor, chorea, dystonia, myoclonus, and tics, all of which can be caused by primary neurologic diseases or occur secondary to structural lesions, systemic illness, or drugs. This chapter covers the clinical features, diagnosis, and treatment of common movement disorders, complementing Chapter 13, which discusses the clinical approach to patients with movement disorders.

DIAGNOSIS AND TREATMENT OF HYPOKINETIC (PARKINSONIAN) DISORDERS

Parkinson Disease

PD (sometimes also referred to as *idiopathic PD*) is the most common cause of parkinsonism. It is the second most common neurodegenerative disorder in the United States after Alzheimer disease and is currently estimated to affect 1% of the population older than age 60. Its prevalence is rising rapidly as the population ages. Most patients first develop symptoms after age 60. Less commonly, patients may develop symptoms before the age of 50, referred to as *young-onset PD*, which is more likely to be hereditary (family history present in ~25% of cases).[1]

The motor symptoms of PD are caused by degeneration of dopaminergic neurons in the midbrain (substantia nigra pars compacta), leading to decreased dopaminergic signaling in the basal ganglia. However, the pathologic changes (Lewy bodies formed of aggregates of the protein α-synuclein) are more widely distributed throughout the nervous system. It is unknown what initiates the neurodegenerative process, but it is likely an interplay between genetic, epigenetic, and environmental factors.

Diagnosis of Parkinson Disease
Clinical features of Parkinson disease

The diagnosis of PD is made clinically based on the presence of characteristic history and examination findings (Table 19.1). Patients develop slowly progressive motor symptoms over months or years, which may be described as slowing, stiffness, "weakness" (although strength is intact on examination), loss of dexterity, or change in gait. Nonmotor symptoms may also be present in the history, including cognitive and psychiatric symptoms, sleep disturbance (rapid eye movement [REM] sleep behavior disorder, in which dreams are enacted physically), gastrointestinal symptoms (most commonly constipation), anosmia (loss of smell), and autonomic symptoms (such as orthostatic hypotension, urinary symptoms, and erectile dysfunction). Other common symptoms at presentation include fatigue, shoulder or back pain, and soft voice (hypophonia). Nonmotor symptoms often predate motor symptoms by many years. Screening for these symptoms in the history—particularly REM sleep behavior disorder, anosmia, and constipation—may provide clues to the diagnosis. For example, in patients with REM sleep behavior disorder, it is estimated that more than 80% will go on to develop a neurodegenerative synucleinopathy (PD, MSA, or DLB) within 16 years.[2]

On examination, the diagnosis of PD requires the presence of bradykinesia, defined as a progressive decrement in speed and/or amplitude of sequential movements of the hands and/or feet (see Chapter 13 for a discussion of how to test for this finding). To diagnose PD, bradykinesia must be accompanied by one or more of three other hallmark features of parkinsonism: rigidity, rest tremor, and postural instability. Approximately 30% of patients with PD do not have tremor at presentation, and the presence of tremor is not required for diagnosis. PD typically presents unilaterally and may remain asymmetric for years even after symptoms become bilateral, but typically becomes more symmetric over time.

Despite these core features, PD is a heterogeneous disorder with different phenotypic subtypes. Approximately half of the patients present with a milder form of the disease that generally starts at a younger age, is often tremor predominant, and progresses more slowly over time. About 10% to 15% of patients present with a more severe phenotype with prominent nonmotor symptoms and gait disturbance, respond less well to dopamine replacement, and progress more rapidly. The remaining patients have an intermediate form of the disease.

Unusual or unexpected features in the history or examination that should lead to consideration of a diagnosis other than PD, such as an atypical parkinsonian syndrome, are listed in Table 19.2.

TABLE 19.2 Red-Flag Features Suggesting Atypical Parkinsonism or Secondary Parkinsonism

Red-flag features	Associated atypical condition
Rapid progression	All atypical parkinsonian syndromes
Early symmetry of examination findings	All atypical syndromes other than corticobasal syndrome (CBS)
Lack of sustained response to levodopa	All atypical parkinsonian syndromes
Early falls	Progressive supranuclear palsy (PSP)
Early cognitive impairment	Dementia with Lewy bodies (DLB)
Profound early autonomic dysfunction	Multiple system atrophy (MSA)
Cerebellar or pyramidal tract findings	MSA
Ocular or hepatic abnormalities	Wilson disease
Prior history of antipsychotic drug use	Drug-induced parkinsonism

TABLE 19.1 Core Clinical Features of Parkinson Disease

Typical motor features	Common associated nonmotor features
Slow progression of at least two of the following: • Bradykinesia • Rigidity • Resting tremor Other typical features: • Asymmetric onset • Shuffling gait with reduced arm swing • Postural instability (initially mild or absent)	• Rapid eye movement (REM) sleep behavior disorder • Anosmia • Constipation • Depression/anxiety • Mild autonomic dysfunction

Examples include early falls (suggestive of PSP), early profound autonomic failure (suggestive of MSA), early dementia (suggestive of DLB), or asymmetric apraxia (difficulty performing skilled movements, suggestive of CBS).

The diagnosis of PD is confirmed by a clear and sustained response to dopamine replacement therapy (usually with levodopa). Since some patients may require higher doses of levodopa for symptomatic improvement, a trial of successively higher doses of levodopa (up to 200-300 mg 3 times per day) may be needed before declaring treatment failure. One exception is tremor-predominant PD since the tremor can be resistant to levodopa and may require alternative medications or interventions. If bradykinesia and rigidity are not responsive to levodopa, or there are other ambiguous or red-flag features in the clinical presentation, then further diagnostic testing should be considered.

Supportive diagnostic tests

PD is a clinical diagnosis made by history, examination, and response to levodopa. Magnetic resonance imaging (MRI) of the brain is normal in PD but may be informative if there is concern for an atypical parkinsonian syndrome since these may have specific imaging findings (see subsequent text). In cases of diagnostic uncertainty, a dopamine transporter single-photon emission computed tomography (SPECT) scan can be obtained. Decreased signal in the basal ganglia on dopamine transporter SPECT is sensitive in diagnosing neurodegenerative parkinsonism but not specific as it is also abnormal in atypical parkinsonian syndromes (MSA, PSP, CBS, and DLB). It is more commonly obtained when trying to differentiate drug-induced parkinsonism from PD or in cases of very asymmetric essential tremor that may be challenging to distinguish clinically from PD. Skin biopsy for α-synuclein (the abnormally aggregated protein in PD) is an emerging diagnostic test for PD.

Treatment of Parkinson Disease

There are currently no curative or disease-modifying therapies for PD, but symptomatic treatments are effective in controlling symptoms and improving quality of life. Because individuals with PD experience different symptoms and are affected differently by them, treatment must be individualized. For example, a patient with a subtle tremor in their nondominant hand that is not causing disability or distress may not need pharmacologic treatment, whereas a patient with the same symptom who is disabled or embarrassed by it may benefit. Pharmacologic therapy is recommended once symptoms are beginning to interfere with day-to-day function and quality of life and should be complemented by modalities such as physical therapy, occupational therapy, speech therapy, social work, psychiatry, and palliative care as appropriate. Exercise has potential benefits for symptomatic improvement as well as slowing disease progression. Table 19.3 provides a summary of the overall treatment approach and modalities of treatment in PD.

Initial pharmacologic therapies

There are three main categories of medication used as initial pharmacologic therapy in PD: levodopa (prescribed in combination pills with carbidopa to reduce side effects), dopamine agonists (pramipexole, ropinirole, and rotigotine), and monoamine oxidase inhibitors (MAOIs; selegiline and rasagiline). Of the three, levodopa is the most effective in improving motor symptoms and has the fewest side effects, but the risk of developing motor complications (dyskinesias) is higher within the first 5 years, especially at higher levodopa doses.

Dopamine agonists carry a lower risk of dyskinesias but are often less well tolerated due to side effects, including impulse control disorders (leading to behavioral changes such as gambling, excessive spending, and hypersexuality), excessive daytime sleepiness, sleep attacks (falling asleep without warning), and withdrawal symptoms if the medication is discontinued. A dopamine agonist may be used as an alternative first-line agent in patients who experience side effects from carbidopa/levodopa but are usually reserved for later in the disease course.

MAOIs are less effective than dopaminergic therapies and, although often well tolerated, may cause side effects such as sexual dysfunction and headaches, and have multiple interactions with other medications and

TABLE 19.3	**Overview of Treatment Approach for Motor Symptoms in Parkinson Disease**		
	Early stage	**Mid stage**	**Advanced stage**
Symptoms	Early motor symptoms that are interfering with day-to-day function	• Motor fluctuations • More severe motor symptoms	• Loss of independence for activities of daily living • Postural instability and falls • Dementia
Efficacy of treatment	• Each dose remains within the therapeutic window. • No wearing off or dyskinesias	• More frequent doses required to prevent wearing off • Some peak-dose dyskinesias	• Frequent doses during the day • Frequent or sudden wearing off • Frequent or persistent dyskinesias
Multidisciplinary team	←———	• Physical therapy • Occupational therapy • Speech-language pathology • Driving rehabilitation/evaluation • Social work • Palliative care • Chaplaincy	———→

Pharmacologic therapies	• Carbidopa-levodopa 25/100 mg
	• Dopamine agonists
	• Anticholinergics (for tremor-predominant disease)
		• Higher dose or frequency of levodopa
		• Extended or fast-release levodopa
		• Addition of adjunctive therapies such as the following:
		  ○ Dopamine agonists
		  ○ Catechol-_O_-methyltransferase (COMT) inhibitors
		  ○ Monoamine oxidase inhibitors
		  ○ Adenosine receptor antagonists
		  ○ Anticholinergics
		  ○ Amantadine (for dyskinesias)	

Continuous dopaminergic therapies		• Transjejunal levodopa infusions • Subcutaneous dopamine (pending U.S. Food and Drug Administration [FDA] approval)	
Interventional therapies	←———	Botulinum toxin injections for dystonia (if present)	———→
Surgical therapies	Deep brain stimulation or magnetic resonance imaging (MRI)-guided focused ultrasound for levodopa-resistant tremor	• Deep brain stimulation to the globus pallidus internus (GPi) or subthalamic nucleus (STN)	

certain foods (including cheese). MAOIs may be used in patients with mild motor symptoms who prefer not to start dopaminergic therapy or experience side effects from carbidopa/levodopa and can be helpful for treating concurrent anxiety or depression.

For most patients requiring treatment for PD, levodopa is the first-line medication and should be used at the lowest effective dose. The medication is generally given 3 times daily during the active portion of the patient's day. One possible exception is younger patients with tremor-predominant PD since tremor may not respond to levodopa. In such patients, an anticholinergic agent (trihexyphenidyl or benztropine) can be considered, although side effects (eg, dry

mouth, blurry vision, constipation, urinary retention, confusion, and cognitive impairment) are common, and these medications should be used with caution in older individuals.

Subsequent pharmacologic therapy

As PD progresses, patients often begin to experience complications from levodopa therapy known as motor fluctuations, including wearing off (decreased time of medication effectiveness) and dyskinesias (involuntary, often choreiform or dystonic movements). For wearing off symptoms, the dose of levodopa may be increased, levodopa may be taken more frequently, extended-release levodopa may be added, or adjunctive medications can be given with levodopa to potentiate its effect (eg, catechol-*O*-methyltransferase [COMT] inhibitors [entacapone] or MAOIs [rasagiline or selegiline], or adenosine receptor antagonists [istradefylline]). Other strategies include adding longer-acting dopamine agonists, or, in cases in which the wearing off is sudden, rapid-acting dopaminergic medications such as inhaled levodopa or subcutaneous injection of apomorphine. Levodopa-induced dyskinesias can be treated by reducing dopaminergic medications (at the risk of worsened motor symptoms) and by adding amantadine (which is available in short-acting and long-acting formulations). Amantadine should be used with caution in older patients as it can cause anticholinergic side effects, including cognitive dysfunction.

Advanced therapies

In patients with motor fluctuations that cannot be adequately controlled with pharmacologic therapy, or tremor unresponsive to medication, surgical approaches can be considered, such as deep brain stimulation (DBS) or focused ultrasound thalamotomy. DBS involves the surgical implantation of a stimulator into basal ganglia or thalamic structures that is controlled from an external device. DBS provides relief comparable to the patient's best symptomatic response to levodopa for bradykinesia and rigidity, although it may exceed the benefit of pharmacologic therapy for medication-refractory tremor. DBS improves symptom control with less wearing off and fewer dyskinesias, and may decrease medication requirements, reducing side effects and pill burden. Symptoms such as freezing of gait, postural instability, and cognitive impairment do not usually improve with DBS and may worsen. The decision of when to pursue DBS requires a multidisciplinary specialized team, including a neurologist, neurosurgeon, and psychologist.

For patients who do not want neurosurgery or for whom neurosurgery would be too high-risk, another option to decrease motor fluctuations is enteral infusion of levodopa gel through a jejunostomy tube. This delivers levodopa directly to its site of absorption in the small intestine, bypassing absorption issues related to slowed gastrointestinal

transit, and has been shown to provide more stable motor benefit with fewer dyskinesias. It requires the patient to wear a portable pump, and adverse effects include complications of device insertion, postoperative wound infection or device blockage, abdominal pain, nausea, and peripheral neuropathy (mechanism unclear; studies suggest abnormalities of B vitamin metabolism related to high enteral doses of levodopa). Continuous subcutaneous infusion of apomorphine (a dopamine agonist) is available for the treatment of motor fluctuations in Europe but is not currently approved for use in the United States. Reported side effects include the typical side effects of dopamine agonists (see preceding text) as well as injection site skin reactions. Continuous subcutaneous carbidopa-levodopa infusion therapy is currently being evaluated in clinical trials.

Management of nonmotor symptoms

Nonmotor symptoms of PD affecting sleep, cognition, mood, and autonomic function may be as or more disabling than the motor symptoms. These should be screened for and treated with symptomatic therapies (Table 19.4).

Atypical Parkinsonian Syndromes

Atypical parkinsonian syndromes are neurodegenerative diseases that are all characterized by the presence of parkinsonism but each have additional neurologic features not typically seen in PD (see Table 19.2). The atypical parkinsonian syndromes are DLB, MSA, PSP, and CBS.

DLB is one of the most common causes of dementia after Alzheimer disease, whereas MSA, PSP, and CBS are rare conditions. DLB and MSA are characterized pathologically by the accumulation of α-synuclein (synucleinopathy), whereas PSP and CBS are characterized pathologically by the accumulation of an abnormal form of a protein called *tau* (tauopathy). Patients with atypical parkinsonian syndromes tend to present in their 60s to 70s.

Dementia With Lewy Bodies

The core diagnostic features of DLB are cognitive impairment that fluctuates from day to day or even within a

TABLE 19.4   Treatment of Nonmotor Symptoms in Parkinson Disease and Other Parkinsonian Syndromes

Nonmotor Symptom	Treatment	Notes
Rapid eye movement (REM) sleep behavior disorder	• Melatonin • Clonazepam	Recommend actively treating this for safety of patient and bed partner (eg, preventing falls out of bed and injury to partner)
Pain	• Depends on underlying cause • Pain may improve with higher dose of levodopa. • For spinal degenerative disease, consider physical therapy, or epidural steroid injections. • Pharmacologic options: acetaminophen, gabapentin, and duloxetine	Very common with many different etiologies, including musculoskeletal (spinal stenosis, radiculopathy, and rotator cuff)
Constipation	• Diet, fluids, exercise • Daily stool softeners • Stimulant laxatives as needed • Guanylate cyclase agonists	Very common; stepwise approach helpful

Orthostatic hypotension	• Diet: 2 L fluids daily, increased salt
	• Conservative measures: abdominal binder, pumping legs before standing, and exercise
	• Pharmacologic options:
	  ○ Lower dose of dopaminergic medication
	  ○ Midodrine, pyridostigmine, fludrocortisone (risk of heart failure exacerbation), and droxidopa
		Stepwise approach

Urinary frequency/urgency	• β-3 adrenergic agonists (mirabegron)—preferred because no cholinergic side effects • Antimuscarinic agents can be used with caution • Intradetrusor botulinum toxin injections	Urodynamic testing can be helpful to distinguish whether there is a component of prostatic hyperplasia or stress incontinence vs. bladder overactivity
Erectile dysfunction	• Phosphodiesterase inhibitors	
Drooling	• Sublingual atropine spray • Parotid and submandibular gland botulinum toxin injections	
Depression/anxiety	• Cognitive behavioral therapy, exercise • Selective serotonin reuptake inhibitors (SSRIs), and serotonin norepinephrine reuptake inhibitors (SNRIs) • Tricyclic antidepressants (TCAs; caution in older patients) • Mirtazapine (consider if patient anxious or weight loss/reduced appetite) • Bupropion (also may help apathy) • Dopamine agonists and monoamine oxidase inhibitors (MAOIs) may also have some antidepressant activity.	There have been no clinical trials specifically assessing the best agent for anxiety in Parkinson disease.
Apathy and fatigue	• Bupropion can be helpful. • Modafinil or methylphenidate can be considered for daytime sleepiness.	There are no specific pharmacologic agents for apathy.
Psychosis	• Discontinue anticholinergic agents. • Consider downtitrating the dose of dopaminergic therapies. • Addition of acetylcholinesterase inhibitors (see later) • If specific antipsychotic medication is indicated, recommend atypical antipsychotics such as pimavanserin, clozapine, or quetiapine.	Mainstay of treatment is avoidance or treatment of triggering etiology (eg, underlying infection or withdrawal of contributory medication).
Cognitive impairment	• Acetylcholinesterase inhibitors, including donepezil or rivastigmine • No clear evidence for the use of memantine in Parkinson disease	Rivastigmine is available in patch form, which can be helpful for patients with swallowing difficulties.

day (most commonly affecting attention, visuospatial function, and executive function), parkinsonism (often bilateral, symmetric, and less responsive to levodopa than in PD), and visual hallucinations (often of small people or animals that the patient knows are not real and that are not disturbing to the patient). In DLB, cognitive impairment occurs prior to or within 1 year of the onset of motor symptoms of parkinsonism, whereas if dementia occurs in PD, it generally follows the onset of motor symptoms by years (typically ≥10 years). Other common features of DLB include REM sleep behavior disorder, postural instability and falls early in the disease course, autonomic dysfunction, sensitivity to neuroleptic agents (causing sudden, severe worsening of parkinsonism), and psychiatric symptoms such as delusions and depression.

There is no specific pattern of brain atrophy on MRI in DLB as in other neurodegenerative dementias (see Chapter 18). An FDG-PET scan in DLB typically shows occipital hypometabolism with relative sparing of the posterior cingulate cortex (called the cingulate island sign, in contrast to the cingulate usually being affected in Alzheimer disease). Dopamine SPECT scan in DLB shows reduced basal ganglia uptake, although this is not specific to the condition and is also seen in other atypical parkinsonian syndromes and in PD. Cardiac scintigraphy in DLB demonstrates reduced cardiac sympathetic innervation, reflecting involvement of the peripheral autonomic nervous system, which is a finding also seen in PD but not in MSA, PSP, or CBS. A sleep study may confirm the presence of REM sleep behavior disorder, which can also be seen in PD and MSA but not in PSP or CBS.

Multiple System Atrophy

MSA is characterized by severe autonomic dysfunction (eg, orthostatic hypotension, urinary retention, urinary incontinence, erectile dysfunction, and impaired temperature regulation) accompanying either cerebellar ataxia (MSA-C), parkinsonism (MSA-P), or both. Rather than a typical parkinsonian rest tremor, patients often have a jerky postural or kinetic tremor. MSA-P is usually poorly responsive to levodopa, and a prominent sustained response to levodopa is considered evidence against the diagnosis. Disease progression is often more rapid than PD, with about half of patients require a walking aid within 3 years of motor

symptom onset, and many patients dying within 6 to 10 years of diagnosis.

Other features of MSA include postural instability and falls, axial dystonia (most commonly forward flexion of the neck, called *anterocollis*), dysarthria, dysphagia, inspiratory stridor (most commonly at night), REM sleep behavior disorder, cold hands and feet, and other neurologic examination findings such as a Babinski sign. Unlike DLB and PD, anosmia is uncommon in MSA.

Brain MRI in MSA may demonstrate atrophy of the putamen, cerebellum, middle cerebellar peduncles, and/or pons, although it may be normal early in the disease. T2 hyperintense cruciform signal change in the pons called the *hot cross bun sign* may be seen, reflecting degeneration of surrounding cerebellar fibers and pontine neurons (Figure 19.1A,B). Autonomic testing demonstrates central autonomic dysfunction, and cardiac scintigraphy may show preserved peripheral cardiac sympathetic innervation (in contrast to PD and DLB, in which this is reduced).

Progressive Supranuclear Palsy

PSP is characterized by progressive impairment of voluntary eye movements and parkinsonism that is typically symmetric and responds poorly to levodopa. Patients with PSP have difficulty with voluntarily vertical gaze, although passive head movements are able to elicit vertical eye movements, known as a *supranuclear gaze palsy*. Slowing of vertical saccades can be an early sign before complete loss of vertical gaze. Postural instability in PSP presents as repeated unprovoked falls early in the disease course, usually described as "going down like a tree"; these falls may cause severe injuries, including facial fractures and subdural hematoma. Cognitive dysfunction in PSP often presents as progressive language or speech deficit (aphasia or apraxia of speech) or change in behavior (such as sudden uncontrollable and inappropriate crying or laughing, known as pseudobulbar affect). Patients with PSP may have an unusual facial expression caused by facial dystonia, which causes them to have an angry or puzzled expression (eg, furrowed brow, deep nasolabial folds).

Brain imaging in PSP is likely to show focal midbrain atrophy on MRI (giving the midbrain a characteristic "hummingbird" appearance) or hypometabolism of the midbrain on FDG-PET (Figure 19.1C).

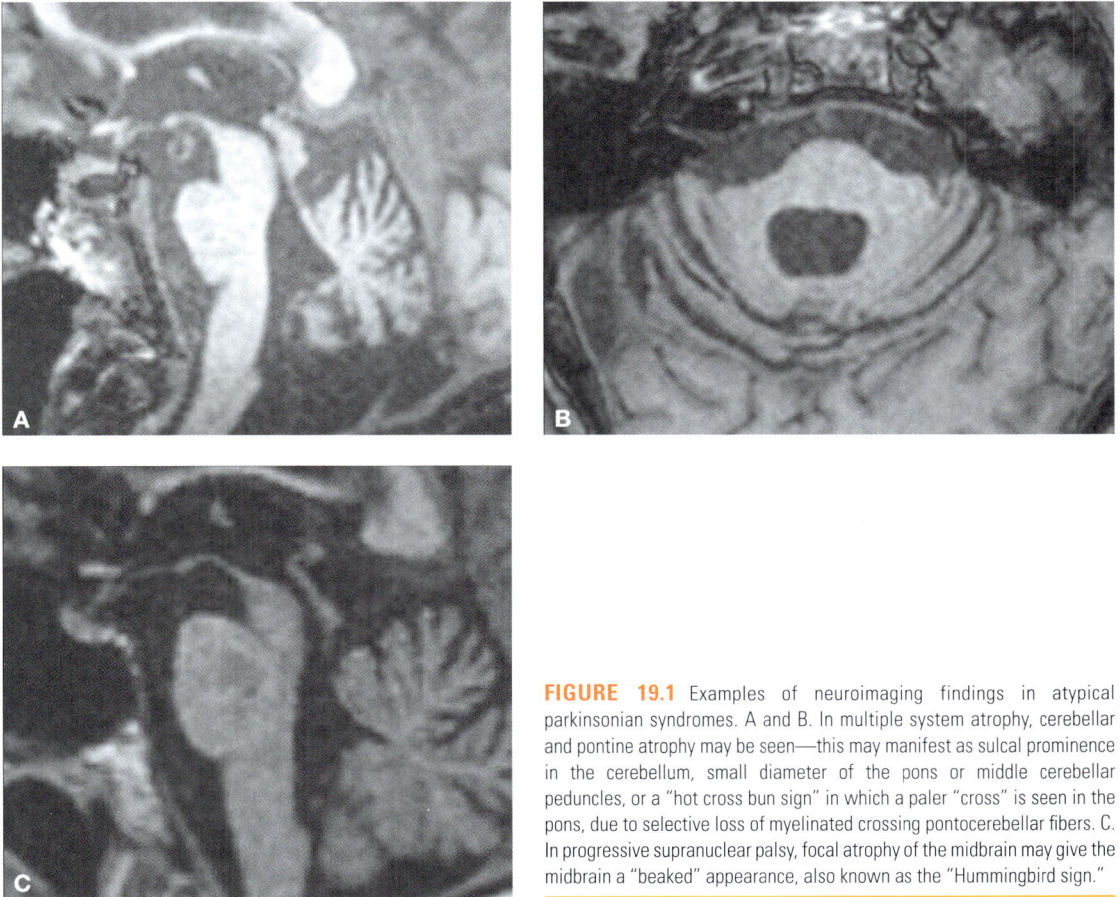

FIGURE 19.1 Examples of neuroimaging findings in atypical parkinsonian syndromes. A and B. In multiple system atrophy, cerebellar and pontine atrophy may be seen—this may manifest as sulcal prominence in the cerebellum, small diameter of the pons or middle cerebellar peduncles, or a "hot cross bun sign" in which a paler "cross" is seen in the pons, due to selective loss of myelinated crossing pontocerebellar fibers. C. In progressive supranuclear palsy, focal atrophy of the midbrain may give the midbrain a "beaked" appearance, also known as the "Hummingbird sign."

Corticobasal Syndrome

CBS presents as progressive asymmetric parkinsonism accompanied by unilateral or asymmetric cortical signs such as limb apraxia (inability to perform or mimic purposeful actions despite intact strength), hemisensory neglect (ignoring sensory information from one side of the body), agraphesthesia (inability to recognize numbers or letters traced on the skin by the examiner despite normal primary sensation), or astereognosis (inability to recognize objects by touch alone). Some patients may experience alien limb phenomena in which a limb may take on a "mind of its own" and make involuntary semi-purposeful movements. CBS can also present with limb dystonia (twisting movements or postures) or myoclonus (sudden, irregular, jerk-like movements of the arms or legs). Other features may include weakness of one side of the body, speech disturbance, dementia, and depression. Patients with CBS tend to have an action tremor or myoclonic tremor rather than a typical parkinsonian resting tremor. The term corticobasal degeneration (CBD) refers to a pathologic entity that can present not only as CBS but also as other neurodegenerative clinical phenotypes such as PSP, behavioral variant frontotemporal dementia, or primary progressive aphasia. The clinical syndrome of CBS may be caused by Alzheimer pathology, frontotemporal lobar degeneration pathology, or CBD pathology.

MRI in CBS will typically show asymmetric cortical atrophy, with more prominent atrophy contralateral to the most affected limb. FDG-PET may show asymmetric cortical hypometabolism.

Treatment of Atypical Parkinsonian Syndromes

There are currently no curative therapies for atypical parkinsonian disorders. Treatment is focused on addressing specific symptoms through a multidisciplinary team, including involvement of palliative care. Carbidopa/levodopa can be trialed for motor symptoms of parkinsonism if tolerated but is often ineffective or only transiently effective. Pharmacologic management of cognitive impairment with acetylcholinesterase inhibitors such as rivastigmine or donepezil may be helpful, especially in DLB, where they are an effective first-line treatment for hallucinations and delusions. Dopamine receptor antagonist antipsychotic medications should be avoided if possible or used at the lowest possible dose to avoid worsening of motor parkinsonism, especially in DLB, in which severe neuroleptic sensitivity is common. Early involvement of physical therapy and prescriptions for walking aids (eg, cane, rolling walker with or without walking cues) for postural instability and freezing of gait are important for fall prevention and patient safety. Occupational therapy can provide helpful strategies for managing activities of daily living and compensating for limb apraxia.

Secondary and Hereditary Parkinsonism

In addition to neurodegenerative diseases, parkinsonism can be caused by medications, toxins, cerebrovascular disease, infections, antibody-mediated conditions (including paraneoplastic disorders), prior head trauma, and hereditary disorders such as Wilson disease (Table 19.5). Drug-induced parkinsonism is a common cause of secondary parkinsonism and is discussed in further detail subsequently. Metabolic or endocrine abnormalities (eg, hypothyroidism and hypoparathyroidism) may cause slowed movements, which can mimic parkinsonism. Chronic subcortical microvascular disease or stroke of the midbrain or basal ganglia can cause parkinsonism, and normal pressure hydrocephalus may produce a gait disorder that can appear parkinsonian.

TABLE 19.5	Causes of Parkinsonism
Category	**Examples**
Idiopathic (primary)	Parkinson disease
Hereditary	Wilson disease
	Huntington disease
	Neurodegeneration with brain iron accumulation (NBIA; eg, pantothenate kinase–associated neurodegeneration [PKAN])
	Neuroacanthocytosis
	Spinocerebellar ataxias (SCAs; eg, SCA3)
	X-linked dystonia parkinsonism
	Hereditary juvenile dystonia-parkinsonism
Acquired (secondary)	
Drugs	Dopamine receptor blockers (antipsychotics, antiemetics/motility agents)
	Dopamine-depleting drugs (vesicular monoamine transporter [VMAT]) inhibitors
	Lithium
	Calcium channel blockers (flunarizine, cinnarizine—these are not FDA approved in the United States)
	Antiseizure medications (sodium valproate)
Toxins	Recreational drug contaminants (historically, MPTP [1-methyl-4-phenyl-1,2,3,6-tetrahydropyridine])
	Carbon monoxide
	Organophosphates
	Manganese
Metabolic/endocrine	Hypothyroidism
	Hypoparathyroidism and hypocalcemia
Vascular	Multiple infarcts (including basal ganglia/midbrain)
	Extensive subcortical microvascular disease (Binswanger disease)
Infectious/parainfectious	West Nile virus (acute and postencephalitic parkinsonism)
	Influenza A virus (postencephalitic parkinsonism)
	Other viruses: Japanese encephalitis virus, Epstein-Barr virus, varicella zoster virus, and HIV
	Prion disease
Autoimmune/ paraneoplastic	Examples include anti-CRMP5, anti-Ma, anti-LGI1, and anti-IgLON5
Neoplastic	Midbrain or basal ganglia tumors
Trauma	Chronic traumatic encephalopathy

CRMP5, collapsin response mediator protein; IgLON5, immunoglobulin-like (cell adhesion molecule); LGI1, leucine-rich glioma inactivated.

Wilson Disease

Wilson disease is a rare, autosomal recessive, inherited condition caused by accumulation of copper in the liver, brain, and other organs. Wilson disease can cause parkinsonism and other movement disorders and should therefore be considered in any patient younger than age 50 with a new-onset movement disorder. In patients who present at a young age (younger than 20), hepatic manifestations are more common, whereas in patients who present in young adulthood (older than 20), neurologic manifestations tend to be more prevalent. Neurologic features can be varied, including tremor (often a proximal postural tremor that can be brought out by asking the patient to hold their arms elevated with hands close to the nose and elbows out to the side [called a *wing-beating tremor*]), dystonia, and parkinsonism; neuropsychiatric symptoms are also common. The slit-lamp ocular examination may reveal green deposits around the iris (Kayser-Fleischer rings). Wilson disease can be diagnosed by low serum ceruloplasmin (<20 mg/dL) and elevated 24-hour urinary copper (>100 pg/24 hours); if these tests are inconclusive, liver biopsy and genetic testing may be necessary. Treatment is with copper-chelating therapy. Symptomatic treatment of parkinsonism with levodopa, dopamine agonists, and anticholinergics can also be symptomatically helpful.

DIAGNOSIS AND TREATMENT OF HYPERKINETIC MOVEMENT DISORDERS

Essential Tremor

Essential tremor causes a postural and kinetic tremor most commonly affecting the hands but also often present in the head and/or voice. The tremor usually affects both hands but can be asymmetric or even unilateral in a small minority of patients, especially early in the disease course. There is a bimodal distribution of age at presentation, with one peak younger than the age of 40 and another peak in older adults aged 50 to 70 years. Some patients may have a mild tremor for decades that progressively worsens in later life. A family history of tremor is often present, but its absence does not exclude the diagnosis. A medication-related tremor can be excluded if no tremor-inducing medications (Table 19.6) were started or increased in dose in the months prior to tremor onset. Essential tremor may improve with alcohol; however, the amount of alcohol required to provide symptomatic benefit varies between individuals. Since the tremor is most prominent with action, essential tremor can interfere with eating, drinking, writing, typing, texting, and other fine motor tasks.

On examination, the tremor is most prominent with posture (eg, holding the hands outstretched) and action (eg, on finger-to-nose testing). Frequency varies between patients from 4 to 12 Hz but is usually very consistent within an individual patient. The amplitude of the tremor can be exacerbated by anxiety, sleep deprivation, hunger, or caffeine. The postural tremor is typically a flexion-extension movement at the wrist (as opposed to the pronation-supination tremor seen in PD) and occurs immediately on holding the arms outstretched (as opposed to the reemergent tremor of PD that appears after a delay of 5-10 seconds after adopting this posture). In long-standing essential tremor, a resting tremor can be seen but is usually lower in amplitude

TABLE 19.6 Secondary Causes of Tremor

Category	Examples
Medications	
Rest (+/− action) tremor	Antipsychotic medications Antiemetic medications (eg, metoclopramide and prochlorperazine).
Action tremor (postural and kinetic)	Caffeine Psychiatric medications (selective serotonin reuptake inhibitors [SSRIs], serotonin norepinephrine reuptake inhibitors [SNRIs], lithium, antipsychotic medications, methylphenidate) Anti-seizure medications (sodium valproate) Asthma medications (β-agonists and theophylline) Immunosuppressive agents (cyclosporin and tacrolimus)
Metabolic/endocrine	Hypoglycemia Hyperthyroidism
Enhanced physiologic tremor	Anxiety/stress Hunger Sleep deprivation

than the action component of the tremor. The severity of the tremor can be assessed by asking the patient to write a sentence, draw an Archimedes spiral (which shows a characteristic sinusoidal tremor waveform; see Figure 13.4), pour water from one cup to another, or hold a pen with the wrist unsupported very close to a dot on a page without touching it (dot approximation test).

The head tremor of essential tremor often begins in the horizontal ("no-no"), vertical ("yes-yes"), or side-side directions but over time can become multidirectional. The presence of a head tremor helps exclude the diagnosis of an enhanced physiologic tremor (which typically has no head involvement). The head tremor in essential tremor improves when lying down (since the supine position is not an antigravity posture for the head), which distinguishes it from a dystonic head tremor, which persists when supine.

A voice tremor may be present during conversation or elicited on examination by asking the patient to produce sustained vowel sounds. A jaw tremor is less common but can be observed with the mouth held open, whereas the jaw tremor of PD is typically present with the mouth closed.

Essential tremor can sometimes be associated with other neurologic features such as mild gait ataxia and, rarely, dystonic postures and sensorineural hearing loss. A minority of patients with essential tremor may go on to develop neurodegenerative parkinsonism, but the association between essential tremor and PD remains unclear. Brain MRI and dopamine transporter SPECT scans are normal in essential tremor. Thyroid function tests should be checked to rule out hyperthyroidism as a secondary cause of tremor (or a contributor to worsening of tremor in patients with essential tremor).

Treatment of Essential Tremor

For mild tremor, occupational therapy can provide individualized tips and strategies to improve function. Adaptive devices such as weighted or tremor-dampening utensils, pens, or modified computer keyboards and mouses can assist in specific tasks.

First-line pharmacologic therapies are indicated when symptoms interfere with day-to-day function. The two first-line medications are propranolol and primidone. These can reduce tremor severity in most patients, although efficacy is often limited by side effects (sedation, lightheadedness, exercise intolerance, mood changes, erectile dysfunction for propranolol; sedation, confusion, ataxia, and nausea for primidone). If patients do not respond adequately to either medication alone, both propranolol and primidone can be used together. In patients who respond inadequately to either of these medications or have unacceptable side effects, second-line pharmacologic therapies include gabapentin, topiramate, clonazepam, and botulinum toxin injections. A noninvasive wearable device that stimulates the median and radial nerves at the wrist may provide temporary tremor suppression in some cases.

For patients with disabling and medication-refractory tremor, DBS or MRI-guided focused ultrasound thalamotomy may be considered. For both interventions, patients can expect significant improvement in their hand tremor and may be able to reduce their medication doses accordingly. Common adverse effects of both interventions include paresthesias, dysarthria, and ataxia, although in the case of DBS, these can be minimized with adjustments in stimulation parameters, and in the case of MRI-guided focused ultrasound thalamotomy, these adverse effects are usually transient. Benefits of surgery from either approach may begin to wane after 5 or more years.

Chorea

Chorea is defined as an involuntary hyperkinetic movement disorder characterized by random and irregular nonpurposeful movements that flow from one part of the body to another. Chorea exists on a spectrum with other involuntary irregular movements, including athetosis (slower writhing movements) and ballism (high-amplitude flinging movements). The velocity and amplitude of chorea can fluctuate within an individual, from low-amplitude movements that resemble fidgeting to high-amplitude reaching or kicking movements. Chorea can involve the face (including the mouth and tongue), limbs, and torso and may affect one side of the body or both depending on the underlying etiology. Patients with chorea often demonstrate motor impersistence, which is the inability to maintain a sustained motor action such as tongue protrusion (leading to the intermittent withdrawal of the tongue into the mouth) or hand grip (leading to milkmaid grip). Patients may be able to partially suppress or disguise choreiform movements by incorporating them into a voluntary movement.

Chorea can be caused by hereditary conditions (eg, Huntington disease) or may be secondary to a focal brain lesion, systemic conditions, or drugs (Table 19.7). The levodopa-induced dyskinesias of PD and the tardive dyskinesias that arise from antipsychotic use are choreiform in phenomenology.

TABLE 19.7   Causes of Chorea and Recommended Initial Diagnostic Tests

Category	Example	Diagnostic tests
Hereditary	Huntington disease	Genetic testing for Huntington disease
	Wilson disease	24-h urinary copper, serum ceruloplasmin, slit-lamp examination, and liver biopsy
	Spinocerebellar ataxias (SCA3 and SCA17)	Genetic testing (repeat expansion panel and whole-exome sequencing)
	Dentatorubral-pallidoluysian atrophy (DRPLA)	Genetic testing
	Neuroacanthocytosis	Peripheral blood smear (for acanthocytes) and MRI brain
	Neurodegeneration with brain iron accumulation (NBIA) diseases (eg, pantothenate kinase–associated neurodegeneration [PKAN] and Fahr disease)	MRI brain and genetic testing
Acquired		
Focal structural lesion	Vascular (subthalamic nucleus infarct) and infectious (toxoplasmosis)	MRI brain and intracranial vessel imaging
Metabolic	Nonketotic hyperglycemia (diabetic striatopathy)	MRI brain, serum glucose, and HbA$_{1c}$
	Hypocalcemia, hypo/hypernatremia, hypomagnesemia, uremia, and hyperthyroidism	Complete metabolic panel and TSH
Infectious/parainfectious	Viral (West Nile virus, varicella zoster virus, Epstein-Barr virus, HIV, and measles)	Viral serology in serum/CSF
	Bacterial (group A streptococcus)—Sydenham chorea	Anti-streptolysin O antibodies, throat swab for group A streptococcus
	Parasitic	Toxoplasma serology in serum/CSF and MRI brain
	Prion disease	Cerebrospinal fluid real-time quaking-induced conversion (RT-QuIC)
Autoimmune/ paraneoplastic/ neoplastic	Systemic lupus erythematosus and antiphospholipid antibody syndrome (APLAS)	C3, C4, antinuclear antibody (ANA), anti-Smith (Sm), anti-double stranded DNA (dsDNA), anti-RNP, anti-SS-A (Ro), anti-SS-B (La), and antiphospholipid antibodies
	Chorea gravidarum	Antiphospholipid testing and throat swab for group A strep
	Paraneoplastic syndrome—commonly small cell lung cancer or ovarian teratoma	Autoimmune encephalopathy panel including anti-NMDAR, anti-Hu, anti-Ma, anti-P/Q Ca channel, anti-LGI1, anti-CASPR2, and anti-CRMP5
	Polycythemia rubra vera	CBC, smear, and bone marrow evaluation
Medications/toxins	Dopamine blocking medications (eg, antipsychotics/ antiemetics)	Medication history
	Levodopa in a patient with a history of Parkinson disease	Medication history
	Toxins (eg, carbon monoxide and organophosphate poisoning)	MRI brain (focal abnormalities of the basal ganglia)

CASPR2, contactin-associated protein-like 2; CBC, complete blood count; CRMP5, collapsin response mediator protein; CSF, cerebrospinal fluid; LGI1, leucine-rich glioma inactivated; MRI, magnetic resonance imaging; NMDAR, *N*-methyl-D-aspartate receptor; TSH, thyroid-stimulating hormone.

The anatomic distribution and symmetry of the chorea provides clues as to the underlying etiology. For example, chorea involving the upper face (including the forehead) is characteristic of Huntington disease, whereas chorea limited to one side of the body (hemichorea or hemiballismus) is usually seen in the setting of a focal lesion (eg, an ischemic or hemorrhagic stroke of the subthalamic nucleus) or nonketotic hyperglycemia (diabetic striatopathy). Chorea of the mouth and tongue (orobuccolingual) is characteristic of tardive dyskinesia caused by antipsychotic medication exposure (see subsequent text).

Laboratory testing to determine the etiology of chorea is summarized in Table 19.7 and includes evaluation for metabolic, infectious, inflammatory, and paraneoplastic etiologies of acquired chorea. In younger individuals (age 50 or younger) with new-onset chorea, laboratory testing for ceruloplasmin and 24-hour urinary copper should be performed to evaluate for Wilson disease. Genetic testing for hereditary chorea should be considered in patients with a family history of chorea. Genetic testing should always be performed in conjunction with genetic counseling; in cases of suspected Huntington disease, the diagnosis has wide-reaching psychological, social, and financial implications for the patient and family. Imaging studies such as brain MRI should be performed to evaluate for a causative structural lesion in cases of unilateral chorea.

Huntington Disease

Huntington disease is the most common hereditary cause of chorea. It is caused by a triplet repeat expansion in the *huntingtin* gene and is inherited in an autosomal dominant manner. Diagnosis is suspected on the basis of the clinical history, examination, and family history suggestive of autosomal dominant inheritance, although the absence of a family history does not rule out the diagnosis as spontaneous de novo mutations can occur.

The classic clinical triad includes motor symptoms (chorea, oculomotor abnormalities, dystonia, tics, myoclonus, and parkinsonism), progressive psychiatric symptoms (including increased risk of suicidality), and cognitive impairment. Once the diagnosis

of Huntington disease is suspected, patients and their families should be referred to genetic counseling for confirmatory testing and to discuss the potential psychological, social, and financial ramifications of a confirmed diagnosis. There is currently no disease-modifying therapy, but symptomatic treatment of chorea and other motor symptoms, and psychiatric, behavioral, and cognitive symptoms, forms the mainstay of management (see subsequent text). This supportive treatment approach requires a multidisciplinary team involving neurologists, psychologists and psychiatrists, genetic counselors, occupational therapists, physical therapists, speech-language pathologists, and social and palliative care workers.

Chorea in Systemic Autoimmune Disease

Chorea may be a presenting neurologic symptom of systemic lupus erythematosus (SLE) and antiphospholipid antibody syndrome. Chorea is the most common movement disorder in SLE and antiphospholipid antibody syndrome, but it is still a rare neurologic feature of these conditions (<2% of cases). The chorea may be asymmetric (hemichorea) or symmetric and can be accompanied by other movement disorders such as tremor, dystonia, or parkinsonism. Diagnostic testing may include serum levels of C3 and C4, antinuclear antibody (ANA), anti-Smith (Sm), anti-double stranded DNA (dsDNA), anti-RNP, anti-SS-A (Ro) and anti-SS-B (La), and antiphospholipid antibodies (lupus anticoagulant, anti-cardiolipin, and anti-β2 glycoprotein-I).

Treatment of Chorea

For some causes of chorea, specific curative treatments may be available, such as antibiotics for streptococcal infection in Sydenham chorea, immune-modulating agents for an autoimmune process, correction of hyperglycemia in the nonketotic hyperglycemic state, or copper chelation therapy in Wilson disease. Other hereditary and acquired causes of chorea are treated symptomatically. For levodopa-induced dyskinesias, the addition of amantadine can be helpful if the levodopa dose cannot be reduced.

For chorea in Huntington disease and tardive dyskinesia, specific anti-chorea agents such as vesicular monoamine transporter (VMAT) inhibitors may be considered. These medications reduce dopamine release in the basal ganglia and suppress hyperkinetic movements. Two VMAT inhibitors are U.S. Food and Drug Administration (FDA) approved for the treatment of Huntington disease: tetrabenazine and deutetrabenazine. Both medications have the potential to cause depression, suicidality, and parkinsonism and should therefore be used with caution in patients with a prior psychiatric history, although deutetrabenazine has fewer side effects overall.

Valbenazine is another VMAT inhibitor that, along with deutetrabenazine, has been approved for the treatment of tardive dyskinesia, and is well tolerated. Second-line or adjunctive therapies for chorea may include dopamine receptor blocking medications (antipsychotics), anti-seizure medications (such as sodium valproate, carbamazepine, levetiracetam, or gabapentin), or long-acting benzodiazepines (such as clonazepam).

Dystonia

Dystonia is involuntary sustained or intermittent co-contraction of muscle groups that leads to repetitive patterned twisting movements, abnormal postures, and/or tremor. Dystonic postures can be accompanied by pain and a sense of pulling. Dystonia can be focal (in one region of the body), multifocal (in multiple regions of the body), or generalized (throughout the body), and it can fluctuate in severity over time. The abnormal posture and tremor of dystonia are characterized by position dependence: They increase when the body part is held in one position and decrease in other positions (the null point). Patients may discover that touching the affected body part transiently alleviates the symptoms (called a *sensory trick* or *geste antagoniste*). For example, twisting of the neck in cervical dystonia may be briefly improved by the patient touching their hand to their cheek.

Dystonic tremor is often jerky and irregular, in contrast to the more sinusoidal oscillations of essential tremor. Dystonic head tremor will persist on lying flat (in contrast to the head tremor of essential tremor, which subsides when the patient lies flat). Dystonia may occur only in the context of specific tasks, such as writing or playing a musical instrument. As with many other movement disorders, dystonia may be exacerbated by anxiety, hunger, or sleep deprivation, and resolves during sleep.

Genetic dystonias typically present in childhood or young adulthood, with generalized dystonia involving multiple (three or more) parts of the body, including the trunk. There is often a family history, although not always, since de novo mutations can occur. The most common genetic dystonias have autosomal dominant inheritance, but others have autosomal recessive inheritance. In genetic dystonias, parkinsonism, chorea, myoclonus, or ataxia may accompany dystonia.

The most common genetic dystonia is DYT-*TOR1A* (also known as DYT1), which is more common in patients with Ashkenazi Jewish heritage. This condition causes childhood-onset dystonia that usually begins focally and later generalizes. DBS is often required for the treatment of DYT-*TOR1A*.

Some genetic dystonias improve with levodopa therapy and are therefore known as dopa-responsive dystonia. Wilson disease is an example of an autosomal recessive inherited cause of dystonia, presenting in childhood or young adulthood, often in combination with tremor, parkinsonism, or chorea, and systemic manifestations (see earlier text).

Idiopathic and secondary dystonias usually present in adulthood with focal, segmental, or multifocal dystonia. Focal dystonia affects just a single body part, such as the eyelids (blepharospasm), oropharynx (oromandibular dystonia), larynx (spasmodic dysphonia), neck (cervical dystonia), hand (writer's cramp, musician's dystonia), foot (runner's or bicycling dystonia), or trunk. Truncal dystonia may cause the body to flex forward (camptocormia), sideways (Pisa syndrome), or backward (opisthotonos). Segmental dystonia affects two or more contiguous body parts, such as the neck and trunk, arm and trunk, or leg and trunk, whereas multifocal dystonia involves two or more noncontiguous body parts. Hemidystonia affects the arm and leg only on one side of the body and is often associated with a focal structural brain or spinal cord lesion. Table 19.8 lists examples of secondary causes of dystonia. Idiopathic dystonia is thought to result from interactions between susceptibility genes and environmental factors (such as a history of overuse or trauma of the affected body part).

TABLE 19.8   Secondary Causes of Dystonia

Category	Examples
Brain pathology	
Trauma	Head trauma
	Perinatal cerebral injury
	Iatrogenic (postthalamotomy)
Vascular	Ischemic stroke (especially in basal ganglia)
	Hemorrhage
	Arteriovenous malformation of basal ganglia
	Hypoxia
Infectious/parainfectious	Brain abscess (eg, in basal ganglia)
	Prion disease
	Mycoplasma pneumoniae
	Tuberculosis
	Japanese B encephalitis
	Reye syndrome
	Subacute sclerosing leukoencephalopathy (measles)
Inflammatory/autoimmune	Multiple sclerosis
	Antiphospholipid syndrome
Neoplastic/paraneoplastic	Brain tumor
	Paraneoplastic encephalitis (eg, anti-LGI1 [leucine-rich glioma inactivated] antibody)
Metabolic	Osmotic demyelination (from inappropriately rapid treatment of hypo/hypernatremia)
	Hepatic encephalopathy
Endocrine	Hypoparathyroidism
Neurodegenerative	Parkinson disease
	Atypical parkinsonian syndromes (multiple system atrophy [MSA], progressive supranuclear palsy [PSP], and corticobasal syndrome [CBS])
Spine pathology	
	Syringomyelia
	Spinal stenosis/compression myelopathy
Peripheral injury	
	Electrocution and ionizing radiation
Medications	
Dopamine blocking medications	Antipsychotics
	Antiemetics (eg, metoclopramide and prochlorperazine)
Levodopa (Parkinson disease)	Carbidopa-levodopa
Antiseizure medications	Sodium valproate
Toxins	
	Carbon monoxide, cyanide, and manganese

The most common adult-onset idiopathic dystonia is cervical dystonia, which usually develops between ages 40 and 60. Symptoms include leaning or rotation of the head to one side, often with a sense of tightness or pulling of the neck muscles. The head may be rotated (torticollis), tilted to one side (laterocollis), flexed forward (anterocollis), extended backward (retrocollis), or there may be a combination. Patients may have sought prior manipulative therapy for neck stiffness, such as chiropractic treatment or massage, and headache is common. Cervical dystonia can cause a head tremor that has an irregular jerky quality that persists when lying flat and has a null-point head position in which the tremor is lessened.

Blepharospasm is the most common cranial dystonia and often starts as brief blinking of both eyes, but when severe can cause the eyes to close for extended periods. Task-specific dystonias such as writer's cramp or musician's dystonia are focal dystonias in which the affected body part begins to form abnormal postures only when a specific task is being performed, such as writing or playing a musical instrument.

Focal dystonia is also seen in neurodegenerative movement disorders such as PD (eg, unilateral foot dystonia), MSA (eg, anterocollis), PSP (eg, retrocollis), and CBS (eg, hemidystonia). Dystonia in PD may vary with dopamine levels, occurring either as levodopa is wearing off or as a peak-dose side effect. Dystonia can also be provoked by medications, such as antipsychotic drugs (ie, tardive dystonia, discussed subsequently). Functional neurologic disorders can sometimes present with symptoms suggestive of dystonia and are characterized by a lack of consistency in the pattern of movements or postures. It is important to note that functional dystonia can coexist with other neurologic diseases; therefore, its presence does not exclude other neurologic diagnoses.

Diagnostic tests for dystonia include laboratory tests to screen for Wilson disease (serum ceruloplasmin, 24-hour urinary copper), genetic testing (with single-gene testing or dystonia panels to assess for inherited dystonias), structural brain and spine imaging (especially in the case of hemidystonia), or tests specific for associated neurodegenerative diseases, such as dopamine transporter SPECT imaging if there is accompanying parkinsonism.

Treatment of Dystonia

Treatment of dystonia may be directed specifically at the underlying etiology, for example, copper chelation therapy with penicillamine or zinc in Wilson disease or levodopa for dopa-responsive dystonia. For medication-induced dystonia (eg, tardive dystonia or levodopa-induced dystonia), withdrawal or reduction of the causative medication is the first-line approach if possible. Symptomatic treatments aim to improve pain, discomfort, and disability and include physical approaches (physical therapy, occupational therapy, speech therapy, and development of sensory tricks), botulinum toxin injection to affected regions, pharmacologic therapies, and neurosurgical interventions (DBS or MRI-guided focused ultrasound).

First-line therapy for focal dystonia is chemodenervation by botulinum toxin injection. This causes weakness of the injected muscles and possibly also alters sensory feedback. It is a highly effective therapy without systemic side effects; however, it cannot be used to treat generalized dystonia and must be repeated every 3 to 4 months since its benefits wear off. Local side effects include excessive weakness and the spread of weakness to nearby nontargeted muscles (these side effects generally wear off after several months). Generalized or severe dystonia can be treated with oral pharmacologic agents such as anticholinergic drugs (eg, trihexyphenidyl, benztropine, or amantadine), VMAT inhibitors (eg, tetrabenazine or deutetrabenazine), baclofen, or benzodiazepines, although many of these may be limited by side effects.

If botulinum toxin or oral pharmacologic agents for dystonia are ineffective or not tolerated, neurosurgical interventions can be considered, such as DBS of the globus pallidus. DBS can be a very effective option for severe generalized dystonia, such as those with childhood onset.

Dystonic storm (status dystonicus) is a rare movement disorder emergency with a high mortality rate (~10%). It is more common in patients with genetic dystonia and is characterized by severe, uncontrolled, continuous hyperkinetic movements (dystonia that may be accompanied by dyskinesia) and can cause rhabdomyolysis leading to renal failure, autonomic instability, respiratory failure, and death. Triggers must be addressed, including treating acute infection, reversing recent medication changes, and ensuring implanted DBS hardware is functioning. Oral anti-dystonic therapies such as anticholinergics or VMAT inhibitors should be administered. If symptoms persist, escalation to intravenous benzodiazepines, barbiturates, or general anesthesia should be initiated in an intensive care unit. In some cases, emergency DBS or pallidotomy may be required.

Myoclonus

Myoclonus is defined as sudden, brief, jerking movements. In contrast to many other movement disorders, the most common cause of myoclonus is usually systemic illness rather than primary neurologic disease. Most frequently, it is seen in the context of toxic or metabolic conditions (eg, renal or hepatic failure) or secondary to medications (see Table 19.9). Less commonly, myoclonus can be seen in infectious, inflammatory, or neoplastic disorders. When occurring in the context of a primary neurologic disease, myoclonus is most often caused by epilepsy syndromes (myoclonic epilepsy, especially in children or adults younger than the age of 30) or neurodegenerative disease (in adults older than the age of 60).

On examination, myoclonus can be distinguished from other involuntary movements by its irregularity (in contrast to the rhythmicity of tremor) and its brief and jerky nature (in contrast to the more flowing movements of chorea or the more sustained contractions and postures of dystonia). Myoclonus can be focal, multifocal, segmental, or generalized, and this may give clues as to the underlying etiology. For example, focal myoclonus may suggest a structural cortical lesion, whereas generalized myoclonus is more suggestive of a brainstem process such as brainstem encephalitis or a multifocal process (cortical and brainstem) such as posthypoxic myoclonus (Lance-Adams syndrome). Segmental myoclonus (affecting muscles innervated by one or a few contiguous spinal levels) is characteristic of a spinal cord etiology.

The examination may reveal provoking factors such as sensitivity to sensory stimuli or movements; for example, post-hypoxic myoclonus can be induced by light touch or a loud sound (eg, a clap) or if the patient makes an intentional action. The examination may also indicate signs of the underlying etiology, such as signs

TABLE 19.9   Causes of Myoclonus and Associated Initial Diagnostic Tests

Category	Examples	Diagnostic testing
Physiologic		
Sleep related	Hypnopompic and hypnogogic jerks	Often not required, sleep study can be performed if diagnostic uncertainty
Startle reflex		None required
Hiccups		None required
Systemic		
Drugs	Many—including opiates, benzodiazepines, antibiotics, anti-seizure medications (eg, gabapentin), and antidepressants (such as selective serotonin reuptake inhibitors [SSRIs], levodopa, and amantadine)	Drug levels, if available (anti-seizure medications and antibiotics)
Metabolic	Liver failure, renal failure, hyponatremia, hypocalcemia, hypomagnesemia, hypo/hyperglycemia, metabolic alkalosis, and hypoxemia	Complete metabolic panel, liver function tests, serum glucose/HbA$_{1c}$, serum ammonia, and arterial blood gas
Endocrine	Hyperthyroidism and hyper/hypoparathyroidism	TSH, serum calcium, and parathyroid hormone
Infectious/parainfectious	HSV, HIV, syphilis, Lyme disease, measles (Subacute sclerosing panencephalitis [SSPE]), and prion disease	Serum/CSF viral serology, treponemal Ab, Lyme serology, and RT-QuIC
Autoimmune/paraneoplastic		Anti-Ri, anti-Hu, anti-mitochondrial antibody
Neurologic		
Primary	Genetic, familial (family history present but no gene identified), or sporadic (no cause identified)	Genetic testing for myoclonic dystonia (eg, DYT-SGCE/DYT11, DYT-KCTD17/DYT26, and DYT-KMT2B/DYT28)
Epileptic	Childhood myoclonic epilepsy (eg, infantile spasms, Lennox-Gastaut syndrome, and Dravet syndrome), idiopathic generalized myoclonic epilepsies (eg, juvenile myoclonic epilepsy and myoclonic absence epilepsy)	EEG
Neurodegenerative	Alzheimer's disease, Parkinson disease dementia, dementia with Lewy bodies, corticobasal syndrome, multiple system atrophy, and Huntington disease	Clinical history and exam, MRI brain, CT-PET brain scan, dopamine transporter SPECT scan may be helpful in some cases, and genetic testing (eg, Huntington disease)
Spinocerebellar ataxias (SCAs)	SCA2, SCA3, and SCA17	Genetic testing, repeat expansion panel, and whole-exome sequencing
Structural CNS lesion	Stroke, tumor, trauma, and abscess	MRI brain and intracranial vessel imaging
Autoimmune	Hashimoto encephalopathy	Antithyroid antibodies
Posthypoxic intention (action) myoclonus	Lance-Adams syndrome	History of anoxic episode (eg, cardiac arrest and MRI brain)

CNS, central nervous system; CSF, cerebrospinal fluid; CT-PET, computed tomography-positron emission tomography; EEG, electroencephalogram; MRI, magnetic resonance imaging; RT-QuIC, real-time quaking-induced conversion; SPECT, single-photon emission computed tomography; TSH, thyroid-stimulating hormone.

of systemic illness (eg, hepatic failure) or neurologic conditions (such as Alzheimer disease or DLB).

Table 19.9 lists examples of causes of primary and secondary myoclonus. The choice of diagnostic tests will depend on information gathered during the history and examination, with particular attention to the medication history. Routine laboratory tests to exclude metabolic etiologies of myoclonus include electrolytes, renal and liver function tests, ammonia, glucose, and thyroid function tests. Electroencephalogram (EEG) should be obtained if myoclonic epilepsy is being considered. In patients with concurrent cognitive decline, brain MRI should be performed to evaluate for Creutzfeldt-Jakob disease or patterns of atrophy suggestive of specific neurodegenerative diseases. If the etiology of myoclonus is not determined by these tests, cerebrospinal fluid (CSF) and/or genetic testing may be considered.

Treatment of Myoclonus

For myoclonus secondary to metabolic, toxic, or other systemic etiologies, treatment is of the underlying etiology or by withdrawal of the offending agent. Epileptic myoclonus is treated with anti-seizure medications. Myoclonus related to brain injury (eg, hypoxic-ischemic) or neurodegenerative disease is generally treated with levetiracetam, sodium valproate, zonisamide, clonazepam, barbiturates, or a combination of these. Other anti-seizure medications, such as carbamazepine and lamotrigine, can paradoxically worsen myoclonus.

DRUG-INDUCED MOVEMENT DISORDERS

Drug-Induced Parkinsonism

Drug-induced parkinsonism is caused by dopamine blocking drugs such as antipsychotics and antiemetics (eg, metoclopramide and prochlorperazine). Drug-induced parkinsonism is more common with first-generation (typical) antipsychotics but can also occur with second-generation (atypical) antipsychotics. Medications more rarely associated with parkinsonism include calcium channel blockers (eg, flunarizine or cinnarizine; neither of these are FDA approved in the United States), lithium, and sodium valproate. The onset of drug-induced parkinsonism can be days to months after initiation or dose increase of a culprit medication. On examination, bradykinesia, rigidity, and tremor are usually symmetric but may be asymmetric. The tremor may be a pill-rolling rest tremor as in idiopathic PD, but often also has a postural or kinetic component.

A common dilemma in older patients with drug-induced parkinsonism is whether the parkinsonism is purely drug induced or represents an unmasking of underlying neurodegenerative parkinsonism. Cases of purely drug-induced parkinsonism may have other "tardive" features, such as tardive dyskinesia or dystonia. Clues that suggest a neurodegenerative etiology include prodromal REM sleep behavior disorder or anosmia. In clinically ambiguous cases, a dopamine transporter SPECT scan can be obtained, which will be normal in patients with purely drug-induced parkinsonism but abnormal in patients with neurodegenerative parkinsonism.

The mainstay of treatment of drug-induced parkinsonism is withdrawal of the offending agent, although improvement can take several months. If the patient requires treatment with a medication from the culprit drug class (eg, antipsychotics for schizophrenia), attempts could be made to reduce the dosage or switch from typical to atypical antipsychotics (eg, clozapine) with careful psychiatric monitoring. If the risk of stopping or changing medications is too high, then anticholinergic agents such as benztropine, trihexyphenidyl, or amantadine may be considered for symptomatic treatment.

Tardive Syndromes

Tardive syndrome is an umbrella term that refers to delayed onset of involuntary hyperkinetic movements caused by dopamine receptor blocking medications such as antipsychotic medications or certain antiemetic medications. A tardive syndrome is suspected when involuntary movements begin within at least a few months of initiating a dopamine receptor blocker (although individuals older than age 60 may develop symptoms with shorter-duration exposure). The movements typically develop slowly over weeks to years, sometimes with a waxing and waning course. Within the tardive syndromes, there are several different types of involuntary movements, the most common being tardive dyskinesi (choreiform movements), but other less common movement disorders may occur, including tardive dystonia (sustained muscle contractions and postures), akathisia (feeling of restlessness, agitation, or jitteriness), stereotypies (eg, frequent leg crossing and uncrossing, wringing of hands, rocking back and forth), tics, myoclonus, tremor, and parkinsonism. An individual may experience a combination of these movements. Tardive dyskinesia refers specifically to choreoathetoid movements that typically involve the lips, tongue, and jaw (orobuccolingual), for example, tongue protrusions, lip smacking, or chewing movements. Tardive dyskinesia can also involve the limbs, trunk, and respiratory muscles, the latter causing irregular or loud breathing.

To diagnose a tardive syndrome, the medication history is particularly important, including a history of prior exposure to a dopamine receptor blocking medication (Table 19.10) within the past

TABLE 19.10 **Examples of Medications With Potential to Cause Tardive Syndromes**

Category	Class	Examples
Psychiatric medications	Typical antipsychotic medications[a]	Chlorpromazine Perphenazine Fluphenazine Haloperidol
	Atypical antipsychotic medications	Olanzapine Aripiprazole Risperidone
	Other psychiatric medications	Tricyclic antidepressants Selective serotonin reuptake inhibitors (SSRIs) Serotonin norepinephrine reuptake inhibitors (SNRIs) Lithium
Gastrointestinal medications	Gastric motility agents or antiemetics	Metoclopramide Prochlorperazine
Cardiac medications	Calcium channel blockers	Cinnarizine Flunarizine (Cinnarizine/Flunarizine are not FDA approved in the United States)

[a]Most common cause of tardive syndromes.

1 to 2 years and any recent dose changes. It is important to ask about any injected medications, as some antipsychotics are given as depot injections on a weekly or monthly basis. Tardive syndromes are more common in patients treated with first-generation antipsychotic medications (annual incidence of 6.5%)[3] such as haloperidol or perphenazine; however, the risk is still present in patients treated with newer generation (atypical) antipsychotic agents (annual incidence of 2.6%)[3], with the exception of clozapine for which the risk is very low. Several nonpsychiatric medications have also been linked to tardive syndromes, including antiemetic and gastric motility medications that block dopamine receptors (eg, metoclopramide and prochlorperazine), and less commonly other drug classes, including anti-arrhythmics, antidepressants, and anti-seizure medications (Table 19.10).

The history, examination, and diagnostic testing should also seek to exclude other causes of dyskinesias or involuntary movements, including PD, Huntington disease, Wilson disease, or infectious, autoimmune, or paraneoplastic causes of hyperkinetic movements. A tardive tremor may clinically mimic a parkinsonian tremor, and a dopamine transporter SPECT scan may therefore be helpful to differentiate it from neurodegenerative PD (normal in tardive tremor and abnormal in PD).

For patients with a history of psychiatric illness, it is helpful to establish communication with the patient's psychiatric provider, both to verify the complete prior psychiatric medication list and for collaboration on future management. If safe and feasible, it is recommended to switch to a nondopamine receptor blocking medication (such as an alternative antiemetic or antidepressant), or if an antipsychotic medication is still required, to switch from a typical antipsychotic to an atypical antipsychotic, such as clozapine. Any withdrawal or switch from a dopamine receptor blocker should be done slowly, as a quick wean or withdrawal can exacerbate tardive symptoms. Withdrawal of the causative agent is associated with an improvement or resolution in tardive symptoms in a minority of cases.

For tardive symptoms that are impacting quality of life, treatment with VMAT inhibitors, which reduce dopamine release, may be indicated. There are two FDA-approved medications for tardive dyskinesia, deutetrabenazine and valbenazine, which are longer acting and have better side effect profiles compared to older VMAT inhibitors (eg, tetrabenazine). Side effects include depression and parkinsonism, and deutetrabenazine carries an FDA boxed warning for risk of suicide. Second-line agents include amantadine, clonazepam, baclofen, levetiracetam, vitamin B_6, and ginkgo biloba extract. Botulinum toxin injections may be used for treatment of focal tardive dystonia. For severe cases of tardive dystonia and dyskinesia, DBS to the globus pallidus interna may be considered.

Acute Dystonic Reaction

An acute dystonic reaction is a severe, sudden-onset dystonia that occurs within hours to a few days of treatment with dopamine antagonists (eg, antipsychotics and antiemetics) or dopamine-depleting medications (VMAT inhibitors). Acute dystonic reactions include deviation of the eyes or forced eye closure (oculogyric crisis and blepharospasm), turning of the neck (torticollis), hyperextension of the neck with arching of the back (opisthotonos), grimacing or locking of the jaw, jaw opening (jaw-opening dystonia), tongue protrusion (buccolingual crisis), or difficulty breathing (laryngospasm). Acute dystonic reactions are treated by withdrawing the causative medication and initiating intravenous anticholinergic medications (eg, benztropine) or intravenous antihistamine (eg, diphenhydramine), followed by ongoing oral treatment for 2 to 3 days.

SUMMARY

Movement disorders are primarily diagnosed by examination findings of either too little movement (hypokinetic) or too much movement (hyperkinetic). Hypokinetic disorders are typically referred to as parkinsonism, which is most commonly due to neurodegenerative disease but can also be caused by medications, toxins, or systemic illness. Hyperkinetic disorders, which include tremor, chorea, dystonia, and myoclonus, have a much broader differential, with many hereditary as well as secondary systemic causes. This chapter outlines the initial diagnostic workup for hypokinetic and hyperkinetic disorders to help guide evaluation and treatment of these conditions.

EDITORS' KEY POINTS

▶ Parkinsonism (bradykinesia accompanied by rigidity, tremor, or both) can be caused by medications (eg, dopamine blocking antiemetics or antipsychotics), neurodegenerative diseases (eg, PD), and toxins (eg, manganese).

▶ Motor symptoms of PD include chronically progressive slowing of movements (bradykinesia), stiffness (rigidity), rest tremor, and postural instability. Bradykinesia, rigidity, and rest tremor are usually unilateral at onset and often remain asymmetric throughout the disease course. The diagnosis of PD is made clinically and confirmed by a clear and sustained response to levodopa therapy.

▶ Nonmotor symptoms of PD include cognitive and psychiatric changes, REM sleep behavior disorder, gastrointestinal symptoms (most commonly constipation), anosmia, and autonomic symptoms. These nonmotor symptoms may predate motor symptoms by many years.

▶ For most patients with PD, levodopa is the first-line medication. As the disease progresses, patients may experience complications known as motor fluctuations, including wearing off and dyskinesias. Treatment of these complications includes alteration of the dose, frequency, or formulation of levodopa administration, adjunctive medications (eg, medications to potentiate the effect of levodopa or medications with other mechanisms), or the use of surgical approaches such as DBS or focused ultrasound thalamotomy.

▶ Atypical parkinsonian syndromes are neurodegenerative diseases that are characterized by the presence of parkinsonism and additional characteristic neurologic features not typically seen in PD. These include DLB (which causes parkinsonism, dementia, hallucinations, and fluctuations in alertness), MSA (which causes parkinsonism and/or cerebellar ataxia with dysautonomia), PSP (which causes parkinsonism with a vertical gaze palsy and early falls), and CBS (which causes parkinsonism with asymmetric cortical signs such as myoclonus, apraxia, and alien hand).

▶ Wilson disease is a rare, autosomal recessive condition caused by the accumulation of copper in the liver, brain, and other organs. Although rare, the diagnosis should be considered in any patient younger than age 50 with a new-onset movement disorder because it is treatable with medications that reduce copper levels.

▶ Essential tremor is a common disorder that causes a symmetric postural and kinetic tremor most commonly affecting the hands; it may also affect the head and voice. Treatment includes the use of adaptive devices, pharmacologic therapy with propranolol or primidone, or in severe medication-refractory cases, surgical therapies (DBS or focused ultrasound thalamotomy) may be considered.

▶ Huntington disease is an autosomal dominant inherited condition caused by a triplet repeat expansion in the *huntingtin* gene; the classic clinical triad includes motor symptoms (chorea, oculomotor abnormalities, dystonia, tics, myoclonus, and parkinsonism), progressive psychiatric symptoms (including increased risk of suicidality), and cognitive impairment. Treatment is symptomatic with dopamine blocking medications.

▶ Dystonia refers to involuntary sustained or intermittent co-contraction of muscle groups that leads to repetitive patterned twisting movements and abnormal postures that may be accompanied by tremor. Dystonia can be focal, multifocal, or generalized. Treatments include botulinum toxin, surgical therapy for severe medication-resistant cases, and levodopa for rare, genetic dopa-responsive dystonias.

▶ Dopamine receptor blocking medications such as antipsychotic medications or certain antiemetic medications may cause drug-induced parkinsonism or tardive syndromes (delayed onset involuntary hyperkinetic movements). Treatment involves changing the medication regimen if safe to do so from a psychiatric perspective.

▶ Acute dystonic reactions (which may include oculogyric crisis, blepharospasm, torticollis, opisthotonos, grimacing or locking of the jaw, or laryngospasm) may occur within hours to a few days of treatment with dopamine antagonists; treatment includes withdrawing the causative medication and initiating intravenous anticholinergic or antihistamine agents.

REFERENCES

1. Tan MM, Malek N, Lawton MA, et al. Genetic analysis of Mendelian mutations in a large UK population-based Parkinson's disease study. *Brain*. 2019;142(9):2828-2844.
2. Högl B, Stefani A, Videnovic A. Idiopathic REM sleep behaviour disorder and neurodegeneration—an update. *Nat Rev Neurol*. 2018;14(1):40-55.
3. Factor SA, Burkhard PR, Caroff S, et al. Recent developments in drug-induced movement disorders: a mixed picture. *Lancet Neurol*. 2019;18(9):880-890.

Multiple Sclerosis and Other Demyelinating Diseases of the Central Nervous System

Monica M. Diaz and Irena Dujmovic Basuroski

INTRODUCTION

Demyelinating diseases are a group of neurologic disorders that lead to dysfunction of the myelin sheath coating nerve fibers, which disrupts signal transmission and neuronal connectivity, leading to a wide spectrum of clinical manifestations. These disorders challenge both clinicians and researchers, as they encompass a range of etiologies, pathogenic mechanisms, and clinical presentations. In this chapter, we review multiple sclerosis (MS) and other central nervous system (CNS) demyelinating diseases, including neuromyelitis optica spectrum disorder (NMOSD), myelin oligodendrocyte glycoprotein (MOG) antibody-associated disease (MOGAD), and acute disseminated encephalomyelitis (ADEM), focusing on pathophysiology, clinical presentation, diagnostic evaluation, and treatment of these conditions.

MULTIPLE SCLEROSIS

Background

MS is a chronic inflammatory disease affecting the myelin of the CNS. Approximately 3 million people live with MS worldwide (prevalence 35.9 per 100,000 population), but this is likely an underestimation given lack of access to neurologists and diagnostic tests in many regions of the world.[1] The prevalence is greater at higher latitudes (ie, further from the equator). The disease usually starts between the ages of 20 and 40, but MS onset can occur in children as well as in older patients. MS is more frequent in women. The precise pathophysiology initiating immune-mediated demyelination in MS is unknown but is hypothesized to involve both environmental factors and genetic predisposition. Risk factors for the development of MS include Epstein-Barr virus (EBV) infection, vitamin D deficiency, low sunlight exposure, childhood obesity, and smoking.

Clinical Features of Multiple Sclerosis

The clinical presentations of MS have classically been divided into relapsing-remitting MS, secondary progressive MS, and primary-progressive MS (PPMS). In relapsing-remitting MS, the patient has distinct periods of relapses (also called flares or attacks) of MS followed by periods of remission (recovery or partial recovery from the preceding relapse). In secondary progressive MS, there is gradual worsening of neurologic disability over time independent of relapses, in a patient who previously had relapsing-remitting MS. PPMS is characterized by progressive worsening of symptoms from the initial onset of the disease without remission, although a relapsing form of PPMS does exist.

Relapsing-Remitting Multiple Sclerosis

Relapses of MS cause symptoms related to demyelination in a particular region of the CNS. Symptoms arise and progress over days, last weeks, and generally improve over months. Common sites of involvement include the optic nerve (causing optic neuritis), spinal cord (causing myelitis), cerebellum, and brainstem.

Optic neuritis in MS is most commonly monocular, causing central vision loss and decreased color vision in one eye with pain upon eye movement. Examination may demonstrate decreased visual acuity in the affected eye, impaired performance on Ishihara color plates, central scotoma on Amsler grid testing (the patient sees distortion of the center of the grid), and relative afferent pupillary defect (both pupils constrict when light is shined in the unaffected eye [normal direct and consensual response to light], but constrict less or not at all when light is moved from the unaffected eye to the affected eye [impaired direct response]), and there may be optic disc edema on fundoscopy. Magnetic resonance imaging (MRI) of the orbit may demonstrate contrast enhancement of the affected optic nerve. Most patients with MS recover vision completely or significantly after the first attack of optic neuritis, but subsequent attacks may have less recovery.

In MS-associated myelitis, patients develop numbness, tingling, and/or weakness on one side or both sides of the body, often accompanied by bladder, bowel, and/or sexual dysfunction. Myelitis is typically not fully transverse in MS as it commonly is in NMO (see later) and is therefore usually less severe.

A relapse involving the cerebellum causes unilateral ataxia, which may be accompanied by vertigo and nystagmus. The most common brainstem symptom of an MS relapse is internuclear ophthalmoplegia due to a lesion of the medial longitudinal fasciculus, causing failure of one or both eyes to adduct on contralateral gaze (ie, impaired adduction of the left eye on right gaze, impaired adduction of the right eye on left gaze, or both, along with nystagmus of the abducting eye). Trigeminal neuralgia may also occur due to demyelination of the trigeminal pathways in the brainstem; unilateral or bilateral trigeminal neuralgia in a young individual should raise suspicion for MS. Speech or swallowing problems may also occur.

Repeated MS relapses over time lead to accumulation of deficits and disability including visual symptoms, sensory symptoms (tingling, numbness, pain, and burning sensation), muscle weakness, spasticity, balance problems, gait dysfunction, neurogenic bladder (hesitancy, incomplete emptying, retention, incontinence, urgency, and frequency), constipation, sexual dysfunction, cognitive impairment, and mood disorders. Patients may report heat sensitivity (called the *Uhthoff phenomenon*) or a sudden, electric shock–like or stabbing sensation traveling down the spine radiating to the limbs, particularly when the neck is flexed (called the *Lhermitte phenomenon*). Examination outside of acute relapses may demonstrate relative afferent pupillary defect and diminished visual acuity from prior episodes of optic neuritis, spasticity and other upper motor neuron signs (eg, hyperreflexia, clonus, and Babinski sign) due to prior episodes of myelitis, as well as areas of numbness and gait dysfunction.

Progressive Multiple Sclerosis

Secondary progressive MS is defined as insidious worsening of neurologic disability over time in a patient with prior relapsing-remitting MS that is independent of relapses.[2] MS disease progression independent of relapses is responsible for irreversible accumulation of disability that occurs in progressive MS. Most patients who begin initially with a relapsing-remitting MS disease course will eventually transition to secondary progressive MS. Disease-modifying treatment for MS (see later) lowers the risk of converting from relapsing-remitting MS to secondary progressive MS.

In PPMS, the patient develops progressive worsening of symptoms from the time of disease onset without remission. PPMS occurs in 10% to 15% of all patients with MS worldwide,[3] and factors usually associated with PPMS are male gender and older age of disease onset (older than age 40).

Diagnosis of Multiple Sclerosis

MS is diagnosed by a combination of clinical features, MRI findings, and, in some cases, the finding of oligoclonal bands on cerebrospinal fluid (CSF) analysis (the latter measuring intrathecal immunoglobulin G [IgG] synthesis, a nonspecific marker of immune activation in the CNS that is present in most patients with MS). MRI in MS demonstrates multiple, small, ovoid lesions in the white matter of the brain, brainstem, cerebellum, and/or spinal cord on T2-weighted and fluid-attenuated inversion recovery (FLAIR) sequences (Figures 20.1, 20.2, and 20.3). Acute lesions may enhance on postcontrast sequences. Rarely, large lesions (known as *tumefactive* lesions) may occur. Over time, T1 hypointensities on MRI called *black holes* may develop at sites of chronic demyelination (Figure 20.4A).

If obtained, CSF parameters (ie, cell count, protein, and glucose) are typically normal in MS, although small elevations in protein and white blood cell count may be seen. CSF-specific oligoclonal bands are present in most patients with MS, although they are not specific for MS and can be seen in other CNS inflammatory conditions as well as in neurologic infections.

Diagnostic criteria for relapsing-remitting MS require clinical and radiologic demonstration of dissemination of lesions in space and time in the appropriate clinical context.[4] Evidence for dissemination in space can be determined by the patient having clinical evidence of lesions affecting different parts of the CNS, or MRI evidence of lesions in two or more distinct locations out of the following four: cortical/juxtacortical (lesions in the cortex or in the white matter adjacent to the cortex), periventricular (in the white matter adjacent to the ventricles), infratentorial (white matter of the brainstem or cerebellum), and spinal cord. Evidence for dissemination in time can be determined by the patient having two or more clinical relapses, or a single clinical attack with MRI evidence of both acute lesions (ie, enhancing with gadolinium; Figure 20.4B) and chronic lesions (ie, nonenhancing), or presence of CSF oligoclonal IgG bands. Since dissemination in space and time can be demonstrated on MRI at a single point in time (ie, by lesions in at least two out of four locations with some enhancing lesions), the diagnosis of relapsing-remitting MS can be made in

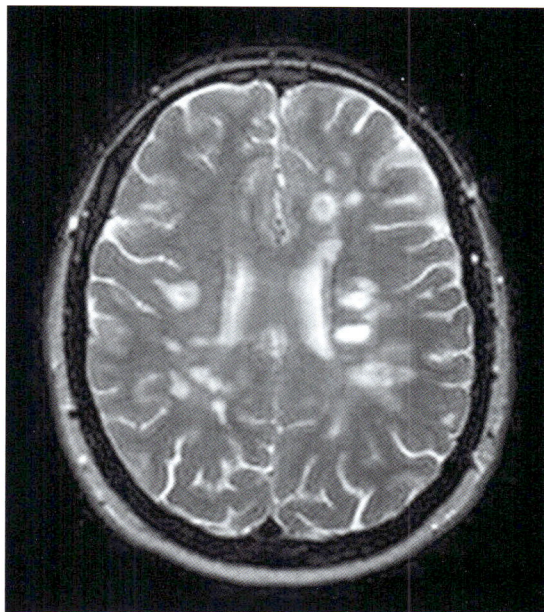

FIGURE 20.1 Axial T2-weighted brain magnetic resonance imaging showing multiple ovoid hyperintensities in the periventricular white matter in a patient with multiple sclerosis.

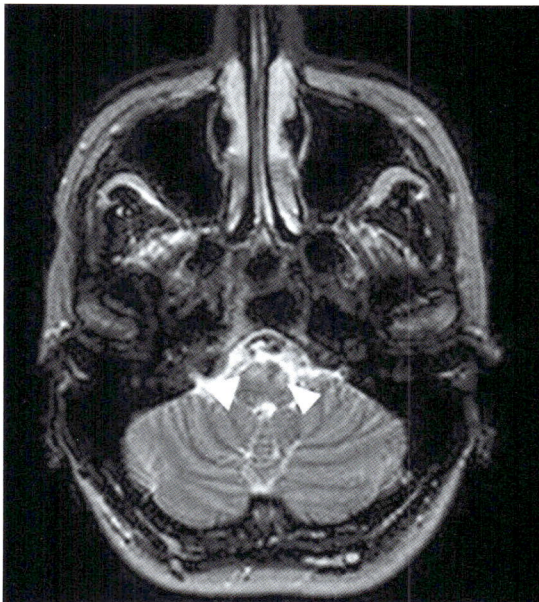

FIGURE 20.2 Axial T2-weighted magnetic resonance imaging showing hyperintensities in the medulla (arrowheads) in a patient with multiple sclerosis.

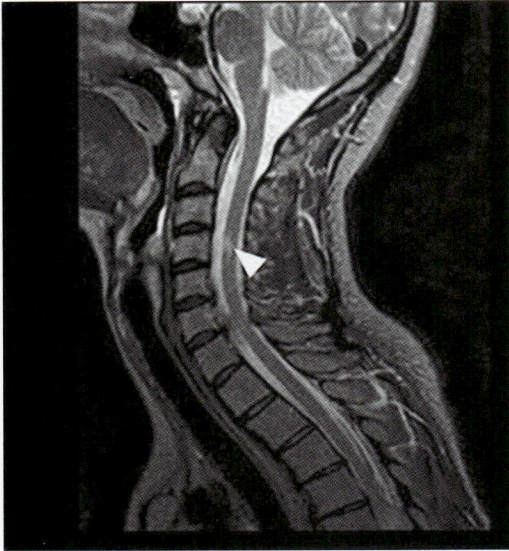

FIGURE 20.3 Sagittal T2-weighted magnetic resonance imaging of the cervical spine demonstrating a T2 hyperintense lesion at the C4 level (arrowhead) in a patient with multiple sclerosis.

some patients at the time of the first attack. This earlier diagnosis of MS at the time of a first attack with the current diagnostic criteria allows for earlier initiation of disease-modifying therapy (DMT) than with previous diagnostic criteria.

The term *clinically isolated syndrome* refers to the first clinical presentation of a classic CNS demyelinating syndrome (eg, optic neuritis or transverse myelitis). Some patients with clinically isolated syndrome do not meet criteria for MS and should be followed clinically for potential development of the disease, whereas others meet the criteria for dissemination in space and time and can be diagnosed with MS at the time of the first attack.

Diagnosis of PPMS requires 1 year of disability progression independent of clinical relapses and two of the following: one or more T2 hyperintense brain MRI lesions characteristic of MS in periventricular, or cortical/juxtacortical, or infratentorial regions; two or more T2 hyperintense MRI lesions in the spinal cord; CSF-specific oligoclonal IgG bands.

Given that many conditions can cause white matter lesions in the brain, the diagnostic criteria for MS—and the diagnosis of MS—should only be considered in patients with a clinical history consistent with the condition. Table 20.1 presents examples of other conditions that can cause CNS dysfunction, many with accompanying white matter lesions. Sometimes called *MS mimics*, an evaluation for these conditions should be considered in patients whose clinical presentation and/or MRI is not typical for MS.

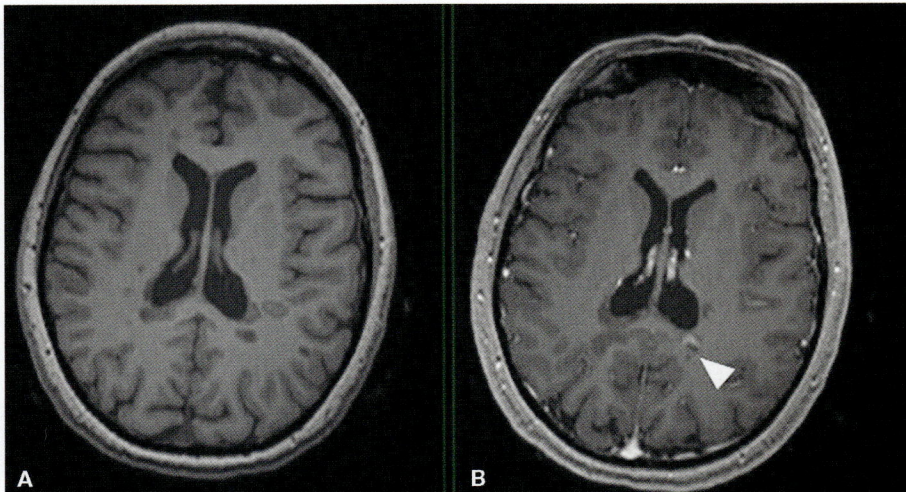

FIGURE 20.4 A. Axial T1-weighted magnetic resonance imaging (MRI) showing periventricular black holes in a patient with multiple sclerosis. B. Axial T1-weighted postcontrast MRI showing enhancement of one of the lesions (arrowhead).

TABLE 20.1	Conditions That Can Mimic MS
Inflammatory/ autoimmune/ rheumatologic	Acute disseminated encephalomyelitis Neurosarcoidosis Primary CNS vasculitis Histiocytosis Systemic lupus erythematosus Sjögren syndrome Behçet disease Susac syndrome Neuromyelitis optica spectrum disorder (NMOSD) Myelin oligodendrocyte glycoprotein antibody-associated disorder Idiopathic transverse myelitis Idiopathic optic neuritis
Infectious	HTLV-1 Lyme disease HIV Neurosyphilis
Vascular	Cerebral small vessel disease/cerebral microvascular disease
Nutritional/ metabolic	Vitamin B_{12} deficiency Copper deficiency
Genetic	CADASIL Leukodystrophies Mitochondrial diseases
Other	Migraine White matter brain lesions due to normal aging Functional neurologic disorder

CADASIL, cerebral autosomal dominant arteriopathy with subcortical infarcts and leukoencephalopathy; CNS, central nervous system; HIV, human immunodeficiency virus; HTLV-1, human T-lymphotropic virus type 1; MS, multiple sclerosis.

Sometimes, MRI obtained for headache or another indication reveals lesions consistent with MS despite the lack of clinical history or exam findings suggestive of the disease. This scenario is called *radiologically isolated syndrome* and carries an approximately 50% risk of future development of MS over 10 years. The risk for conversion from radiologically isolated syndrome to MS is higher in patients who are younger than 37 years of age, have CSF-specific oligoclonal bands, have infratentorial and spinal cord lesions, and/or have gadolinium-enhancing lesions on MRI.[5] Some MS specialists may consider offering patients with radiologically isolated syndrome disease-modifying treatment for MS when one or more of these high-risk features is present.

Treatment of Multiple Sclerosis

Treatment of MS involves disease-modifying treatment, treatment of acute relapses, and symptomatic management.

Disease-Modifying Therapy

DMT in relapsing-remitting MS reduces the risks of relapse, long-term disability, and conversion to secondary progressive MS. Practice guidelines therefore recommend initiation of treatment at the time of MS diagnosis and discussing the benefits and risks of DMT for people with a single clinical demyelinating event.[6] Given the large number of treatment options available, factors to be considered in choosing a treatment include: patient-related factors (eg, patient preference, risk tolerance, comorbidities, pregnancy plans, and lifestyle), disease-related factors (eg, disease course, disease severity/activity, and prognostic factors), treatment-related factors (eg, drug efficacy, safety, tolerability, monitoring requirements, frequency, and route of administration), and system-related factors (eg, access to medical care, cost, and insurance coverage).

Some patients ask whether treatment needs to be initiated after a first attack or whether it would be safe to wait until a second relapse. While it is recommended that all patients diagnosed with MS initiate DMT, patients can be counseled on the risk of relapse and disease progression based on their particular demographic, clinical, and radiologic data; factors associated with poorer prognosis are listed in Table 20.2. If the patient prefers to defer initiation of treatment, clinicians generally recommend serial imaging at least annually for the first 5 years and close follow-up if the patient has a clinically isolated syndrome not meeting criteria for MS or has relapsing-remitting MS but has not had relapses in the preceding 2 years and does not have active new MRI lesion activity on recent imaging.

MS disease-modifying treatments are categorized by mode of administration (eg, injectable, oral, and infusion) and level of efficacy. Injectable treatments, such as glatiramer acetate, interferon β-1a, and interferon β-1b, are considered low/moderate-efficacy DMT but have a good safety profile and have been in use since the early 1990s; ofatumumab is a

TABLE 20.2   Prognostic Factors Associated With Poorer Clinical Outcomes in MS

Demographic and clinical features	Older age at onset
	Male sex
	Black, Latino, Middle Eastern, North African, and Asian ancestry compared with Northern European ancestry
	Cardiovascular comorbidities (eg, hypertension, diabetes, hypercholesterolemia)
	Psychiatric comorbidities (eg, depression)
	Smoking
MS clinical disease characteristics	More frequent relapses during initial years of disease onset
	Brief intervals between attacks
	Poor recovery following first relapse
	Type of clinical symptom during first attack: pyramidal, cerebellar, bladder/bowel symptoms, cognitive symptoms
	Clinical presentation other than optic neuritis
	Multifocal presentation at onset
	Progression at onset
	Rapid progression of disability
Radiographic features	New T2 lesions over time
	Gadolinium contrast-enhancing lesions at baseline
	Infratentorial (cerebellar, brainstem) lesions at baseline
	Spinal cord lesions at baseline
Laboratory measures	CSF-specific oligoclonal IgG bands

CSF, cerebrospinal fluid; IgG, immunoglobulin G; MS, multiple sclerosis.

high-efficacy injectable treatment (described later under B-cell–depleting agents). Patients with lower disease severity based on clinical (infrequent relapses), radiographic (lower T2 lesion burden and/or no spinal cord lesions), or other risk factors considered to be associated with less frequent relapses (older age and less disability) may be considered for a low/moderate-efficacy injectable treatment, if appropriate. Patients must be counseled on injection fatigue and side effects (listed in Table 20.3).

Traditionally, MS has been treated with a stepwise escalation approach using low/moderate- or moderate-efficacy DMT and subsequently escalating to higher-efficacy treatment if there is clinical or radiographic disease activity. Patients with moderate disease activity based on clinical and radiographic indicators (relapse frequency, relapse severity, MRI lesion burden, and presence of spinal cord lesions) could be considered for a moderate-efficacy DMT, but the risks, benefits, and side-effect profiles should be discussed with patients prior to a decision on DMT. There may be some benefit to initiating a higher-efficacy DMT earlier in the disease course, weighing the risks of higher-efficacy treatment. The infusions ocrelizumab, ublituximab-xiiy, natalizumab, and alemtuzumab; the injectable ofatumumab; and the oral medication cladribine are generally considered higher-efficacy DMTs. These higher-efficacy DMTs could be considered in patients with more severe disease (more frequent clinical relapses, more severe relapses, high MRI brain lesion burden, several spinal cord lesions, and infratentorial lesions) and other risk factors known to be associated with more severe disease activity (see Table 20.2).

Most of the oral DMTs are considered to be moderate-efficacy treatments: teriflunomide, dimethyl fumarate, diroximel fumarate, monomethyl fumarate, and the sphingosine-1-phosphate (S1P) receptor modulators fingolimod, siponimod, ozanimod, and ponesimod. Some of these oral DMTs have notable side effects that must be discussed with the patient when considering starting a new DMT. Notably, teriflunomide may be teratogenic and should always be taken with effective birth control in women of childbearing age. Teriflunomide is detected in human semen, so men taking teriflunomide who wish to father a child should discontinue use of teriflunomide and undergo an accelerated elimination procedure to reduce plasma concentrations of the medication first. Potentially serious side effects associated with fingolimod include bradycardia and bradyarrhythmia; therefore, all patients must be observed by a health care professional for a period of at least 6 hours after taking the first dose of fingolimod. Newer S1P modulators (siponimod, ponesimod, and ozanimod) are more selective with less cardiac side effects than fingolimod, and therefore, do not usually require first dose monitoring (see Table 20.3).

Mode of administration	Generic drug name	Clinical indications (per FDA label)	Mechanism of action	Adverse effects	Drug safety monitoring[a,b,c]
Injectables	Glatiramer acetate	CIS, RRMS, active SPMS in adults	Inhibition of activation of autoreactive T cells leading to anti-inflammatory effects	Immediate postinjection reactions (flushing, chest pain, palpitations, tachycardia, anxiety, dyspnea, constriction of the throat), chest pain, potential effects on the immune system, allergic reactions, injection site reactions including lipoatrophy and skin necrosis, hepatic injury	Prior to treatment initiation: no laboratory tests are required except when known/suspected liver pathology (LFTs) While on treatment: no laboratory monitoring is required except when liver injury is suspected (LFTs)
	Interferon β-1a, peginterferon β-1a	CIS, RRMS, active SPMS in adults	Interferes with secretion of pro and anti-inflammatory cytokines, suppresses T cell activation, reducing cell trafficking across blood-brain barrier	Injection site reactions including skin necrosis, flu-like symptoms, transaminitis, decreased peripheral blood counts, allergic reactions, mood changes	Prior to treatment initiation: CBC/diff, LFTs, TSH While on treatment: monitoring CBC/diff, LFTs, TSH
	Interferon β-1b	CIS, RRMS, active SPMS in adults	Same as for interferon β-1a	Injection site reactions, flu-like symptoms, fatigue, nausea, transaminitis, leukopenia or thrombocytopenia (rare), allergic reactions, mood changes, thrombotic microangiopathy, pulmonary arterial hypertension, seizures, secondary autoimmune disorders (idiopathic thrombocytopenia, hyper- and hypothyroidism, and rare cases of autoimmune hepatitis), congestive heart failure	Prior to treatment initiation: CBC/diff, LFTs, TSH While on treatment: CBC/diff, LFTs, TSH
	Ofatumumab	CIS, RRMS, active SPMS in adults	Fully human monoclonal antibody that binds to CD20 on CD20+ B cells, and CD20+ T cells, mostly acts as a B-cell-depleting agent	Injection-related reactions, infections (including PML that can occur), hepatitis B reactivation, fetal harm, reduced vaccine effectiveness	Prior to treatment initiation: CBC/diff, LFTs, hepatitis B screening, quantitative immunoglobulin levels, up-to-date on vaccines While on treatment: CBC w/diff, IgM, IgG

(continued)

TABLE 20.3 **Currently Available Disease-Modifying Treatments for MS Approved by the FDA** (*continued*)

Mode of administration	Generic drug name	Clinical indications (per FDA label)	Mechanism of action	Adverse effects	Drug safety monitoring[a,b,c]
Oral	Teriflunomide	CIS, RRMS, active SPMS in adults	Pyrimidine synthesis inhibitor, reduces proliferation of T and B lymphocytes	Liver toxicity, teratogenic, bone marrow toxicity (WBC decrease, ANC or ALC decrease, thrombocytopenia), increase in creatinine, infections, hair thinning, peripheral neuropathy, increased blood pressure, hypersensitivity and allergy, interstitial lung disease	Prior to treatment initiation: CBC w/diff, LFTs, serum creatinine, pregnancy test, tuberculosis screening, blood pressure. While on treatment: CBC w/differential, LFTs, serum creatinine, blood pressure
	Dimethyl fumarate	CIS, RRMS, active SPMS in adults	Modulates the immune response and has antioxidant properties	Lymphopenia, flushing, skin itching, infections (including PML), gastrointestinal symptoms (nausea, vomiting, diarrhea, abdominal pain), increase in AST, allergy	Prior to treatment initiation: CBC w/diff, LFTs. While on treatment: CBC/diff, LFTs
	Monomethyl fumarate	CIS, RRMS, active SPMS in adults	Oral fumarate with the same mode of action as dimethyl fumarate and diroximel fumarate	Same adverse effect profile as dimethyl fumarate and diroximel fumarate	Same as for dimethyl fumarate
	Diroximel fumarate	CIS, RRMS, active SPMS in adults	Oral fumarate with the same active metabolite as dimethyl fumarate	Same adverse effect profile as dimethyl fumarate, but has been shown in a randomized clinical trial to have lower gastrointestinal adverse effects compared with dimethyl fumarate	Same as for dimethyl fumarate
	Fingolimod	CIS, RRMS, active SPMS in patients 10 y of age and older	S1P modulator: sequester lymphocytes within the lymph nodes, preventing lymphocyte egress from lymph nodes, leading to the reduction in circulating lymphocytes and therefore limiting inflammatory cell migration into the CNS	Bradycardia or bradyarrhythmia and atrioventricular blocks; infections (including PML), macular edema, liver injury, PRES, respiratory effects, fetal harm, increase in disability after drug discontinuation (disease rebound), increased blood pressure, malignancies (BCC, melanoma, lymphoma), hypersensitivity reactions	Prior to treatment initiation: • screen for infections and skin cancer • concomitant medication review for medications that could slow heart rate or affect AV conduction • VZV IgG/VZV vaccination of VZV IgG negative patients • up-to-date on other vaccinations—CBC w/diff, LFTs, ECG-ophthalmologic examination with OCT • FDO required While on treatment: • CBC w/differential, LFTs—OCT—pulse, blood pressure, signs of infection at each follow-up • skin cancer screening

Siponimod	CIS, RRMS, and active SPMS in adults	Same mechanism of action as in fingolimod, a more selective S1P modulator than fingolimod	Similar adverse events as for fingolimod, except less cardiac side effects	Prior to treatment initiation: CYP2C9 genotype • In most patients, no FDO is required, except if the patient has certain preexisting cardiac conditions • CBC/diff and LFTs • OCT • other screening is the same as for fingolimod While on treatment: same as for fingolimod, except OCT is required in case of worsening vision
Ozanimod	CIS, RRMS, active SPMS in adults	Same mechanism of action as in fingolimod, a more selective S1P modulator than fingolimod	Same adverse events as for fingolimod, except less cardiac side effects	Prior to treatment initiation: • screening is the same as for fingolimod, except OCT is required only in people with history of uveitis and diabetes mellitus • FDO could be considered in patients with cardiovascular comorbidities While on treatment: same as for fingolimod, except OCT is required in case of worsening vision
Ponesimod	CIS, RRMS, active SPMS in adults	Same mechanism of action as fingolimod, a more selective S1P modulator than fingolimod, siponimod, and ozanimod	Same adverse events as for fingolimod, except less cardiac side effects	Prior to treatment initiation: screening is the same as for fingolimod a 4-h FDO is recommended for patients with certain cardiac conditions While on treatment: same as for fingolimod, except OCT is required in case of worsening vision

(continued)

TABLE 20.3 Currently Available Disease-Modifying Treatments for MS Approved by the FDA (*continued*)

Mode of administration	Generic drug name	Clinical indications (per FDA label)	Mechanism of action	Adverse effects	Drug safety monitoring[a,b,c]
	Cladribine	RRMS, active SPMS in adults	A purine analogue that selectively suppresses T and B lymphocytes; immune reconstitution therapy	Malignancies, teratogenicity, infections (PML may occur), headaches, hematologic toxicity (lymphopenia, neutropenia, thrombocytopenia, anemia), graft-vs-host disease with blood transfusion, hair thinning, liver toxicity, hypersensitivity, cardiac failure	Prior to the first treatment course: • administer all immunizations according to immunization guidelines • VZV IgG (VZV vaccination in VZV IgG negative patients) • brain MRI for PML screening Prior to the first and second treatment course: • screen for contraindications: current malignancy, pregnancy in females on childbearing potential, acute infection, breast-feeding, HIV, hepatitis B and C, tuberculosis • CBC/diff, LFTs After receiving treatment: • standard cancer screening • CBC/diff
Intravenous	Natalizumab	CIS, RRMS, active SPMS in adults	Humanized monoclonal antibody that inhibits leukocyte migration across the BBB into CNS tissue, thus reducing inflammation and preventing formation of new MS lesions	PML, HSV, and VZV infections; other infections, hepatotoxicity, laboratory abnormalities (increases in circulating lymphocytes, monocytes, eosinophils, basophils), infusion reactions, allergy	Prior to treatment initiation: JC virus antibody, LFTs, screening for pregnancy While on treatment: JC virus antibody, LFTs, screening for pregnancy
	Ocrelizumab	CIS, RRMS, active SPMS in adults PPMS in adults	Humanized monoclonal antibody that targets CD20+ B lymphocytes; B-cell-depleting agent	Infusion reactions; hypogammaglobulinemia (increasing risk of infection), infections (including PML), malignancy (including breast cancer), immune-mediated colitis	Prior to treatment initiation: CBC/diff, hepatitis B screening, quantitative serum immunoglobulin levels • up-to-date on vaccinations • screening for acute infections • screening for pregnancy Prior to each maintenance infusion: • screening for active infection • pregnancy test • IgG and IgM, CBC/diff,CD19 count

Drug	Indications	Mechanism	Adverse effects	Monitoring
Ublituximab-xiiy	CIS, RRMS, active SPMS in adults	Chimeric anti-CD20 monoclonal antibody, B-cell-depleting agent	Similar to ocrelizumab	Same as for ocrelizumab
Alemtuzumab	RRMS, active SPMS in adults Because of its toxicities generally used only in patients who have not adequately responded to two or more MS DMTs	Humanized monoclonal antibody that targets CD52 antigen (expressed on several immune cell types), immune reconstitution therapy	Thyroid cancer, other malignancies (melanoma, lymphoproliferative diseases), secondary autoimmunity (autoimmune thyroid disorders, immune cytopenias, autoimmune hepatitis, glomerular nephropathies), hemophagocytic lymphohistiocytosis infusion reactions, infections (including PML), thrombotic thrombocytopenic purpura, acquired hemophilia A, acute acalculous cholecystitis, pneumonitis, ischemic or hemorrhagic stroke, cervicocephalic arterial dissection	Prior to treatment initiation: CBC/diff, pregnancy test, creatinine, urinalysis with urine cell counts, TSH • consider screening patients at high risk of hepatitis B and C infection • HIV screening • VZV IgG in patients without documented history of varicella vaccine or prior VZV infection, consider VZV vaccination in VZV IgG negative patients • up-to-date on vaccines • Skin cancer screening While on treatment: CBC/diff, LFTs, creatinine, TSH, CD4 count, urinalysis with urine cell counts, skin cancer screening
Mitoxantrone	Active SPMS, worsening RRMS	Chemotherapy agent that causes inhibition of DNA synthesis; suppresses activity of T and B cells	Cardiac toxicity, myelosuppression, leukemia, nausea/vomiting, alopecia, mouth ulcers, darkening of the skin and nails, changes in menstrual cycle, infertility, liver toxicity, fetal harm	Prior to each course of therapy: CBC w/diff, LFTs, pregnancy test, echocardiogram (for LVEF), urine culture, echocardiogram yearly after final treatment

As of 2024.

ALC, absolute lymphocyte count; ANC, absolute neutrophil count; AST, aspartate aminotransferase; AV, atrioventricular; BBB, blood-brain barrier; BCC, basal cell carcinoma; CBC/diff, complete blood count with differential; CIS, clinically isolated syndrome suggestive of multiple sclerosis (MS); CNS, central nervous system; DMT, disease-modifying therapy; ECG, electrocardiogram; FDA, U.S. Food and Drug Administration; FDO, first dose observation (predose electrocardiogram [ECG] and vitals, hourly vitals, and observed by a health care professional for a period of at least 6 hours after taking their first dose, +6h postdose ECG); HIV, human immunodeficiency virus; HSV, herpes simplex virus; Ig, immunoglobulin; LFTs, liver function tests; LVEF, left ventricular ejection fraction; MAO, monoamine oxidase; OCT, optical coherence tomography; PML, progressive multifocal encephalopathy; PPMS, primary-progressive MS; PRES, posterior reversible encephalopathy syndrome; RRMS, relapsing-remitting MS; S1P, sphingosine-1-phosphate; SPMS, secondary progressive MS; TSH, thyroid-stimulating hormone; VZV IgG, varicella zoster virus IgG; WBC, white blood count.

[a]Required in most cases, some additional tests may be needed in an individual case based on lifestyle factors and comorbidities.

[b]Screening for contraindications prior to the start on treatment is necessary for all medications.

[c]Annual brain magnetic resonance imaging study as a part of MS monitoring also serves as a PML screening in patients treated with MS DMT that theoretically might be associated with PML risk. PML risk is associated with all MS DMTs listed earlier except with glatiramer acetate and interferon β, and is less likely with teriflunomide (PML was reported in a single patient with prior exposure to natalizumab who was subsequently treated with teriflunomide).

Ocrelizumab, ublituximab, and ofatumumab are high-efficacy DMTs that deplete B cells. Side effects include infusion or injection reactions, and these agents are contraindicated in patients with active hepatitis B virus (HBV) infection. Rituximab, a well-known B-cell-depleting agent, has been used off-label as a high-efficacy MS DMT. Prior to every treatment with B-cell-depleting agents, it is important to determine whether there is an active infection and, if so, delay treatment until the infection resolves. Other reported side effects include hypogammaglobulinemia, malignancy (including breast cancer, specifically for ocrelizumab), and immune-mediated colitis. In PPMS, ocrelizumab was associated with lower rates of clinical and MRI progression compared with placebo and is the only U.S. Food and Drug Administration (FDA)-approved treatment for PPMS.

Natalizumab is another high-efficacy DMT. It has a risk of progressive multifocal leuko encephalopathy (PML), a potentially lethal opportunistic CNS infection of 0.1% overall over 18 months of treatment, but is higher in patients with positive virus antibody, prior immunosuppression use, and longer duration of treatment.[7] Monitoring of JC virus antibodies in the serum is necessary in order to assess the risk of developing PML while on natalizumab treatment.

Autologous hematopoietic stem cell transplant is being actively investigated in clinical trials as a potential treatment option for highly active relapsing-remitting MS.

Management of Multiple Sclerosis Relapses

Acute MS relapses are treated with 3 to 5 days of high-dose intravenous (IV) corticosteroids, which shortens the duration of symptoms and also may reduce the severity of a relapse. Corticosteroids are not used for chronic long-term treatment of MS. In patients unable to tolerate corticosteroids, adrenocorticotropic hormone (ACTH) injection may be considered. In rare cases of severe relapses that do not respond to steroids, plasma exchange may be considered.

Symptomatic Management

Chronic symptoms associated with MS increase disability and decrease quality of life. Therefore, symptoms such as spasticity, bladder and bowel dysfunction, sexual dysfunction, pain, changes in mood, and fatigue should be screened for and treated with symptomatic therapies. Cognitive dysfunction should be addressed with cognitive rehabilitation. Multimodal rehabilitation strategies may be useful in improving functionality in people with MS.

Other Aspects of Treatment

High-dose vitamin D3 is generally recommended in patients with MS and low vitamin D levels, although data on efficacy are conflicting. Lifestyle modification including dietary changes is usually recommended to lower body mass index as an adjunct to pharmacologic treatment of MS. Many patients with MS ask about diet. The Mediterranean diet has been associated with less disability from MS, and other diets may reduce fatigue and improve quality of life, but data are limited.

NEUROMYELITIS OPTICA SPECTRUM DISORDER

NMOSD is an inflammatory disease of the CNS often associated with antibodies against aquaporin-4 (AQP4), a water channel in the CNS that is expressed on astrocytes and pial and ependymal cells. As the name indicates, optic neuritis (inflammation of the optic nerve) and myelitis (inflammation of the spinal cord) are common in NMOSD, but the condition can also cause a variety of other neurologic presentations related to sites of disease activity that tend to cluster in areas of high AQP4 expression such as the regions surrounding the third and fourth ventricle (Figure 20.5). NMOSD can occur at any age, but onset is most common between ages 30 and 50. However, 3% to 5% of patients with NMOSD have a pediatric onset,[8] and the disease can also occur in older patients. NMOSD affects women more often than men. Unlike MS, there is no geographical prominence related to latitude, although the disease is more prevalent in some parts of the world (eg, East Asia and Martinique).

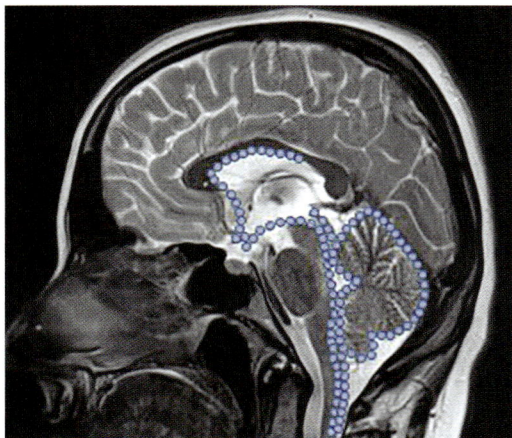

FIGURE 20.5 Brain areas (outside of the optic nerves) with high aquaporin-4 (AQP4) expression (blue dots).

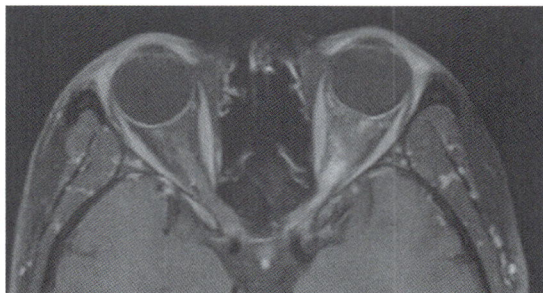

FIGURE 20.6 Axial T1-weighted postcontrast magnetic resonance imaging demonstrating extensive enhancement of the left optic nerve in a patient with neuromyelitis optica spectrum disorder.

Clinical Features of Neuromyelitis Optica Spectrum Disorder

Like MS, NMOSD is typically a relapsing disease, presenting with flares of symptoms (disease attacks) arising and progressing over days. NMOSD can also be a monophasic disease, but categorizing NMOSD as "monophasic" depends on the duration of follow-up since disease relapses after more than 10 years from the first attack have been reported. In NMOSD, deficits during an acute attack are often more severe than in MS, and recovery from flares is often incomplete.

Optic neuritis in NMOSD is usually more severe than optic neuritis in MS, often causing complete blindness. It may be bilateral at onset. On MRI with contrast, enhancement of the optic nerve may be extensive, involving the nerve from orbit to optic chiasm, and more often affects the posterior portion of the optic nerve (Figure 20.6).

Myelitis in NMOSD is typically longitudinally extensive, meaning that it extends the length of three or more vertebral segments of the spinal cord (called *longitudinally extensive transverse myelitis*) and may extend up to the entire length of the spinal cord (Figure 20.7). However, lesions affecting less than three vertebral segments may also be seen in NMOSD. Spinal cord lesions in NMOSD are typically localized in the central

cord. This is in contrast to the smaller, more peripheral spinal cord lesions seen in MS-associated myelitis. Patients present with extremity weakness and sensory impairment below the level of the lesion with bowel, bladder, and/or sexual dysfunction and may also have balance problems and dysautonomia.

In addition to the optic neuritis and transverse myelitis that are part of its name, NMOSD can cause a number of other clinical manifestations. In area postrema syndrome, patients present with intractable hiccups and/or nausea and vomiting without other known etiology. This is caused by a lesion in the area postrema of the dorsal medulla (Figure 20.8). In acute brainstem syndrome, patients present with one or more symptoms related to the brainstem (eg, vertigo, diplopia, hearing loss, ataxia, weakness, and trigeminal neuralgia). In acute diencephalic clinical syndrome, patients can develop symptoms related to involvement of the thalamus and hypothalamus (including a narcolepsy-like syndrome, changes in appetite causing anorexia or obesity, hypothermia or fever, syndrome of inappropriate antidiuretic hormone secretion, and other endocrine dysfunction). In symptomatic cerebral syndrome, patients develop symptoms and signs referable to the cerebral hemispheres (eg, encephalopathy, hemiparesis, cortical visual loss, and seizures). Brain lesions in NMOSD can have variable appearance on MRI, including large confluent tumor-like lesions, lesions spanning the corpus callosum, lesions extending along the corticospinal tracts, and periependymal lesions surrounding the third, fourth, and lateral ventricles.

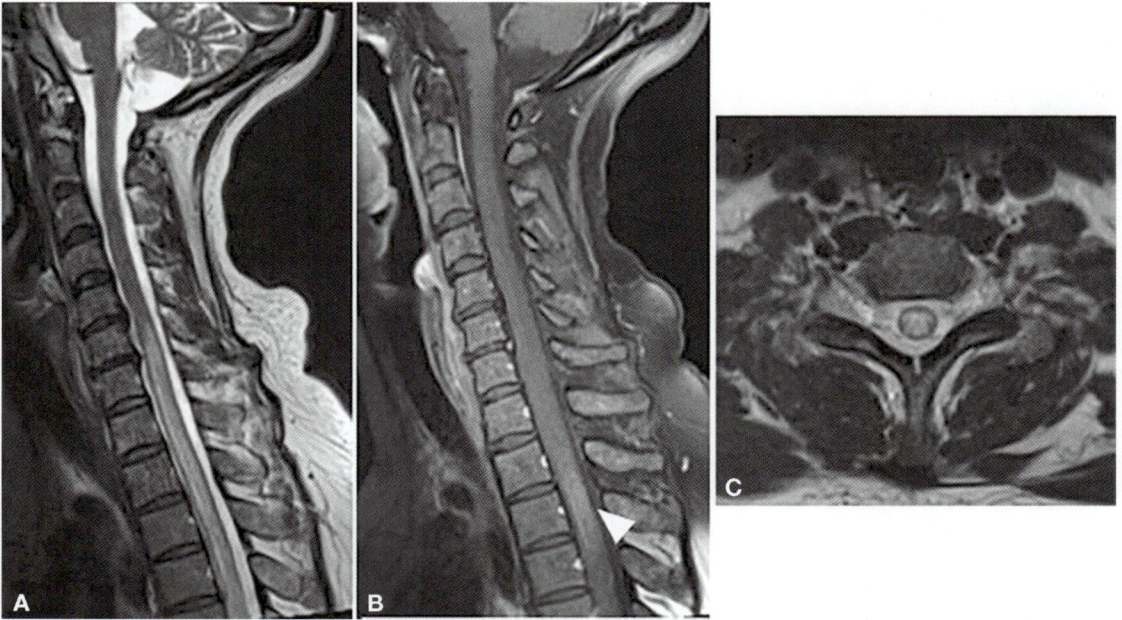

FIGURE 20.7 A. Sagittal T2-weighted magnetic resonance imaging (MRI) of the cervical spine showing longitudinally extensive T2 hyperintensity spanning from C6 through the upper thoracic spinal cord in a patient with neuromyelitis optica spectrum disorder. B. Sagittal T1-weighted postcontrast MRI demonstrating enhancement at the T3 level in the lesion shown in A. C. Axial T2-weighted MRI of the cervical spine demonstrating central hyperintensity in this patient.

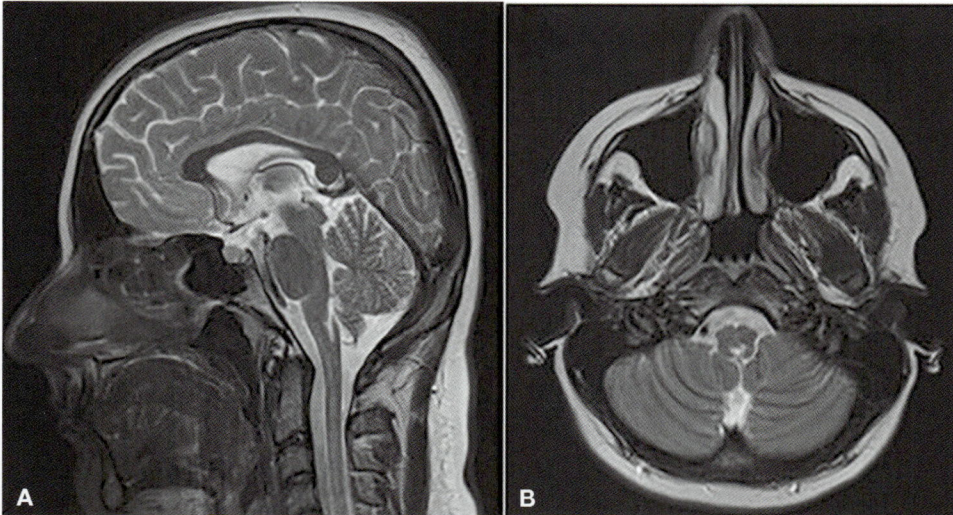

FIGURE 20.8 A. Sagittal T2-weighted magnetic resonance imaging demonstrating a lesion in the area postrema of the dorsal medulla in a patient with neuromyelitis optica, also shown on an axial image (B).

Diagnosis of Neuromyelitis Optica Spectrum Disorder

The diagnosis of NMOSD is made by serum NMO-IgG (AQP4-IgG) in the context of at least one of the typical (core) clinical syndromes (optic neuritis, transverse myelitis, area postrema syndrome, acute brainstem syndrome, acute diencephalic clinical syndrome, or symptomatic cerebral syndrome with characteristic MRI lesions). NMO-IgG should be tested for using the best available detection method, with a cell-based assay being strongly recommended. The standard reference test for the detection of serum NMO-IgG is a live cell-based flow cytometric assay, which has 80% sensitivity and more than 99% specificity. CSF testing for NMO-IgG is significantly less sensitive than serum testing. Per the last (2015) revision of the NMOSD diagnostic criteria,[9] NMOSD can also be diagnosed in patients without seropositivity for NMO-IgG (called *seronegative NMOSD*) if they have at least two different clinical syndromes (of the six core syndromes listed earlier, at least one must be optic neuritis, longitudinally extensive transverse myelitis, or area postrema syndrome), they meet MRI criteria for lesion characteristics typical for NMOSD, and alternative diagnoses are excluded.[9]

NMOSD may co-occur with systemic autoimmune diseases such as systemic lupus erythematosus (SLE) and Sjögren syndrome or with other organ-specific autoimmune diseases such as autoimmune thyroid disease or myasthenia gravis. If patients with these or other primary rheumatologic diseases develop CNS manifestations, they should be evaluated for concurrent NMOSD. Rarely, NMOSD can occur as a paraneoplastic condition, so cancer screening should be performed in patients in whom the disease develops at a later age or in whom there is clinical suspicion for malignancy.

Treatment of Neuromyelitis Optica Spectrum Disorder

Treatment of NMOSD involves treating acute relapses, maintenance treatment to prevent future relapses, symptomatic treatment, and multimodal rehabilitation.

Acute attacks are treated with IV corticosteroids for 3 to 5 days, followed by a steroid taper until maintenance treatment is initiated and reaches its optimal efficacy (this timing of which is different for different maintenance treatments). In moderate to severe NMOSD attacks, early administration of plasma exchange should be considered since this approach may improve NMOSD outcomes. Severe NMOSD attacks not responsive to steroids or plasma exchange may be treated with IV cyclophosphamide.

Given the severity of NMOSD attacks and often incomplete recovery from these attacks, all patients with NMOSD should be treated with lifelong maintenance therapy. As of 2024, FDA-approved treatment options include eculizumab, inebilizumab, ravulizumab and satralizumab. Rituximab has been approved in Japan for NMOSD and ravulizumab in the European Union and Japan, and is currently under FDA review in the United States. Where these labeled treatments are unavailable, off-label immunomodulatory treatments can be considered.

Eculizumab is a humanized monoclonal antibody that acts as terminal C5 complement inhibitor (complement-mediated mechanisms play a significant role in CNS tissue damage in NMOSD). Ravulizumab has the same mode of action as eculizumab but is engineered as a long-acting humanized monoclonal antibody. The main safety concern associated with eculizumab and ravulizumab treatment is meningococcal infections, and therefore, patients should receive the meningococcal vaccine prior to treatment. Inebilizumab is a humanized anti-CD19 monoclonal antibody that depletes B cells. Other B-cell-depleting agents (rituximab, ocrelizumab, and ofatumumab) can also be used in NMOSD. Potential safety risks associated with B-cell depletion may include infections (including hepatitis B reactivation), immunoglobulin deficiency with prolonged use, and reduced response to vaccines. Interleukin-6 (IL-6) is a cytokine that significantly contributes to inflammatory processes in NMOSD, and therefore, medications targeting IL-6 receptor (satralizumab, FDA labeled; tocilizumab and sarilumab used off-label) can be maintenance treatment options in

NMOSD. Potential safety concerns associated with IL-6-targeted therapy includes infections, neutropenia, thrombocytopenia, and hepatotoxicity.

Other off-label NMOSD maintenance treatment options that can be considered include prednisone, azathioprine, mycophenolate mofetil, cyclophosphamide, cyclosporin A, tacrolimus, methotrexate, mitoxantrone, monthly intravenous immunoglobulin (IVIg), or monthly plasma exchange. Combination therapies can be considered in certain patients. Therapeutic strategies that promote immune tolerance are in development.

Symptomatic treatment in NMOSD is similar to symptomatic treatment used in MS. Physical, occupational, and speech therapy, as well as psychosocial support are extremely important in an effort to improve functionality and quality of life of patients with NMOSD.

MYELIN OLIGODENDROCYTE GLYCOPROTEIN ANTIBODY-ASSOCIATED DISEASE

MOGAD is a demyelinating condition of the CNS associated with antibodies to MOG. MOGAD affects males and females with similar prevalence, and the disease is more common in children than in adults. MOGAD can present as ADEM, optic neuritis, myelitis, cortical encephalitis, or a brainstem or cerebellar syndrome. While many of these clinical entities can be seen in MS and NMOSD, there are distinct clinical and radiologic features of them that suggest MOGAD (Table 20.4). For example, the most common presenting phenotype is ADEM in children and optic neuritis in adults. MOGAD may be monophasic or relapsing; relapses are more common in patients with persistent seropositivity for MOG-IgG. Features of MOGAD

TABLE 20.4	Clinical and Radiographic Features Distinguishing MOGAD, MS, and NMOSD		
Clinical presentation	**MOGAD**	**MS**	**NMOSD**
Optic neuritis	• Clinical: ○ Unilateral or bilateral simultaneous involvement ○ Often severe vision loss • Radiographic: ○ Usually a longitudinal optic nerve involvement (>50% length of the optic nerve) ○ Perineural optic nerve sheath enhancement ○ Predominantly anterior optic nerve involvement ○ May be recurrent on the same eye or on alternate eyes	• Clinical: ○ Unilateral (most common), bilateral simultaneous is not typical but can occur ○ May affect any portion of the optic nerve ○ May be recurrent on the same eye or on alternate eyes ○ Often mild to moderate vision loss • Radiographic: ○ Usually MRI enhancement does not affect >50% of the optic nerve length.	• Clinical: ○ Unilateral or bilateral simultaneous involvement, may be recurrent on the same eye or on alternate eyes ○ Often severe vision loss • Radiographic: ○ T2 hyperintense lesion or T1-weighted gadolinium-enhancing lesion extending over >50% optic nerve length or involving optic chiasm ○ Posterior optic nerve involvement is more typical.
Transverse myelitis	• Clinical: usually symmetric presentation (but may be asymmetric) with sensory changes, extremity weakness, bladder/bowel control problems, balance problems • Radiographic: LETM (≥3 contiguous segments) or short-segment transverse myelitis ○ Central cord lesion or H-sign ○ May involve any spinal cord level, conus medullaris lesions are common.	• Clinical: usually asymmetric presentation (but may be symmetric) with sensory changes, extremity weakness, bladder/bowel control problems, balance problems • Radiographic: "short-segment" lesion usually involving one to two vertebral segments, usually ovoid or round	• Clinical: usually symmetric presentation (but may be asymmetric) with sensory changes, extremity weakness, bladder/bowel control problems, balance problems • Radiographic: • Acute myelitis: in most cases presents as LETM (lesion extending over ≥3 contiguous segments), but may be a short-segment lesion • Focal cord atrophy in chronic stage may occur.

TABLE 20.4 Clinical and Radiographic Features Distinguishing MOGAD, MS, and NMOSD (*continued*)

Clinical presentation	MOGAD	MS	NMOSD
Cerebral/cerebellar syndrome	• Clinical: ADEM-like presentation with encephalopathy, often with seizures, focal or multifocal deficits, encephalitis, hemiencephalitis, cerebellitis • Radiographic: 　○ Ill-defined T2/FLAIR hyperintense lesions in supratentorial and often infratentorial white matter 　○ Deep gray matter involvement 　○ Variable enhancement patterns of active lesions on postcontrast sequences 　○ Cortical lesion(s) with or without lesional and overlying leptomeningeal enhancement 　○ Partial or complete resolution of lesions	• Clinical: heterogeneous clinical involvement localizing to the brain, often suggestive of multifocal lesions, seizures may occur • Radiographic: 　○ Hyperintense on T2/FLAIR/STIR 　○ Hypointense on T1 sequences (if chronic—are considered a black hole) 　○ Variable enhancement patterns of active lesions on postcontrast sequences 　○ Typical shape of an MS lesion is ovoid or round, size >3 mm up to several centimeters, well-defined or ill-defined edges 　○ The lesions may also appear fingerlike, as is the case in "Dawson's fingers," projections that extend outward oriented perpendicular to the ventricle, that can be visualized on sagittal T2 FLAIR imaging on MRI of the brain. 　○ Typical locations include: periventricular (abutting the walls of the ventricle and in corpus callosum), juxtacortical lesions (at the gray-white junction), cortical, infratentorial (brainstem or cerebellum), and the spinal cord. 　○ Leptomeningeal enhancement is possible. 　○ Lesion resolution may occur.	• Clinical: symptomatic narcolepsy or acute diencephalic clinical syndrome; heterogenous clinical presentations of symptomatic cerebral syndrome: 　○ Radiographic: usually well-defined T2/FLAIR hyperintense lesion(s), in brain hemispheres, white matter (often extensive lesions), internal capsule, diencephalon, periependymal lesions surrounding ventricles, corpus callosum (splenium), cerebellum 　○ Variable enhancement patterns of active lesions on postcontrast sequences 　○ Cortical, juxtacortical involvement and leptomeningeal enhancement is very rare. 　○ Lesion resolution is infrequent.
Brainstem syndrome	• Clinical: brainstem symptoms may be similar to those of MS or NMOSD. • Radiographic: 　○ Ill-defined T2/FLAIR hyperintensity involving pons, midbrain, cerebellar peduncles, or medulla 　○ Variable enhancement pattern of acute lesions on postcontrast images	• Clinical: one of multiple brainstem symptoms/signs can be present. • Radiographic: 　○ One or multiple lesions in brainstem, >3 mm up to several centimeters, well-defined or ill-defined edges 　○ Variable enhancement pattern of acute lesions on postcontrast images	• Clinical: area postrema syndrome (episode of otherwise unexplained hiccups or nausea and vomiting) • Acute brainstem syndrome with variable presentation • Radiographic: 　○ Dorsal medulla/area postrema lesions, periependymal brainstem lesions 　○ Other brainstem lesions may occur. 　○ Variable enhancement pattern of acute lesions on postcontrast images
Laboratory features	• Positive MOG-IgG antibody test using cell-based assay in serum. CSF testing is promising but requires further studies. • CSF-restricted oligoclonal IgG bands are present in up to 20% of cases.	• CSF-restricted oligoclonal IgG bands are present in 90%-95% of patients	• Positive test for serum AQP4-IgG using best available detection method (live cell-based assay strongly recommended). Seronegative cases are possible. Routine CSF testing of AQP4-IgG is not recommended but might be considered in selected seronegative cases. • CSF-restricted oligoclonal IgG bands may be present in up to 37% of cases.

ADEM, acute disseminated encephalomyelitis; AQP4, aquaporin-4; CSF, cerebrospinal fluid; FLAIR, fluid-attenuated inversion recovery; Ig, immunoglobulin; LETM, longitudinally extensive transverse myelitis; MOGAD, myelin oligodendrocyte glycoprotein antibody-associated disease; MRI, magnetic resonance imaging; MS, multiple sclerosis; NMOSD, neuromyelitis optica spectrum disorder; STIR, short tau inversion recovery.

attacks are highly heterogeneous. Common presentations include: bilateral optic neuritis, ADEM (presenting with altered mental status, focal neurologic deficit, and/or T2 hyperintense lesions in the brain and/or spinal cord), cortical encephalitis (presenting as headache, seizures, altered mental status, fevers, focal neurologic deficits), and/or transverse myelitis (presenting as limb weakness, sensory loss, and bowel/bladder dysfunction) (Figure 20.9).

MOGAD attacks develop over the course of days, and recovery may occur over the course of weeks to months. MOG-IgG is a biomarker of MOGAD, and NMO-IgG (AQP-4 antibody) is a highly specific biomarker for NMOSD. However, some NMO-IgG negative patients with clinical and imaging features suggestive of NMOSD are MOG-IgG positive and may meet criteria for both MOGAD and seronegative NMOSD.

MOGAD diagnosis is confirmed by positive serum MOG-IgG antibody test using a cell-based assay. Using a live cell-based assay, a positive MOG-IgG titer is defined as at least two doubling dilutions above the assay cutoff; using a fixed cell-based assay, a titer ≥1:100 is considered positive. Fixed or live assay results are considered to be low positive if in the low range of the individual live assay or if the titer is positive but <1:100 for fixed cell-based assays. Low-titer false positives can be seen in patients with MS and in the general population.

If CSF analysis is performed, pleocytosis and elevated protein may be seen, and oligoclonal bands may be present but are less common in MOGAD (5%-20%) compared to MS in which they are nearly always present (95%). MRI typically demonstrates only symptomatic lesions (ie, no silent lesions as are common in MS), and lesions often resolve on repeat imaging after acute MOGAD attacks. Radiologic signs that may distinguish MOGAD from MS and NMOSD are listed in Table 20.4.

Treatment of MOGAD attacks is similar to treatment of MS attacks in that 3 to 5 days of high-dose IV or oral corticosteroids are utilized, but in MOGAD, a steroid taper that may last up to several months is often utilized following the high-dose initial treatment (which is not typically done for MS flares). In severe

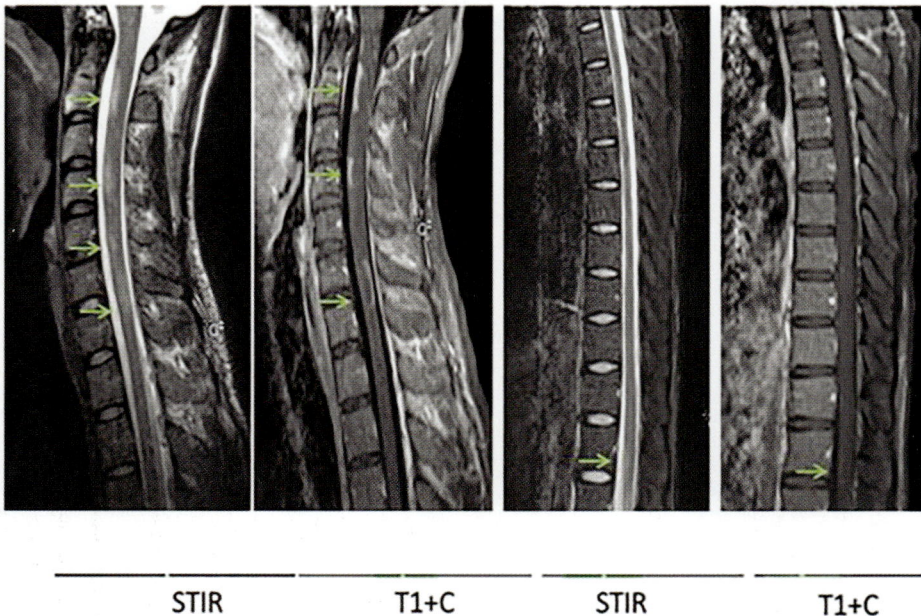

STIR   T1+C   STIR   T1+C

FIGURE 20.9 Typical spinal cord lesions in myelin oligodendrocyte glycoprotein antibody-associated disease in an adult patient. STIR, short tau inversion recovery; T1 + C, T1 sequences with intravenous gadolinium contrast.

flares refractory to steroids, IVIg or plasma exchange may be considered. In patients with more than one attack regardless of attack severity or a more severe attack with or without incomplete recovery, long-term immunomodulatory treatment can be considered to prevent relapses. Although there are currently no evidence-based guidelines for how long to administer maintenance treatment, therapies that may be considered include oral prednisone, mycophenolate mofetil, mycophenolic acid, azathioprine, methotrexate, rituximab, or monthly IVIg.

ACUTE DISSEMINATED ENCEPHALOMYELITIS

ADEM is an acute immune-mediated demyelinating disorder of the CNS most common in children and young adults, but it may rarely occur in older patients. The condition most commonly follows weeks after an infection. The most common preceding infections are viruses (eg, Epstein-Barr, measles, mumps, rubella, coxsackie B, herpes simplex virus, human herpes virus-6, influenza, HIV, and COVID-19), but cases associated with preceding bacterial infection may occur (eg, *Mycoplasma pneumoniae* and *Legionella pneumophila*). The vaccinations that have been most commonly reported to be associated with postvaccination ADEM are measles, mumps, and rubella, but ADEM has also been reported following other vaccines, including the COVID-19 vaccine. However, a causal association between vaccination and ADEM remains controversial.

The most common symptoms of ADEM are headache, fever, altered mental status (ranging from confusion to coma), focal neurologic signs referable to the brain and/or spinal cord, and optic neuritis. Seizures may occur. Symptoms arise over days and report of a febrile illness (or less often a vaccine) in the preceding weeks is common.

Brain MRI demonstrates multifocal, bilateral, large lesions in the white matter of the brain and/or spinal cord that may enhance. Deep gray matter involvement may also be seen (Figure 20.10). A severe hemorrhagic variant called acute hemorrhagic leukoencephalitis or acute hemorrhagic encephalomyelitis is rare but can be fatal. CSF analysis in ADEM demonstrates a lymphocytic pleocytosis (generally fewer than 100 cells/mm³) and elevated protein, and CSF-specific

oligoclonal bands are generally absent. Children with ADEM may have serum antibodies to MOG, but this is uncommon in adults who develop the condition.

Treatment of ADEM is with high-dose IV corticosteroids followed by an oral prednisone taper over 4 to 6 weeks. In severe cases with no response to steroids, IVIg or plasma exchange may be considered. Most patients recover completely. If MRI is repeated in the first 3 months following the onset of ADEM, additional lesions may be seen to emerge as part of the same ADEM episode. In most cases, the condition is monophasic with complete clinical recovery. MRI lesions resolve on MRI studies obtained more than 3 months after onset. In rare instances, ADEM may recur (called *multiphasic disseminated encephalomyelitis*) or represent the first presentation of MS or MOGAD.

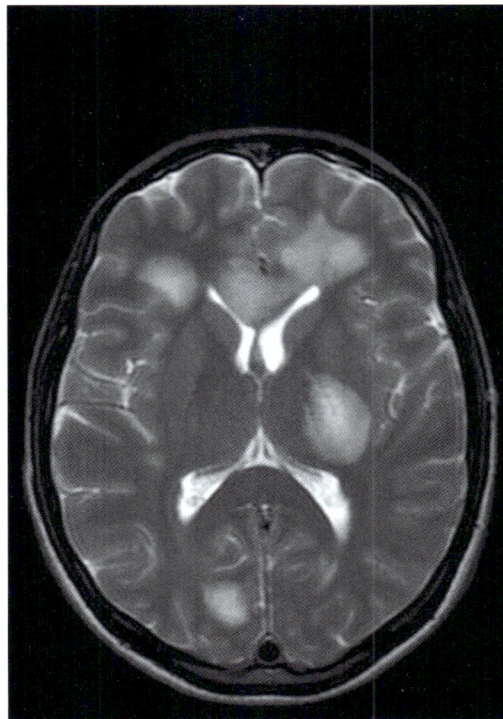

FIGURE 20.10 Axial T2-weighted magnetic resonance imaging demonstrating multifocal fluffy, bilateral, asymmetric hyperintense lesions in the bilateral white matter and deep gray matter in a patient with acute disseminated encephalomyelitis.

SUMMARY

CNS demyelinating diseases should be considered when neurologic symptoms and signs localizing to the CNS (eg, optic neuritis, myelitis, brainstem or cerebellar symptoms) emerge and evolve over days. Recent advances have demonstrated specific biomarkers associated with NMOSD (anti-AQP4 antibodies) and MOGAD (anti-MOG antibodies) that are treated distinctly from MS. Establishing the correct diagnosis early in the disease course is a crucial step toward achieving the best long-term treatment outcomes. Patients with these conditions should be referred to a neurologist for accurate diagnosis and selection of appropriate disease-modifying treatment.

EDITORS' KEY POINTS

▶ MS most commonly presents with relapses (flares) of symptoms affecting the CNS evolving over days, such as optic neuritis, myelitis, or cerebellar ataxia. Some patients with this relapsing-remitting phenotype evolve into a secondary progressive form over time. Less commonly, patients present with a progressive course from onset (called PPMS).

▶ MS is diagnosed by the finding of dissemination of lesions in space and time demonstrated by a combination of neuroimaging features (and, in some instances, CSF oligoclonal bands) and a characteristic clinical syndrome. Multifocal white matter lesions on MRI are often a nonspecific finding, and MS should only be diagnosed when a patient has a clinical syndrome consistent with MS and MRI findings meet published criteria for the condition.

▶ Acute attacks of MS are treated with IV corticosteroids. Disease-modifying treatments for prevention of relapse in MS include injectable agents, oral agents, and intermittent infusions, each of which has particular risks and benefits.

▶ NMOSD is an immune-mediated condition of the CNS caused by antibodies against AQP-4. Common presentations include optic neuritis (often severe and/or bilateral), transverse myelitis (often severe and longitudinally extensive), and area postrema (medullary) syndrome (causing acute nausea, vomiting, and/or hiccups). Diagnosis is made by serum AQP-4 antibody, although seronegative cases can occur. Treatment of acute attacks is with IV corticosteroids, and treatment to prevent relapses is with immunomodulatory therapy.

▶ MOGAD is an antibody-mediated condition of the CNS that can present as ADEM, optic neuritis, or transverse myelitis. Diagnosis is made by the presence of serum anti-MOG antibody. Treatment of acute attacks is with IV corticosteroids, and treatment to prevent relapses (if indicated) is with immunomodulatory therapy.

▶ ADEM is an acute, usually monophasic, immune-mediated demyelinating disorder of the CNS that is most common in children and young adults. It is characterized by headache, fever, altered mental status, and focal neurologic signs referable to the brain and/or spinal cord. ADEM most commonly occurs after a febrile illness, or less commonly a vaccination. Treatment of ADEM is with high-dose corticosteroids.

REFERENCES

1. Walton C, King R, Rechtman L, et al. Rising prevalence of multiple sclerosis worldwide: insights from the Atlas of MS, third edition. *Mult Scler.* 2020;26(14):1816-1821.

2. Ziemssen T, Bhan V, Chataway J, et al. Secondary progressive multiple sclerosis: a review of clinical characteristics, definition, prognostic tools, and disease-modifying therapies. *Neurol Neuroimmunol Neuroinflamm.* 2023;10(1):e200064.

3. McKay KA, Jahanfar S, Duggan T, Tkachuk S, Tremlett H. Factors associated with onset, relapses or progression in multiple sclerosis: a systematic review. *Neurotoxicology.* 2017;61:189-212.

4. Thompson AJ, Banwell BL, Barkhof F, et al. Diagnosis of multiple sclerosis: 2017 revisions of the McDonald criteria. *Lancet Neurol.* 2018;17(2):162-173.

5. Lebrun-Frénay C, Rollot F, Mondot L, et al. Risk factors and time to clinical symptoms of multiple sclerosis among patients with radiologically isolated syndrome. *JAMA Netw Open.* 2021;4(10):e2128271.

6. Rae-Grant A, Day GS, Marrie RA, et al. Practice guideline recommendations summary: disease-modifying therapies for adults with multiple sclerosis: report of the guideline development, dissemination, and implementation subcommittee of the American Academy of Neurology. *Neurology.* 2018;90(17):777-788.

7. Yousry TA, Major EO, Ryschkewitsch C, et al. Evaluation of patients treated with natalizumab for progressive multifocal leukoencephalopathy. *N Engl J Med.* 2006;354(9):924-933.

8. Tenembaum S, Yeh EA, Guthy-Jackson Foundation International Clinical Consortium (GJCF-ICC). Pediatric NMOSD: a review and position statement on approach to work-up and diagnosis. *Front Pediatr.* 2020;8:339.

9. Wingerchuk DM, Banwell B, Bennett JL, et al. International consensus diagnostic criteria for neuromyelitis optica spectrum disorders. *Neurology.* 2015;85(2):177-189.

Neurologic Infections

Anna Cervantes-Arslanian

INTRODUCTION

Neurologic infections need to be recognized quickly since prompt treatment can reduce the risk of morbidity and mortality. Some neurologic infections present acutely (eg, bacterial meningitis and viral encephalitis), whereas others may present subacutely or chronically (eg, fungal and mycobacterial infections, neurosyphilis, neurologic complications of HIV, and parasitic infections). It is therefore essential to be familiar with the symptoms, signs, and diagnostic evaluation of the most common types of neurologic infections. This chapter focuses on meningitis, brain abscess and spinal epidural abscess, encephalitis, and the neurology of HIV infection, including opportunistic infections and neurologic complications of HIV.

MENINGITIS

Meningitis refers to inflammation of the outer coverings of the brain and spinal cord, which consist of the dura mater, arachnoid, and pia mater. When severe, meningitis may lead to inflammation of the underlying brain parenchyma (encephalitis). Meningitis can be caused by infection, autoimmune conditions (eg, sarcoidosis and IgG4-related disease), neoplasia (referred to as *leptomeningeal carcinomatosis* or *carcinomatous meningitis*), or medications (eg, nonsteroidal anti-inflammatory drugs [NSAIDs] and intravenous immunoglobulin [IVIG]). Infectious meningitis can be viral, bacterial, fungal, tubercular, or parasitic. Viral and noninfectious meningitis are sometimes referred to as *aseptic meningitis*. The underlying cause of meningitis is suggested by the cerebrospinal fluid (CSF) profile and confirmed with CSF microbiologic studies (Table 21.1).

TABLE 21.1	Typical CSF Profiles in CNS Infection			
	WBC (cells/mm³)	**Protein (mg/dL)**	**Glucose (mg/dL)[a]**	**Other**
Viral meningitis or encephalitis	100s	<200	Normal[b]	Clear, lymphocytic predominance; in HSV encephalitis may see 10-500 RBCs per mm³
Bacterial meningitis	100s to 10,000s	>100	Low	Turbid, neutrophilic predominance
Fungal meningitis	100s to 1,000s	>100	Low	Lymphocytic predominance
Tuberculous meningitis	100s to 1,000s	>100	Low	Lymphocytic predominance

CNS, central nervous system; CSF, cerebrospinal fluid; HSV, herpes simplex virus; RBC, red blood cell; WBC, white blood cell.
[a]Cerebrospinal fluid (CSF) glucose is low when CSF/blood glucose ratio is less than 0.4 and/or the value is less than 40 mg/dL.
[b]Rarely, viral infections may be associated with low glucose.

Epidemiology and Microbiology

Viral Meningitis

The annual incidence of viral meningitis is estimated at 8 to 14 per 100,000 persons in the United States.[1] The most commonly identified causes are enteroviruses, herpesviruses (eg, herpes simplex virus [HSV]-2, varicella zoster virus [VZV]), and arboviruses (eg, West Nile virus [WNV]). Other causes include lymphocytic choriomeningitis virus (LCMV; associated with exposure to rodents) and HIV (particularly at the time of seroconversion). Prior to widespread vaccination, paramyxovirus (mumps) was a notable cause of viral meningitis, most frequently following parotiditis. Viral meningitis incidence demonstrates a seasonal pattern, with more infections in the summer and fall in temperate climates, likely driven by the predominance of enterovirus infections. HSV-2 may cause recurrent meningitis (known as Mollaret meningitis). Viral meningitis, without associated encephalitis, is generally a self-limited illness with a good prognosis in immunocompetent children and adults.

Bacterial Meningitis

The incidence of acute bacterial meningitis in the United States has declined significantly with the availability of vaccinations against the most common pathogens (Streptococcus pneumoniae, Neisseria meningitidis, and Haemophilus influenzae), reported at 1.38 per 100,000 patient-years.[2] This is in stark contrast to lower-income countries where epidemics of acute bacterial meningitis (usually caused by N. meningitidis) still occur regularly with an incidence of more than 100 per 100,000 patient-years.[3] Despite vaccination, nonvaccine serotype strains (strains of bacteria resistant to the vaccine) have emerged, and S. pneumoniae accounts for the majority of community-acquired acute bacterial meningitis in adults. N. meningitidis is the leading cause of acute bacterial meningitis in children and the second most common cause in adults.

A patient's risk factors and associated medical conditions may suggest a specific pathogen. Local infections (otitis media, sinusitis, and mastoiditis) and basilar skull fractures may cause acute bacterial meningitis via contiguous spread, typically with S. pneumoniae or H. influenzae. Systemic infections such as pneumonia may occur with S. pneumoniae or N. meningitidis meningitis. Asplenia predisposes patients to invasive infections, including acute bacterial meningitis with encapsulated organisms (S. pneumoniae, N. meningitidis, and H. influenzae). Staphylococcus aureus (and other skin flora) should be considered as a potential etiology of acute bacterial meningitis in patients following penetrating head trauma or a recent neurosurgical operation. Similarly, injection drug use may lead to acute bacterial meningitis with or without associated infective endocarditis.

In patients who are older than 50, pregnant, or immunocompromised, or who have alcohol use disorder or diabetes, Listeria monocytogenes should also be considered. In addition to meningitis, Listeria can also cause encephalitis predominantly affecting the brainstem, called rhombencephalitis.

Mortality of acute bacterial meningitis in higher-income countries has decreased with prompt administration of antibiotics and supportive care. However, complications may occur even with appropriate initiation of antibiotic therapy, especially if the presentation for medical care is delayed. The severity of the infection and risk of death vary by pathogen, with the highest mortality associated with S. pneumoniae.[2,4]

Chronic Meningitis

A patient is considered to have chronic meningitis when clinical symptoms last more than 1 month with inflammatory CSF. Many infectious pathogens have been identified in chronic meningitis, including fungal, tubercular, syphilitic, viral, and parasitic etiologies. In addition, noninfectious conditions such as neoplastic and autoimmune conditions must be considered. Chronic meningitis occurs with a frequency similar to that of acute bacterial meningitis in the United States. Host factors, including geographic location, comorbid illness, and immune status, are important considerations for determining the cause of chronic meningitis. Tuberculous meningitis should be considered in patients from endemic countries. In patients who are immunocompromised, especially those with CD4 count less than 100 cells/mm^3, the most commonly identified pathogen is Cryptococcus neoformans. Cryptococcus gattii infection may occur in persons who are immunocompetent, particularly in the Pacific Northwest.

Clinical Presentation

The cardinal features of acute bacterial meningitis include fever, altered mental status, headache, and nuchal rigidity (neck stiffness). However, only a minority of patients will display all these symptoms or signs on presentation. Most patients will have at least two of these signs, and if all are absent, acute bacterial meningitis is unlikely.[5] These cardinal features are most highly associated with acute bacterial meningitis, but a similar presentation may be seen with acute viral meningitis, although typically milder. Fever may be absent, especially in patients who are older or immunocompromised, although the majority of patients with bacterial or viral meningitis will have a temperature above 100 °F (37.7 °C). There are no features of the headache that reliably indicate meningitis, although the accompanying nuchal rigidity is suggestive when present. Most patients with acute bacterial meningitis will have some alteration in mental status, although it may be mild, and up to a third may have normal mental status at presentation.[6] Impaired consciousness is much less common with viral meningitis and typically does not occur with fungal or tubercular meningitis unless the intracranial pressure is elevated or hydrocephalus has developed.

Meningismus may be elicited on examination with Brudzinski and Kernig signs. The Brudzinski sign is involuntary flexion of the hips and knees with passive flexion of the neck in the supine position. The Kernig sign occurs when extension of the knee with the hip flexed in the supine position leads to pain and/or spasm of the hamstring muscle. It is important to note that these classic signs are insensitive, less frequent in chronic meningitis, and not specific to infectious meningitis since they can be seen with other causes of meningeal irritation such as subarachnoid hemorrhage.

Meningitis may present with other symptoms and signs, including photophobia, nausea, vomiting, and cranial nerve palsies. Common cranial nerve palsies include cranial nerve 6 palsy (causing diplopia on lateral gaze) that may occur as a result of elevated intracranial pressure; cranial nerve 7 palsy (causing facial weakness), particularly common in Lyme disease (and mumps in previous eras); and cranial nerve 8 palsy (causing sensorineural hearing loss; occurs most commonly in children). Papilledema may be present due to elevated intracranial pressure but may be absent early in the disease course. Focal neurologic deficits, such as aphasia, visual field deficit, weakness, or sensory loss, can be caused by brain involvement by the infection (cerebritis or abscess) or by stroke due to infectious vasculitis. Focal or generalized seizures may occur in meningitis, occasionally as the presenting symptom.

The symptoms and signs of chronic meningitis are similar to those of acute bacterial meningitis but often less fulminant. Patients often describe a new, persistent, and unrelenting headache that continues to worsen. Fever is not always present. Alterations in mental status are less abrupt than in acute meningitis, but cognitive decline can occur.

Systemic complications may also occur, with severe acute illness occurring more often with acute bacterial meningitis than viral meningitis. Maculopapular rash is common with viral meningitis but may also occur in bacterial meningitis; purpuric rash is classically described with *N. meningitidis*, although it is not always present and can be seen with other bacteria. Acute bacterial meningitis may cause shock due to Waterhouse-Friderichsen syndrome (adrenal hemorrhage) associated with *N. meningitidis*. Concomitant infections that may be seen with acute bacterial meningitis include otitis media, rhinofacial sinusitis, pneumonia, endocarditis, septic arthritis, and spinal epidural abscess.

Diagnosis

A clinical history suggestive of meningitis should lead to emergency room referral for rapid evaluation and treatment. If acute bacterial meningitis is being considered, empiric antibiotics (Table 21.2) and corticosteroids should be initiated immediately since delays in antibiotic administration are associated with worsened outcomes, including death. Definitive microbiologic diagnosis is made by lumbar puncture (LP), but antibiotic initiation should not be delayed since CSF cultures are often still diagnostic

TABLE 21.2   Empiric Antibiotic Regimens for Suspected Acute Bacterial Meningitis[15,32]

Host factor	Antimicrobial therapy
Age	
<1 mo	Ampicillin plus cefotaxime or ampicillin plus aminoglycoside
Between 1 mo and 2 y	Vancomycin plus third-generation cephalosporin
2-50 y	Vancomycin plus third-generation cephalosporin
>50 y	Vancomycin plus third-generation cephalosporin plus ampicillin
Immunocompromised	Vancomycin plus third-generation cephalosporin plus ampicillin
Penetrating head trauma or neurosurgery	Vancomycin plus fourth-generation cephalosporin or vancomycin plus meropenem

Tunkel AR, Hartman BJ, Kaplan SL, et al. Practice guidelines for the management of bacterial meningitis. *Clin Infect Dis.* 2004;39:1267-1284 by permission of Oxford University Press; Tunkel AR, Hasbun R, Bhimraj A, et al. 2017 Infectious Diseases Society of America's Clinical Practice Guidelines for healthcare-associated ventriculitis and meningitis. *Clin Infect Dis.* 2017;64:e34-e65 by permission of Oxford University Press.

up to 2 hours following antibiotic initiation.[7] Blood cultures should also be obtained and are positive in a significant proportion of patients with acute bacterial meningitis (50%-90% in *H. influenzae*, 75% in *S. pneumoniae*, 40%-60% in *N. meningitidis*).[3] Additional laboratory testing should include complete blood cell count (CBC), comprehensive metabolic panel (CMP), coagulation studies, and HIV serology. Serum procalcitonin is useful to distinguish between bacterial and viral meningitis (elevated in the former; normal in the latter).[8] Hyponatremia is common in bacterial meningitis due to the syndrome of inappropriate secretion of antidiuretic hormone (SIADH). An arterial blood gas and lactate should be sent in patients with sepsis. A chest x-ray may be helpful in identifying a concomitant pneumonia. Urine antigen testing may be helpful for microbiologic diagnosis.

LP for CSF analysis and microbiologic testing is necessary for the diagnosis of meningitis. Brain imaging (usually emergent noncontrast head CT) should be obtained prior to LP if the patient is older than 60 years, immunocompromised, has a history of a central nervous system (CNS) mass lesion, or if there are symptoms or signs suggestive of elevated intracranial pressure or focal neurologic deficits. CT and LP should not delay immediate empiric antibiotics and steroids if there is suspicion

of acute bacterial meningitis. For most patients with acute bacterial meningitis, the head CT finding may appear normal or may show nonspecific signs such as sulcal effacement with slight hyperattenuation (due to brain inflammation) and leptomeningeal enhancement (if contrast is given). Magnetic resonance imaging (MRI) may demonstrate meningeal hyperintensity or contrast enhancement. In fungal and tubercular meningitis, hydrocephalus, cranial nerve enhancement, and/or cerebral infarction may be seen.[9]

CSF parameters to analyze include opening pressure, protein, glucose, and cell count. Very high opening pressure is common in fulminant bacterial meningitis (as may occur with *S. pneumoccus* and *N. meningitidis*), fungal meningitis (especially cryptococcal meningitis), and tuberculous meningitis. CSF protein is elevated in all forms of meningitis but is often particularly high in bacterial, fungal, and tubercular meningitis. CSF glucose should be compared to a simultaneously obtained serum glucose measurement. Hypoglycorrhachia (low CSF glucose) most frequently suggests a bacterial, fungal, or tubercular meningitis but can be rarely seen with some viral infections (eg, cytomegalovirus [CMV]) and can also be seen in noninfectious etiologies (such as carcinomatous meningitis and neurosarcoidosis). Factors such as immune status, season, geography, and animal exposures aid in guiding selection of diagnostic testing. In patients with chronic meningitis, a large volume of CSF should be sent (>30 mL), and multiple LPs may be needed to obtain sufficient CSF for diagnosis.

Microbiologic testing may include viral polymerase chain reaction (PCR); IgM serology for arboviruses; Gram stain and culture for bacteria; culture, antibody, and antigen testing for fungi; and culture and PCR (Xpert MTB/RIF assay) for tuberculosis. The yield of Gram stain varies by bacterium and burden of infection and is often higher for *S. pneumoniae* than for *N. meningitidis* or *Listeria*. CSF cultures are highly specific, but sensitivity varies by pathogen. Antibiotic pretreatment may decrease the yield of CSF cultures by up to 50%, usually occurring within 2 hours for *N. meningitidis* and within 8 hours for *S. pneumoniae*.[10] Cultures for fungi and tuberculosis take time to grow and may be less sensitive than other modalities such as antigen testing for fungi and PCR for tuberculosis.

A multiplex PCR panel (BioFire Film Array Meningitis/Encephalitis) simultaneously tests for six bacteria (*Escherichia coli* K1 capsular subtype, *Haemophilus influenzae*, *Listeria monocytogenes*, *Neisseria meningitidis*, *Streptococcus agalactiae*, and *Streptococcus pneumoniae*), seven viruses (HSV-1, HSV-2, VZV, CMV, human herpes virus 6 [HHV-6], enterovirus, and parechovirus), and one fungus (*Cryptococcus neoformans* and *gattii*). Although multiplex PCR facilitates rapid screening for the most common etiologies of meningoencephalitis, it cannot replace CSF culture as it does not provide any information regarding antibiotic sensitivity. Furthermore, the sensitivity of detection of the individual pathogens varies, with high sensitivity for bacterial pathogens but low sensitivity for *Cryptococcus* (52%).[11] Cryptococcal antigen testing is the most sensitive test for *Cryptococcus,* and India ink staining is insensitive. The multiplex panel detection of viral pathogens, in particular HSV-1 and HSV-2, is less sensitive than the stand-alone PCR for individual viruses, so in patients in whom there is high concern for viral encephalitis, appropriate targeted PCR testing should also be sent.

Metagenomic next-generation sequencing (NGS) holds promise for diagnosis of less common infectious agents for which culture, serology, and PCR may be insensitive. Metagenomic NGS is hypothesis-free, meaning it looks for any potential infectious pathogen rather than requiring a pretest hypothesis and sending particular microbiologic tests for specific organisms.[12]

If an infectious cause is not found in a case of chronic meningitis, autoimmune causes should be considered.[13] Despite exhaustive workup, the cause remains unknown in approximately a third of cases of chronic meningitis.[13] Table 21.1 outlines the CSF profiles expected in different CNS infections.

Treatment

Treatment of viral meningitis is supportive, apart from meningitis caused by herpesviruses, which is treated with acyclovir. Patients with viral meningitis should be monitored for development of complications such as encephalitis or seizures.

As discussed earlier, in patients with suspected acute bacterial meningitis, empiric antibiotics and corticosteroids should be initiated immediately based on likely pathogens determined by age and past medical history (eg, immunocompromise, prior neurosurgery, or open head trauma; Table 21.2).

Steroids decrease mortality from acute bacterial meningitis due to *S. pneumoniae* in adults and decrease the risk of hearing loss in children with *H. influenza* meningitis.[14,15] Dexamethasone should therefore be administered before or concomitant with the first dose of antibiotics and continued if testing reveals *S. pneumoniae or H. influenza* in children. Steroids are also commonly used in tuberculous meningitis.

Patients with acute bacterial meningitis are often systemically ill and may develop sepsis, requiring fluid resuscitation and vasopressors. Although hyponatremia is very common and usually due to SIADH, fluid restriction is not advised due to the risk of decreased cerebral perfusion pressure. Cerebral edema, seizures, intracranial hypertension, hydrocephalus, and stroke can occur and should be monitored for and treated accordingly.

Prognosis

Outcomes following acute viral meningitis are generally good, with very low mortality. This is in stark contrast to acute bacterial meningitis, where mortality is still 6% to 30% in high-income countries depending on the pathogen (highest mortality with *S. pneumoniae*); risk factors for adverse outcomes include older age, hypotension, seizures, concomitant pneumonia, purpuric rash, tachycardia, lower Glasgow Coma Scale (GCS) score at admission, focal neurologic deficits, CSF white blood cell (WBC) count of less than 1,000, positive blood cultures, high serum C-reactive protein (CRP), and not receiving antibiotics before hospital admission.[16]

CENTRAL NERVOUS SYSTEM ABSCESS

Brain Abscess

Brain abscesses are relatively uncommon, with an incidence of 0.4 to 0.9 per 100,000 persons per year.[17] Brain abscess can be caused by hematogenous spread (eg, from endocarditis or pneumonia) or contiguous spread of infection (eg, from sinusitis or otitis) or by direct infection from head trauma or neurosurgery. Bacterial etiology is most common in immunocompetent patients and may be polymicrobial (commonly *Staphylococcus aureus*, *Streptococcus* species, and *Bacteroides* species). Fungi (eg, *Candida* and *Aspergillus*), parasites (eg, *Toxoplasma*), and atypical/opportunistic bacteria (eg, *Nocardia*) should be considered in patients who are immunocompromised. Tuberculous brain abscess (tuberculoma) is common in endemic regions.

Clinical Presentation

Symptoms of brain abscess include headache, fever, and focal neurologic deficits, although the complete triad is often absent at presentation. Headache is the most common feature, occurring in up to 70% of patients, whereas fever and focal deficits occur in only about half of patients.[18] Symptoms and signs of elevated intracranial pressure (nausea, vomiting, diplopia, depressed level of consciousness, and papilledema) may occur with large abscesses or if there is a rupture into the ventricles (ventriculitis). Seizures occur in 25% of patients with brain abscess and may be the presenting symptom.[18] Symptoms and signs of a potential systemic source should be sought on examination (eg, otitis, sinusitis, pneumonia, or endocarditis).

Diagnosis

Brain abscess is diagnosed by neuroimaging, which reveals a ring-enhancing lesion with surrounding edema that usually shows central diffusion restriction on MRI diffusion-weighted imaging (DWI) sequences. HIV testing should be performed, since if positive, this expands the differential diagnosis for the underlying pathogen. Blood cultures should be obtained but are rarely positive unless there is a concurrent systemic infection. Body imaging (eg, chest x-ray and CT) for the source of infection should be considered. LP is often contraindicated due to mass effect, and CSF analysis is often unremarkable since the abscess is typically walled off within the brain parenchyma. In patients who are immunocompromised, or in those who are immunocompetent and do not respond to empiric antibiotics, stereotactic aspiration for culture may be necessary for microbiologic diagnosis.

Treatment

In patients who are immunocompetent, empiric antibiotic treatment regimens to cover the most common culprit bacteria should include a third- or fourth-generation cephalosporin (for broad-spectrum coverage of most gram-positive and gram-negative bacteria except *Enterococcus*), vancomycin (for coverage of most gram-positive cocci and bacilli including penicillin-resistant *Streptococcus*, methicillin-resistant *Staphylococcus*, and most *Enterococcus* species), and metronidazole (to cover anaerobes). If there is mass effect or proximity to the ventricular system, surgical drainage should be considered. In patients who are immunocompromised, stereotactic aspiration for diagnosis is often necessary, given the broad microbiologic differential diagnosis. In patients with HIV and one or more ring-enhancing lesions, toxoplasmosis should be considered and empiric treatment initiated (see subsequent text).

Prognosis

Mortality from brain abscess remains as high as 20% to 30% in some populations; abscess rupture leading to ventriculitis and hydrocephalus is associated with the highest mortality (27%-85%), and neurologic sequelae occur in 30% of patients.[17]

Spinal Epidural Abscess

Spinal epidural abscesses are infectious collections between the dura and the vertebrae, either posterior or anterior to the spinal cord. The majority of cases of spinal epidural abscess are bacterial, most commonly caused by *Staphylococcus aureus* and gram-negative bacilli. Epidural abscesses may arise from contiguous spread from vertebral osteomyelitis/discitis, hematogenous spread from systemic infection, or direct infection from open trauma or neurosurgical procedures. Risk factors for the development of epidural abscess include alcohol use disorder, diabetes, immunodeficiency, preexisting spinal abnormality or recent intervention, and local/systemic infections.[19]

Clinical Presentation

Spinal epidural abscesses cause neck or back pain and symptoms related to spinal cord compression. This may cause motor weakness and/or sensory loss below the level of the lesion, as well as bowel, bladder, and sexual dysfunction. Fever is present in only half of cases.[20]

Diagnosis

The diagnosis of spinal epidural abscess is made by neuroimaging. MRI is more sensitive than CT. MRI demonstrates a T2 hyperintense contrast-enhancing lesion in the epidural space that often spans multiple levels. Serum erythrocyte sedimentation rate (ESR) and CRP are commonly elevated, but leukocytosis may be absent. Blood cultures should be obtained but the result may be negative, requiring surgical drainage for microbiologic diagnosis. If there is no contiguous source of infection identified on spinal imaging, an echocardiogram should be obtained to evaluate for endocarditis as a potential source. LP should be avoided, given the risk of spreading the infection from the epidural space to the subarachnoid space.

Treatment

Empiric antibiotic treatment for spinal epidural abscess is with vancomycin and a third- or fourth-generation cephalosporin. Surgical evacuation should be considered if there is spinal cord or cauda equina compression. Antibiotics alone or with percutaneous aspiration without decompression may be considered in patients with small abscesses or who are high-risk surgical candidates. Surgery may still be needed if there is worsening of initial mild symptoms despite antibiotics, as this may suggest inadequate source control.

Prognosis

Mortality due to spinal epidural abscess is low and mostly related to associated sepsis and/or meningitis. The most important predictor of neurologic outcome is the patient's status immediately prior to surgery. Early surgical intervention before sensorimotor deficits develop improves the prognosis for neurologic function.[19]

ENCEPHALITIS

Encephalitis refers to inflammation of the brain parenchyma, which may be caused by infection (most commonly viral) or autoimmunity (most commonly antibody mediated). Encephalitis may occur in isolation or concurrently with meningitis (meningoencephalitis). Viral encephalitis affects an estimated 3.4 to 7.4 per 100,000 patients per year worldwide.[21] A large number of viruses may cause encephalitis, including herpesviruses (eg, HSV and VZV), enteroviruses, arboviruses (eg, West Nile Virus and Japanese encephalitis virus), and in patients who are immunocompromised, CMV, and HHV-6. Worldwide, HSV is the most commonly identified sporadic pathogen, and Japanese encephalitis is the most common endemic viral encephalitis.[22]

Clinical Presentation

Infectious encephalitis should be suspected in patients with fever, headache, and altered mental status evolving over days. Other features may include seizures, focal neurologic deficits, movement disorders (particularly with arbovirus infection), or cerebellar signs (eg, in encephalitis caused by VZV or Powassan virus). Unlike meningitis, viral encephalitis is less frequently associated with systemic features at presentation, although patients may be severely neurologically ill, requiring intubation and mechanical ventilation, and may subsequently develop systemic complications of critical illness. Fever is present in the majority of cases of HSV encephalitis (>90% in a series of 112 biopsy-proven HSV encephalitis cases)[23] but is not universally present in all causes of viral encephalitis. Therefore, lack of fever does not exclude infectious encephalitis if other features are supportive, especially in the case of immunocompromise. The presence of nuchal rigidity in encephalitis suggests concomitant meningitis (meningoencephalitis).

Diagnosis

Diagnosis is made by neuroimaging and CSF findings. On brain MRI, affected regions are T2 hyperintense and may demonstrate contrast enhancement, diffusion restriction, and, in the case of HSV, hemorrhage. HSV and HHV-6 tend to affect limbic regions (temporal and inferior frontal cortex), whereas arboviruses tend to affect the deep gray matter (basal ganglia and thalamus). Arboviral encephalitis may also cause a concomitant myelitis (ie, spinal cord involvement) specifically involving the anterior horns, resulting in acute flaccid paralysis.

If there is no concern for mass effect on neuro-imaging, LP should be pursued (see Table 21.1 for expected CSF profiles in viral CNS infections). Viruses may be diagnosed by CSF PCR, CSF antibodies, and/or serum antibody titers (in the acute and convalescent periods, meaning at the time of initial infection and 1 to 4 weeks following initial testing). If no etiology is determined through PCR and serology, metagenomic NGS can be performed on CSF to evaluate for rarer infections. Autoimmune etiologies should be considered in patients with encephalitis in whom no infectious cause is identified; autoimmune encephalitis can be diagnosed with commercially available autoantibody panels.

Electroencephalogram (EEG) should be obtained if there is concern for seizures, recognizing that subclinical seizures/nonconvulsive status epilepticus may manifest as isolated fluctuations in mental status or coma without tonic-clonic movements. Periodic sharp waves can be seen on EEG in HSV, although they are neither sensitive nor specific.

Treatment

In all cases of presumed viral encephalitis, acyclovir should be started immediately for empiric HSV coverage while awaiting MRI and CSF results. VZV encephalitis is treated with valacyclovir. Both CMV and HHV-6 encephalitis (seen exclusively in patients who are immunocompromised) may be treated with ganciclovir or foscarnet. Treatment of other infectious etiologies is largely supportive.

Prognosis

The prognosis of encephalitis is highly varied depending on the etiology and degree to which the patient was initially impacted. Without treatment, HSV encephalitis has an associated mortality of 70%.[24] Even with early acyclovir, HSV encephalitis is a highly morbid illness, with the majority of the survivors having some degree of neurologic impairment, most often neurocognitive and psychiatric sequelae.[25] Some arboviral infections have high mortality (up to 50% in Japanese encephalitis virus); up to 50% of

survivors of Japanese encephalitis have residual severe neurologic disability.[26]

NEUROLOGIC COMPLICATIONS OF HIV

Neurologic complications of HIV can be due to direct effects of HIV on the nervous system, opportunistic infections due to immunocompromise, and side effects of antiretroviral treatment (ART).

Direct effects of HIV on the nervous system seen at the time of seroconversion include viral meningitis and a Guillain-Barré-like syndrome (distinguished from classic Guillain-Barré syndrome [GBS] by the presence of WBCs in the CSF). HIV antibody will be normal at the time of seroconversion, and so if there is concern for HIV seroconversion based on clinical presentation and risk factors, serum viral load should be obtained.

Direct effects of HIV on the nervous system seen later in the disease course include peripheral neuropathy, HIV-associated neurocognitive disorder (HAND), and HIV-associated myelopathy.

HIV neuropathy is common even in patients with suppressed viral load and typically presents as a chronic, sensory-predominant, distal symmetric polyneuropathy (HIV-DSP) causing numbness, tingling, and burning pain beginning in the toes that slowly progresses proximally. Other causes of neuropathy should be screened for, including vitamin B_{12} deficiency, diabetes, and paraprotein-related disorders (via serum protein electrophoresis [SPEP]/immunofixation electrophoresis [IFE]).

Neuropathic pain in HIV-DSP is treated with gabapentinoids (eg, gabapentin and pregabalin), tricyclic antidepressants (eg, amitriptyline or nortriptyline), and SNRIs (eg, duloxetine). Several first-generation antiretrovirals (the "d" drugs: didanosine, stavudine, and zalcitabine) were associated with peripheral neuropathy, but this is rare with newer generation antiretrovirals.

HAND includes a spectrum of conditions with varying degrees of cognitive impairment: asymptomatic neurocognitive impairment, mild neurocognitive disorder, and HIV-associated dementia. The prevalence of HIV-associated dementia has declined with the use of antiretrovirals, but as patients live longer with HIV, the prevalence of milder forms of cognitive impairment has increased. The pattern of cognitive impairment in HAND is most commonly subcortical, causing psychomotor slowing, delayed information processing, and impairment of executive functioning and memory. Patients may show extrapyramidal signs, although this is now less common among patients on ART.[27] Neuroimaging, syphilis serology testing, vitamin B_{12} level, thyroid-stimulating hormone (TSH), and depression screening should be performed to evaluate for alternative and potentially reversible causes of dementia. Treatment of HAND is supportive.

A wide variety of CNS opportunistic infections can occur in patients who are immunocompromised from HIV infection. Here, three of the most common are discussed: toxoplasmosis, cryptococcal meningitis, and progressive multifocal leukoencephalopathy (PML).

Toxoplasmosis

Toxoplasmosis is the most common parasitic infection in humans; latent infection is present in a third of the world's population.[28] CNS toxoplasmosis occurs with reactivation in immune compromise, with the highest risk for patients with a CD4 count below 100 cells/mm³. It is the most common opportunistic infection in patients with HIV, previously seen in up to 40% of patients with AIDS before the advent of ART.[29]

CNS toxoplasmosis presents with subacute headache, confusion, seizures, and/or focal deficits depending on the location and number of lesions. Neuroimaging demonstrates one or more ring-enhancing lesions with surrounding edema with a predilection for the deeper regions of the cerebral hemispheres, including the basal ganglia and subcortical white matter. The main differential diagnosis in high-income countries is primary central nervous system lymphoma (PCNSL), and the two are challenging to distinguish radiologically. Advanced imaging with single-photon emission computed tomography (SPECT) or FDG-PET may be helpful in distinguishing between toxoplasmosis and PCNSL.

Since a significant proportion of the population has latent toxoplasmosis, positive toxoplasma serology does not confirm the diagnosis, but negative serology makes the diagnosis unlikely (although not impossible: some patients with severe immunocompromise may have CNS toxoplasmosis with negative serology). CSF PCR is highly sensitive but often unobtainable due to mass effect from one or more brain lesions precluding LP. Therefore, empiric treatment with pyrimethamine/sulfadiazine (with leucovorin) or trimethoprim-sulfamethoxazole should be started in suspected cases with close clinical and radiologic follow-up. If there is clinical and radiologic improvement after 2 weeks of treatment, the diagnosis of toxoplasmosis is presumed; if symptoms or radiologic lesions progress, brain biopsy should be considered for the possibility of PCNSL or abscess caused by another organism, including tuberculosis in endemic countries.

Primary Central Nervous System Lymphoma

The clinical presentation of PCNSL may be indistinguishable from toxoplasmosis, with patients often presenting with seizure, headache, and focal deficits, although neuropsychiatric presentation may also occur. Neuroimaging is also similar to toxoplasmosis with ring-enhancing lesions most often located in the subependymal and periventricular regions or corpus callosum (note that PCNSL in patients who are not immunocompromised has a different radiologic appearance; see Chapter 26). Positive CSF Epstein-Barr virus (EBV) PCR is highly suggestive of PCNSL, but CSF cytology or tissue diagnosis via brain biopsy is needed to confirm the diagnosis. If a patient who is immunocompromised is undergoing empiric treatment for toxoplasmosis due to ring-enhancing lesions, steroids should be avoided as they may lead to clinical and radiologic improvement of PCNSL, making it challenging to distinguish the two.

Cryptococcal Meningitis

Cryptococcus, a yeast form of fungus, is most associated with meningitis (described earlier) but may also cause intracranial mass lesions known as *Cryptococcomas*. *Cryptococcus neoformans* infections occur most often when CD4 count is less than 100 cells/mm³. Like other meningitides, cryptococcal meningitis may present with headache, fever, and altered mental status. The onset of cryptococcal meningitis is often insidious, sometimes with progressive worsening over months, followed by acute decompensation due to evolving elevated intracranial hypertension.

Neuroimaging in cryptococcal meningitis may show meningeal enhancement or may demonstrate *Cryptococcomas* (cystic lesions with a predilection for the basal ganglia). Hydrocephalus may also be seen. Diagnosis of cryptococcal meningitis is made by CSF cryptococcal antigen testing. The opening pressure during LP may be very high, necessitating repeated CSF drainage as part of treatment. Antimicrobial therapy for cryptococcal meningitis consists of three components: induction therapy with dual antifungals (usually amphotericin B and flucytosine), consolidation therapy with fluconazole, and maintenance therapy with lower dose fluconazole once CSF cultures no longer detect *Cryptococcus*.

Progressive Multifocal Leukoencephalopathy

PML is a disease affecting the white matter of the brain caused by reactivation of the JC virus in patients who are immunocompromised when the CD4 count is less than 200 cells/mm^3. PML was rarely seen before the HIV era and rose to an incidence of 3.3 cases per 1,000 patient-years before declining after the widespread adoption of ART.[30] PML usually presents with subacute development of focal neurologic deficits. Initial symptoms vary depending on the location of the lesion(s) and can include alterations in mental status, aphasia, visual changes, sensory or motor deficits, or ataxia. Brain imaging typically shows T2 hyperintense foci in the white matter adjacent to the cerebral cortex that do not enhance or cause mass effect. Less commonly, JC virus can cause a cerebellar syndrome called granule cell neuronopathy.[31] There is no specific treatment for PML except restoration of immune function with ART, although this can lead to immune reconstitution inflammatory syndrome (IRIS).

Immune Reconstitution Inflammatory Syndrome

IRIS refers to paradoxical worsening after initiation of treatments that reconstitute the immune system. In patients with HIV, this can occur after initiation of ART in patients with active or latent opportunistic infection. For CNS opportunistic infections such as cryptococcal meningitis and tuberculosis, initiation of ART in patients who present with a CNS opportunistic infection (or resumption of ART in patients who have gone off treatment) is generally delayed for weeks while the infection is treated. IRIS is generally treated with steroids.

SUMMARY

Neurologic infections should be considered in the differential diagnosis of some of the most common neurologic presentations, including headache, altered mental status, and seizure. Diagnosis of CNS infections relies on a combination of clinical features, neuroimaging, and cerebrospinal fluid analysis. Since culture, PCR, and serology results often take days to weeks to return, empiric treatment based on the most likely infectious pathogen(s) is generally required while awaiting a specific diagnosis.

EDITORS' KEY POINTS

▶ Meningitis can be caused by infection (viral, bacterial, fungal, tubercular, syphilitic, and parasitic), immune-mediated conditions, or neoplasm.

▶ In patients with possible bacterial meningitis (eg, presenting with headache, fever, neck stiffness, and/or altered mental status), empiric antibiotic coverage for bacterial meningitis should be initiated immediately before obtaining CSF by LP for diagnosis. Early initiation of antibiotics improves outcomes and will not alter CSF results obtained within 24 to 48 hours of antibiotic initiation.

▶ The type of meningitis can be determined by analyzing CSF protein, glucose, and white cell count, and by obtaining CSF Gram stain, culture, PCR, and antigen/antibody testing.

▶ Brain and spinal abscesses in patients who are immunocompetent are usually polymicrobial, requiring antibiotic coverage for gram-positive, gram-negative, and anaerobic organisms. If there is significant mass effect or proximity of a brain abscess to the ventricles, surgical drainage should be considered.

▶ Encephalitis can be infectious (most commonly viral) or immune mediated (eg, anti-*N*-methyl-D-aspartate [NMDA] receptor encephalitis). Diagnosis is made by neuroimaging and CSF analysis (including PCR). In patients with presumed viral encephalitis, empiric treatment with acyclovir should be initiated while awaiting CSF PCR results.

▶ HIV can affect any level of the nervous system either directly (HIV neuropathy and HAND) or due to opportunistic infection (eg, cryptococcal meningitis, toxoplasmosis, PML due to JC virus, and EBV-associated PCNSL).

▶ One or more ring-enhancing brain lesions in a patient with HIV and low CD4 count are commonly due to toxoplasmosis or PCNSL. Patients are generally treated with empiric therapy for toxoplasmosis and reevaluated clinically and with neuroimaging at 2 weeks. If there is no clinical or radiologic improvement, biopsy should be considered.

REFERENCES

1. Wright WF, Pinto CN, Palisoc K, Baghli S. Viral (aseptic) meningitis: a review. *J Neurol Sci*. 2019;398:176-183.

2. Thigpen MC, Whitney CG, Messonnier NE, et al. Bacterial meningitis in the United States, 1998–2007. *N Engl J Med*. 2011;364(21):2016-2025.

3. Brouwer MC, Tunkel AR, van de Beek D. Epidemiology, diagnosis, and antimicrobial treatment of acute bacterial meningitis. *Clin Microbiol Rev*. 2010;23(3):467-492.

4. Durand M, Calderwood S, Weber D, et al. Acute bacterial meningitis in adults: a review of 493 episodes. *N Engl J Med*. 1993;328(1):21-28.

5. Attia J, Hatala R, Cook DJ, Wong JG. Does this adult patient have acute meningitis? *JAMA*. 1999;282(2):175-181.

6. Weisfelt M, Van De Beek D, Spanjaard L, et al. Community-acquired bacterial meningitis in older people. *J Am Geriatr Soc*. 2006;54(10):1500-1507.

7. Kanegaye JT, Soliemanzadeh P, Bradley JS. Lumbar puncture in pediatric bacterial meningitis: defining the time interval for recovery of cerebrospinal fluid pathogens after parenteral antibiotic pretreatment. *Pediatrics*. 2001;108(5):1169-1174.

8. Velissaris D, Pintea M, Pantzaris N, et al. The role of procalcitonin in the diagnosis of meningitis: a literature review. *J Clin Med*. 2018;7(6):148.

9. Abdalkader M, Xie J, Cervantes-Arslanian A, Takahashi C, Mian AZ. Imaging of intracranial infections. *Semin Neurol*. 2019;39(3):322-333.

10. Kanjilal S, Cho TA, Piantadosi A. Diagnostic testing in central nervous system infection. *Semin Neurol*. 2019;39(3):297-311.

11. Liesman RM, Strasburg AP, Heitman AK, Theel ES, Patel R, Binnicker MJ. Evaluation of a commercial multiplex molecular panel for diagnosis of infectious meningitis and encephalitis. *J Clin Microbiol*. 2018;56(4):e01927-17.

12. Ramachandran PS, Wilson MR. Metagenomics for neurological infections—expanding our imagination. *Nat Rev Neurol*. 2020;16(10):547-556.

13. Baldwin KJ, Avila JD. Diagnostic approach to chronic meningitis. *Neurol Clin*. 2018;36(4):831-849.

14. Brouwer MC, McIntyre P, Prasad K, van de Beek D. Corticosteroids for acute bacterial meningitis. Cochrane Acute Respiratory Infections Group, editor. *Cochrane Database Syst Rev [Internet]*. 2015;2015(9):CD004405. doi:10.1002/14651858.CD004405.pub5

15. Tunkel AR, Hartman BJ, Kaplan SL, et al. Practice guidelines for the management of bacterial meningitis. *Clin Infect Dis*. 2004;39(9):1267-1284.

16. Weisfelt M, van de Beek D, Spanjaard L, Reitsma JB, de Gans J. A risk score for unfavorable outcome in adults with bacterial meningitis. *Ann Neurol*. 2008;63(1):90-97.

17. Brouwer MC, Tunkel AR, McKhann GM, van de Beek D. Brain abscess. *N Engl J Med*. 2014;371(5):447-456.

18. Brouwer MC, Coutinho JM, van de Beek D. Clinical characteristics and outcome of brain abscess: systematic review and meta-analysis. *Neurology*. 2014;82(9):806-813.

19. Darouiche RO. Spinal epidural abscess. *N Engl J Med*. 2006;355(19):2012-2020.

20. Long B, Carlson J, Montrief T, Koyfman A. High risk and low prevalence diseases: spinal epidural abscess. *Am J Emerg Med*. 2022;53:168-172.

21. Granerod J, Crowcroft NS. The epidemiology of acute encephalitis. *Neuropsychol Rehabil*. 2007;17(4-5):406-428.

22. Venkatesan A, Michael BD, Probasco JC, Geocadin RG, Solomon T. Acute encephalitis in immunocompetent adults. *Lancet Lond Engl*. 2019;393(10172):702-716.

23. Whitley RJ, Soong S-J, Linneman C Jr, Liu C, Pazin G, Alford CA. Herpes simplex encephalitis: clinical assessment. *JAMA*. 1982;247(3):317-320.

24. Whitley RJ. Herpes simplex encephalitis: adolescents and adults. *Antiviral Res.* 2006;71(2-3):141-148.

25. Thakur KT, Motta M, Asemota AO, et al. Predictors of outcome in acute encephalitis. *Neurology.* 2013;81(9):793-800.

26. Labeaud AD, Bashir F, King CH. Measuring the burden of arboviral diseases: the spectrum of morbidity and mortality from four prevalent infections. *Popul Health Metr.* 2011;9(1):1.

27. Sacktor N. Changing clinical phenotypes of HIV-associated neurocognitive disorders. *J Neurovirol.* 2018;24(2):141-145.

28. Garcia HH, Nath A, Del Brutto OH. Parasitic infections of the nervous system. *Semin Neurol.* 2019;39(3):358-368.

29. Vidal JE. HIV-related cerebral toxoplasmosis revisited: current concepts and controversies of an old disease. *J Int Assoc Provid AIDS Care.* 2019;18:2325958219867315.

30. Engsig FN, Hansen AB, Omland LH, et al. Incidence, clinical presentation, and outcome of progressive multifocal leukoencephalopathy in HIV-infected patients during the highly active antiretroviral therapy era: a nationwide cohort study. *J Infect Dis.* 2009;199(1):77-83.

31. Koralnik IJ, Wüthrich C, Dang X, et al. JC virus granule cell neuronopathy: a novel clinical syndrome distinct from progressive multifocal leukoencephalopathy. *Ann Neurol.* 2005;57(4):576-580.

32. Tunkel AR, Hasbun R, Bhimraj A, et al. 2017 Infectious Diseases Society of America's clinical practice guidelines for healthcare-associated ventriculitis and meningitis. *Clin Infect Dis.* 2017;64(6):e34-e65.

CHAPTER 22

Vestibular Disorders

Justin L. Hoskin and Terry D. Fife

INTRODUCTION

The differential diagnosis of dizziness is broad, including vestibular, neurologic, cardiovascular, psychological, and systemic conditions. An approach to the patient with dizziness is presented in Chapter 9, classifying dizziness into one of four clinical syndromes: episodic triggered vestibular syndrome (recurrent episodic dizziness provoked by a trigger), episodic spontaneous vestibular syndrome (recurrent episodic dizziness without a provoking trigger), acute vestibular syndrome (sudden-onset continuous dizziness), and chronic vestibular syndrome (chronic continuous dizziness for months). In this chapter, the diagnosis and treatment of disorders in each category are discussed individually, with a brief summary of each condition in Table 22.1.

EPISODIC TRIGGERED VESTIBULAR SYNDROMES

Benign Paroxysmal Positional Vertigo

Benign paroxysmal positional vertigo (BPPV) is one of the most common causes of dizziness. BPPV is caused by otoconial debris from the utricle entering one of the semicircular canals (called *canaliths*). This may be the result of preceding head trauma or inner ear inflammation (eg, vestibular neuritis), but is most commonly idiopathic. The condition most often occurs unilaterally. The most commonly affected of the three semicircular canals is the posterior semicircular canal (75%-80%). Less often, the horizontal semicircular canal (10%-20%), anterior semicircular canal (<5%), or multiple semicircular canals may be affected. BPPV is most common in adults aged 40 to 65 years old and occurs more commonly in women than in men.

BPPV is the quintessential example of the episodic triggered vestibular syndrome. The trigger is changes in head position, which may occur when rolling over in bed, turning one's head quickly, or extending the neck (eg, while in the shower or reaching into a high cupboard). The duration of dizziness episodes is brief, lasting less than a minute. Dizziness in BPPV may be accompanied by nausea, although emesis is rare. Patients with BPPV may also have less severe dizziness between episodes.

Posterior canal BPPV is diagnosed by the Dix-Hallpike maneuver, as illustrated in Chapter 9. Starting with the patient seated on an examination

TABLE 22.1   Clinical Features Distinguishing Selected Causes of Dizziness and Vertigo

Disorder	Onset	Timing and duration	Triggers	Associated features
Episodic triggered vestibular syndrome				
Benign paroxysmal positional vertigo (BPPV)	Acute	5-60 s	Tilting head back, rolling in bed, straightening after bending	Vertigo and nystagmus with Dix-Hallpike maneuver on affected side
Superior canal dehiscence syndrome	Chronic dizziness with superimposed episodes	Often chronic dizziness with short-duration triggered nystagmus and vertigo	Pressure-induced or sound-induced	Autophony, pulsatile tinnitus; downbeat and torsional nystagmus with triggers
Episodic spontaneous vestibular syndrome				
Ménière disease	Acute or evolving over 30 min with some variability	30 min-12 h	No trigger in most cases	Unilateral tinnitus and hearing loss that may fluctuate on the affected side; worse during head motion; low-frequency hearing loss on the affected side
Vestibular migraine	Acute or more gradual, sometimes discrete spells, sometimes constant but varying in intensity	Spinning, tilting, rocking, floating; may vary from brief quick spins lasting a few seconds recurrently to spells lasting minutes to much of the day; visually induced vertigo/dizziness, motion sensitivity may be nearly constant	No trigger	Migraine headache history; periodic photophobia or phonophobia; examination is usually normal.
Acute vestibular syndrome				
Vestibular neuritis	Acute or evolving over 30 min with some variability	Days to weeks	No reliable trigger, 15% with antecedent upper respiratory infection symptoms	Worse with any head motion; nausea, direction-constant nystagmus, abnormal head impulse test to the side affected
Posterior circulation ischemia	Acute	Sudden in onset; duration of symptoms depends on size of stroke	No trigger	Normal head impulse test; direction-changing nystagmus, skew deviation, and ataxia may be present.
Chronic vestibular syndrome				
Persistent postural-perceptual dizziness (PPPD)	Gradual after inciting event	Chronic, daily	Visually-induced worsening (grocery store aisles and busy patterns), anxiety or stress	Anxiety, depression; minimal nausea
Mal de débarquement syndrome	Acute after prolonged motion exposure	Chronic, daily	No trigger after initial exposure	Anxiety, improvement with motion

table, the patient's head is turned 45° toward the side to be tested. The patient is then rapidly brought into the supine position with the neck slightly extended over the head of the bed while the patient's head is held by the examiner during the maneuver to avoid turning or neck hyperextension. If the patient has posterior semicircular canal BPPV, when the Dix-Hallpike maneuver is performed on the affected side, the patient experiences dizziness and develops transient upbeat-torsional nystagmus with the top pole of rotation of the eye beating toward the downward (affected) ear. Symptoms and nystagmus usually come on after a brief latency period of a few seconds. After a few seconds, both symptoms and nystagmus abate. If the Dix-Hallpike test finding is normal on one side, the opposite side should be assessed. If a patient with episodic vertigo triggered by head position develops vertigo during the Dix-Hallpike maneuver but without nystagmus, it is reasonable to proceed with treatment for presumed BPPV. If BPPV is suspected but the side is unclear, there is no harm in treating both sides sequentially.

Treatment of BPPV can be performed at the bedside using canalith repositioning procedures that move the canalith(s) from the affected semicircular canal into the utricle. The Epley maneuver is an effective method to treat posterior semicircular canal BPPV (Figure 22.1). The first step of the maneuver is the

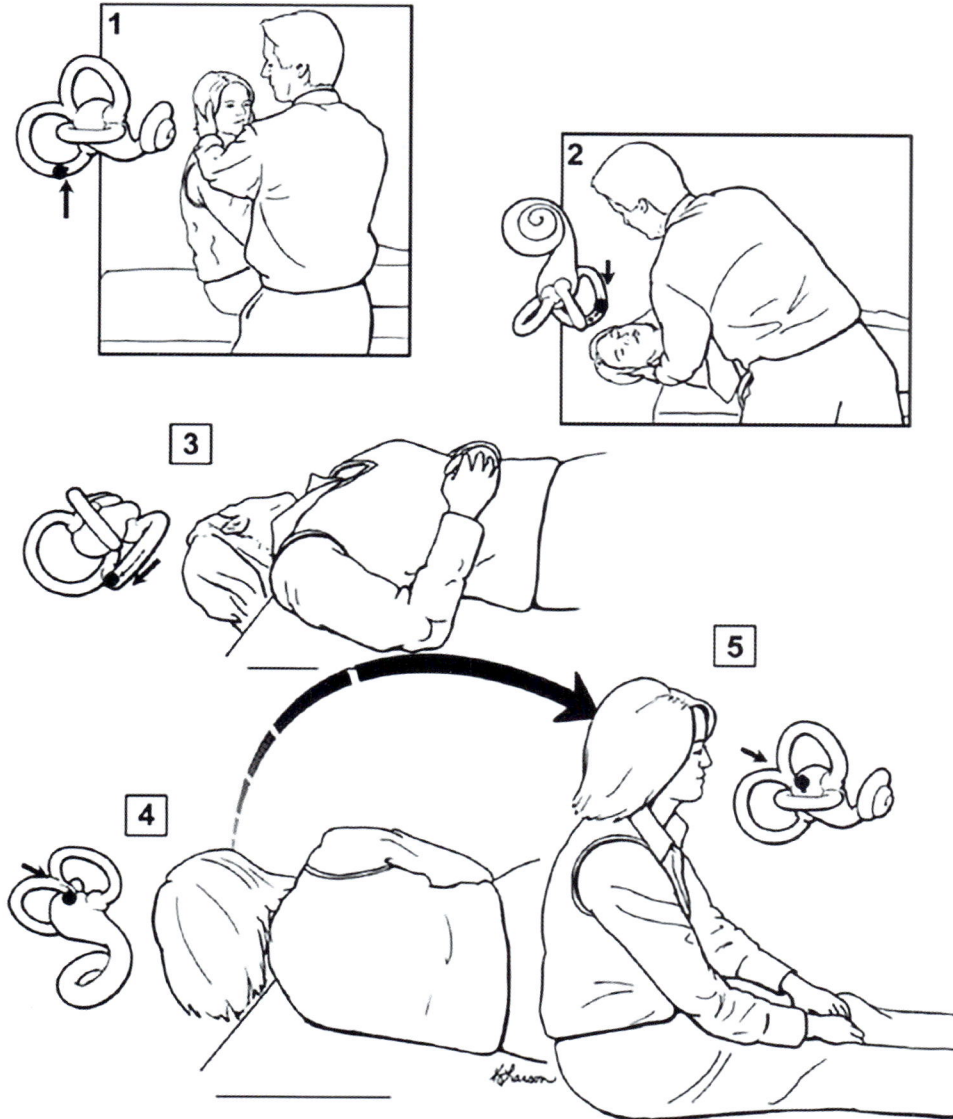

FIGURE 22.1 Canalith repositioning procedure (Epley maneuver) for treatment of right-sided posterior canal benign paroxysmal positional vertigo (BPPV). Positions 1 and 2 are the same as the Dix-Hallpike maneuver. Positions 2 to 4 are movements that use the effect of gravity to move the otoconial debris (arrow), and positions 4 and 5 induce the otoconial debris to pass from the semicircular canal into the main vestibule. Treatment of the left side is the mirror image of this figure (Used with permission from Barrow Neurological Institute, Phoenix, Arizona.).

same as the Dix-Hallpike maneuver: the patient's head is turned 45° toward the affected side, and the patient is rapidly brought into the supine position with the neck extended (this often triggers vertigo with accompanying upbeat and torsional nystagmus as observed during the Dix-Hallpike maneuver). After 30 seconds in this position, the patient's head is turned 90° toward the unaffected ear. After 30 seconds in this position, the patient then rolls their body toward the affected ear such that they are they lying on their side and looking down at the floor. After holding this position for 30 seconds, the patient sits up, keeping their head turned over their shoulder (toward the unaffected side).

The Epley maneuver is a highly effective treatment, with many patients experiencing immediate resolution of symptoms.[1] Some patients may need to perform the maneuver again at home or with a vestibular-trained physical therapist. The Semont maneuver is another effective canalith repositioning procedure that the patient can perform at home for the treatment of posterior canal BPPV (Figure 22.2). If there is no improvement

with repeated repositioning maneuvers, another diagnosis should be considered. In rare instances, BPPV may rarely be caused by otoconial debris in the horizontal or anterior canal. BPPV affecting either of these canals has a different pattern of nystagmus and requires different canalith repositioning maneuvers; these patients should be evaluated and treated by a vestibular-trained medical provider or physical therapist. There is usually no need for vestibular suppressant medications in the treatment of BPPV, although they can be considered prior to canalith repositioning for patients with anxiety or severe motion sickness.

Superior Canal Dehiscence Syndrome and Perilymphatic Fistula

Superior canal dehiscence syndrome and perilymphatic fistula are rare otologic conditions. Superior canal dehiscence syndrome occurs in a small segment of the population with a congenitally thin temporal bone overlying the top part of the labyrinth. Over time, or with strain

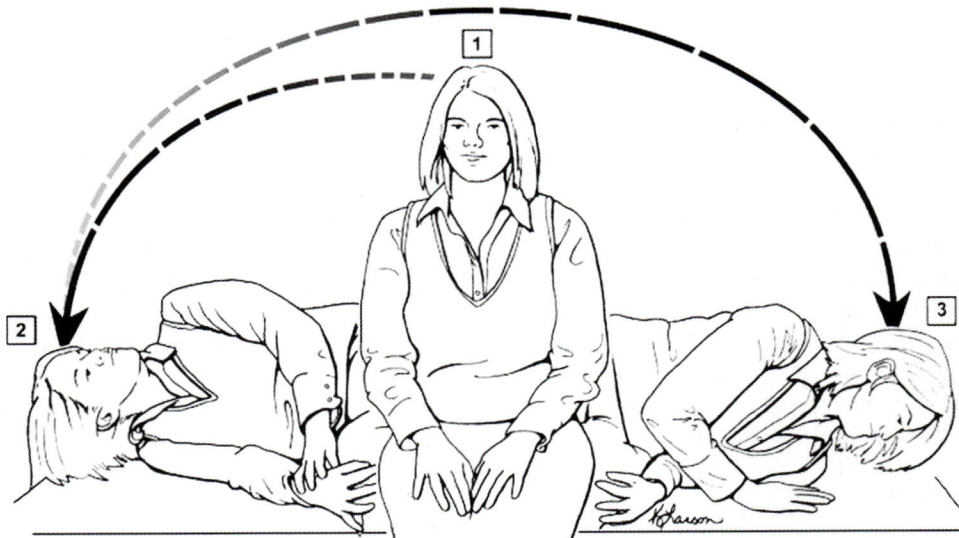

FIGURE 22.2 The Semont (liberatory) maneuver for right-sided posterior semicircular canal benign paroxysmal positional vertigo (BPPV). Positions 1 and 2 are similar to the Dix-Hallpike maneuver, except the patient is on their side rather than their back. The position is held for 20 seconds, and then in one large quick movement, the patient is taken from position 2 to 3, keeping the angle of the head unchanged and 45° toward the left shoulder. After 15 seconds, the patient may sit up. Treatment of left-sided posterior canal BPPV would be the mirror image of this figure. This may also be used for nightly home exercises (Used with permission from Barrow Neurological Institute, Phoenix, Arizona.).

or Valsalva, the paper-thin bone dehisces, causing a syndrome in which the patient has recurrent brief dizziness, mild hearing loss in the affected ear, pulsatile tinnitus, and hypersensitivity to sound, referred to as *autophony* (increased volume of one's own voice and hearing one's own heart sounds or eyelids). Diagnosis is by computed tomography (CT) of the temporal bone and vestibular myogenic evoked potential (VEMP) testing. Treatment, if needed, is surgical.

A perilymphatic fistula is a defect in the membranes separating the middle and inner ear, usually in the round window or the oval window. Perilymphatic fistula is most common after ear surgery but occasionally occurs spontaneously, causing hearing loss, ear fullness, and dizziness. In some patients this may resolve spontaneously, but others require surgical repair.

Patients suspected of either of these conditions should be referred to an otolaryngologist or neuro-otologist for diagnosis and treatment.

EPISODIC SPONTANEOUS VESTIBULAR SYNDROMES

Ménière Disease

Ménière disease is a rare condition caused by recurrent spells of elevated endolymphatic fluid pressure, although the etiology of this is unclear. The age of onset is usually between 30 and 60 years old. Episodes of vertigo occur without trigger, last hours, and are associated with hearing loss, tinnitus, and aural fullness in the affected ear. Over time, patients develop low-frequency hearing loss (in contrast to the more common high-frequency hearing loss that can occur with aging). Rarely, patients may develop drop attacks in which they suddenly lose postural control, causing them to fall to the ground with retained awareness (called *otolithic crises of Tumarkin*).

Examination of patients with Ménière disease may be normal aside from hearing loss, although nystagmus may be present during an attack, and some patients may have gait imbalance.

Treatment involves lifestyle modifications, including reducing dietary sodium and minimizing alcohol intake. Treatment may also include thiazide diuretics and betahistine (this medication must be compounded or obtained outside of the United States).[2] In severe cases, surgical procedures may be considered, such as intratympanic injection of glucocorticoids or gentamicin, or labyrinthectomy. Intratympanic glucocorticoid treatment appears to have relatively few risks but may be ineffective. Intratympanic gentamicin may provide some benefit but can lead to hearing loss in some patients. These more invasive measures should be offered only when less invasive treatments have not led to symptomatic improvement. For symptomatic treatment of acute episodes, antihistamines and antiemetics can be used.

Vestibular Migraine

Vestibular migraine is a common cause of the episodic spontaneous vestibular syndrome. Patients with vestibular migraine may present with vertigo accompanying typical migraine headaches (unilateral, throbbing, severe, accompanied by photophobia, phonophobia, nausea, and vomiting).[3] However, many patients present with episodic vertigo without concurrent headache, and some may have no headaches at all. Episodes generally last minutes to days. In addition, some patients present primarily with severe constant motion intolerance with nausea, and worsened dizziness when seeing objects in motion around them. The examination is generally normal, although mild nystagmus may be seen during episodes.

Acute treatments with analgesics used for migraine seem to provide little benefit for vestibular migraine. Medications such as promethazine, diazepam, meclizine, and ondansetron can sometimes provide short-term symptom relief. Lifestyle changes and migraine prophylactic agents are the mainstay of treatment of vestibular migraine (see Chapter 15).

ACUTE VESTIBULAR SYNDROME

Acute vestibular syndrome refers to sudden-onset unprovoked vertigo lasting at least 24 hours, usually with nausea, vomiting, and imbalance. The two most common conditions causing this syndrome are vestibular neuritis and posterior circulation stroke.

Vestibular Neuritis

Vestibular neuritis is thought to be caused by inflammation of the vestibular nerve (cranial nerve 8) due to a viral infection, although the precise etiology is unknown. The condition is most common in patients aged 30 to 50 years old.

Vestibular neuritis is a clinical diagnosis based on the history and examination. Patients describe acute onset of severe vertigo with nausea, vomiting, and gait imbalance. During ambulation, patients may fall toward the side of the affected ear. By definition, hearing is not affected. When hearing is affected, this suggests labyrinthitis. If a patient presents with acute vertigo accompanied by unilateral hearing loss, viral labyrinthitis or infarction in the territory of the anterior inferior cerebellar artery should be considered. If there is ipsilateral facial paresis, hearing loss, and visible painful vesicles in or around the ear, Ramsay Hunt syndrome (herpes zoster oticus) should be considered.

Patients with vestibular neuritis present similarly to patients with posterior circulation stroke, with acute continuous dizziness. These two conditions can be distinguished by a series of three bedside physical examination maneuvers: head impulse, nystagmus, and test of skew, known as the HINTS (*h*ead *i*mpulse, *n*ystagmus, *t*est of *s*kew) examination. The performance and interpretation of the HINTS examination is discussed in Chapter 9. In vestibular neuritis, patients have a peripheral pattern of findings: abnormal head impulse test on one side, unidirectional nystagmus with the fast phase in the same direction on all positions of gaze, and absent skew deviation.

Vestibular neuritis may be treated with a short course of oral corticosteroids, although the evidence is limited.[4,5] Symptomatic treatment can include vestibular suppressants (eg, antihistamines such as meclizine) or antiemetics (eg, prochlorperazine), but these should only be used for a few days since prolonged use of vestibular suppressants can delay adaptive recovery through central compensation. Vestibular rehabilitation therapy is recommended.[6] The condition is usually severe for several days and then improves, although patients may note residual dizziness with head movement for weeks to months. About half of patients recover fully within about 2 months. Some patients may go on to develop BPPV or persistent postural-perceptual dizziness (PPPD); see subsequent text.

Vertebrobasilar Ischemia

Vertebrobasilar disease can present as episodic spontaneous vertigo from transient ischemic attacks (TIAs), or a more acute vestibular syndrome from ischemic stroke. Posterior circulation stroke often causes ataxia and focal neurologic signs referable to the brainstem in addition to acute-onset vertigo. However, some patients with brainstem or cerebellar stroke may present with isolated vertigo and imbalance, similar to the presentation of vestibular neuritis. In such patients with acute vestibular syndrome, the HINTS examination is highly sensitive and specific in helping to distinguish stroke from vestibular neuritis—more sensitive and specific than magnetic resonance imaging (MRI) in the first 24 hours when performed by experienced specialists. The HINTS examination is discussed in Chapter 9. In patients with posterior circulation stroke, head impulse testing is normal, and direction-changing nystagmus and/or skew deviation may be observed. Diagnosis and treatment of stroke is discussed in Chapter 16.

CHRONIC VESTIBULAR SYNDROME

Chronic vestibular syndrome refers to months or years of dizziness.

Persistent Postural-Perceptual Dizziness

PPPD is characterized by a continuous or near continuous sense of dizziness, often described as rocking, swaying, floating, or lightheadedness. The dizziness is provoked or worsened when the patient is standing or walking. Along with dizziness, patients experience visual disturbances such as blurred vision, difficulty focusing, dizziness worsened when looking at complex visual patterns (eg, carpet, tiling, or pictures on the wall), or a heightened sensitivity to crowded environments (eg, grocery stores).

The cause of PPPD is not fully understood, but it is thought to result from a combination of physical and psychological factors.[7] Patients often describe an inciting initial event that is vestibular or balance related. However, the event does not have to involve the vestibular or neurologic systems, and PPPD can also be seen after a medical illness, surgical intervention, psychological distress, or other traumatic event. It is thought that ongoing sensitization of the central nervous system and maladaptive behavioral patterns contribute to the persistence of symptoms. Patients often have a history of anxiety, depression, or other psychiatric conditions. The diagnosis of PPPD is made by clinical evaluation and by using the clinical criteria described by the International Classification of Vestibular Disorders.[8]

Treatment of PPPD involves a multidisciplinary approach addressing both the physical and psychological aspects of the condition. The first step is educating and counseling the patient regarding the condition. Patients may benefit from vestibular rehabilitation, selective serotonin reuptake inhibitors (SSRIs) or serotonin and norepinephrine reuptake inhibitors (SNRIs), and cognitive behavioral therapy.

Mal de Débarquement Syndrome

Mal de débarquement syndrome, also known as *land sickness*, refers to dizziness that develops after a prolonged period of motion (riding on a boat, airplane, car, or bus). Patients describe feeling like they are still in motion after their journey has ended and often note improvement in their dizziness when they are back in the inciting means of transportation. The condition is thought to be due to disruption of the normal function of the vestibular system by prolonged exposure to movement. The condition usually lasts for months, but for some it can persist for years.

The diagnosis is made by history. The examination is generally normal. Patients should be referred for vestibular therapy, but this is not universally effective. SSRI, SNRI, or benzodiazepine treatment may be considered in severe cases, although evidence is lacking.

SUMMARY

Patients with dizziness can be classified as having one of four clinical syndromes, each of which has a distinct differential diagnosis. Most of these conditions can be diagnosed clinically based on the history and examination. In addition to the neurologic disorders

discussed in this chapter, providers should consider medical and medication-induced etiologies of dizziness (see Chapter 9).

EDITORS' KEY POINTS

▶ BPPV causes positionally triggered episodic vertigo, occurring due to otoconial debris in a semicircular canal; this common syndrome can be diagnosed and treated by easily performed bedside maneuvers (eg, the Dix-Hallpike maneuver for diagnosis and the Epley maneuver for treatment).

▶ Ménière disease, superior canal dehiscence syndrome, and perilymphatic fistula are otologic causes of vertigo with auditory symptoms that require otolaryngologic assessment and management.

▶ Episodic vertigo can occur as a migrainous symptom (vestibular migraine) with or without a concomitant headache.

▶ The acute vestibular syndrome can be due to vestibular neuritis (eg, from vestibular nerve inflammation, possibly viral) or posterior circulation (eg, brainstem or cerebellar) stroke. The clinical presentations of these two conditions may be indistinguishable from each other, and bedside and other clinical investigations should be performed with this important dichotomy in mind.

▶ PPPD is a chronic vestibular disorder felt to be due to both vestibular and psychological factors, requiring a multidisciplinary approach to treatment.

▶ Mal de débarquement syndrome is characterized by a chronic (months to years) feeling of persistent motion after a journey has ended (eg, by boat, plane, or car), and typically transiently improves while resuming the same transportation.

REFERENCES

1. Fife TD, Iverson DJ, Lempert T, et al. Quality Standards Subcommittee, American Academy of Neurology. Practice parameter: therapies for benign paroxysmal positional vertigo (an evidence-based review): report of the Quality Standards Subcommittee of the American Academy of Neurology. *Neurology*. 2008;70(22):2067-2074.

2. Hoskin JL. Ménière's disease: new guidelines, subtypes, imaging, and more. *Curr Opin Neurol*. 2022;35(1):90-97. doi:10.1097/WCO.0000000000001021

3. Lempert T, Olesen J, Furman J, et al. Vestibular migraine: diagnostic criteria1. *J Vestib Res.* 2022;32(1):1-6.
4. Yoo MH, Yang CJ, Kim SA, et al. Efficacy of steroid therapy based on symptomatic and functional improvement in patients with vestibular neuritis: a prospective randomized controlled trial. *Eur Arch Otorhinolaryngol.* 2017;274(6):2443-2451. doi:10.1007/s00405-017-4556-1
5. Fishman JM, Burgess C, Waddell A. Corticosteroids for the treatment of idiopathic acute vestibular dysfunction (vestibular neuritis). *Cochrane Database Syst Rev.* 2011;(5):CD008607. doi:10.1002/14651858.CD008607.pub2
6. Hall CD, Herdman SJ, Whitney SL, et al. Vestibular rehabilitation for peripheral vestibular hypofunction: an updated clinical practice guideline from the Academy of Neurologic Physical Therapy of the American Physical Therapy Association. *J Neurol Phys Ther.* 2022;46(2):118-177.
7. Holle D, Schulte-Steinberg B, Wurthmann S, et al. Persistent postural-perceptual dizziness: a matter of higher, central dysfunction? *PLoS One.* 2015;10(11):e0142468.
8. Staab JP, Eckhardt-Henn A, Horii A, et al. Diagnostic criteria for persistent postural-perceptual dizziness (PPPD): consensus document of the committee for the classification of vestibular disorders of the Bárány society. *J Vestib Res.* 2017;27(4):191-208. doi:10.3233/VES-170622

CHAPTER 23

Spinal Cord and Nerve Root Disorders

Shamik Bhattacharyya

INTRODUCTION

Disorders of the spinal cord (referred to as *myelopathies*) and nerve roots (referred to as *radiculopathies*) are common in clinical practice, presenting with symptoms such as sensory changes, weakness, gait disorders, and pain. Correlating symptoms and signs with neuroimaging findings can be challenging, leading to misdiagnosis, unnecessary testing, and referral for spine surgery that may not benefit the patient. Structural spine disease (ie, degenerative changes to the structures of the spinal column) is the most common cause of myelopathy and radiculopathy; therefore, after reviewing the approach to the diagnosis of myelopathy and radiculopathy and their different etiologic diagnoses, this chapter focuses on the approach to diagnosis and treatment of structural etiologies of myelopathy and radiculopathy.

MYELOPATHY

The term *myelopathy* refers to any disease of the spinal cord. Anatomically, the spinal cord consists of gray matter (neuronal structures) in the center and white matter (axonal projections) surrounding the gray matter (Figure 23.1). Although there are multiple ascending and descending white matter tracts, the most clinically relevant pathways are the lateral corticospinal tracts, dorsal columns (also known as the posterior columns), and spinothalamic tracts (also known as the anterolateral tracts).

Each lateral corticospinal tract is located postero laterally in the spinal cord and contributes to motor control in the ipsilateral half of the body (eg, a lesion in the right corticospinal tract within the spinal cord would cause right-sided weakness below the level of the lesion). The dorsal columns are in the posterior spinal cord, and each carries vibratory and proprioceptive sense from the ipsilateral half of the body (eg, a right dorsal column lesion results in loss of vibratory and proprioceptive sense in the right side of the body below the level of the lesion). In contrast, the spinothalamic tracts carry pain and temperature sensation from the contralateral side of the body (eg, a lesion in the right spinothalamic tract causes pain and temperature sensation deficits in the left half of the body below the level of the lesion).

Due to the involvement of the tracts listed, myelopathy can cause symptoms of weakness, numbness, and gait imbalance (resulting from weakness and/or diminished proprioception). Impaired bladder and bowel sphincter control is also common in myelopathy, although not universally present. Patients with cervical myelopathy may report a sensation of electricity that runs down the spine when they flex the neck forward (known as *Lhermitte sign*).

On examination, patients with chronic myelopathy have upper motor neuron signs, including spasticity, hyperreflexia, ankle clonus, and an upgoing toe upon stimulation of the sole of the foot (known as a

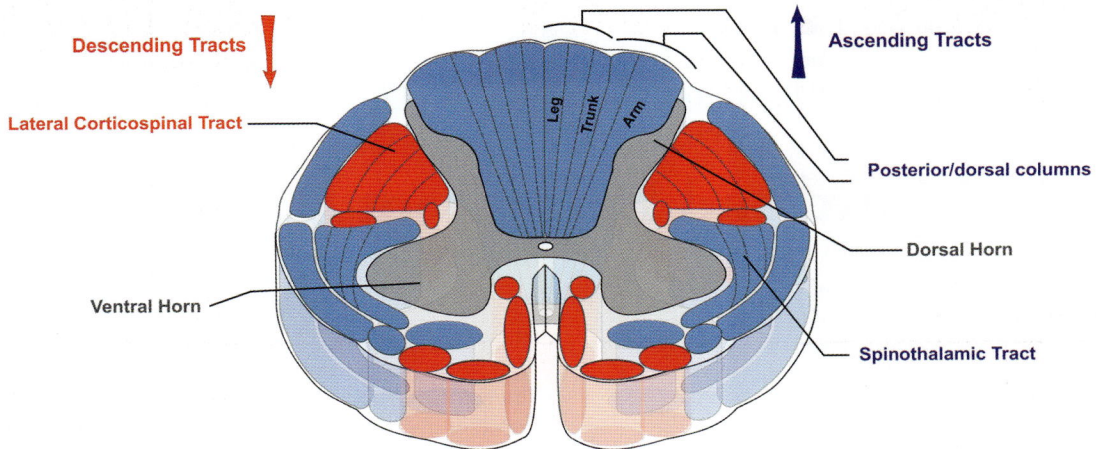

FIGURE 23.1 Axial cross section of spinal cord. Descending tracts are shown in red and ascending tracts are shown in blue. The most clinically relevant pathways are the lateral corticospinal tracts for motor control, dorsal columns for vibration and joint position sense, and spinothalamic tracts for pain/temperature perception. (This work is licensed under a Creative Commons Attribution 2.0 Generic License from Shamik Bhattacharyya.)

Babinski sign). Spasticity of the lower extremities can lead to abnormal gait with circumduction of the legs and scuffing of the toes with each step. If there is not complete paralysis, the pattern of weakness may be one in which the extensor muscles in the arms and flexor muscles in the legs are weaker than the flexors of the arms and extensors of the legs. Notably, some patients may have spasticity and upper motor neuron signs without weakness. Upper motor neuron signs are not immediately present in acute spinal cord injury and take time to emerge; the presence of flaccid paralysis with areflexia in acute spinal cord injury is referred to as *spinal shock*.

Decreased sensation to pain and/or vibration/proprioception can be seen below the level of the spinal cord lesion. A sensory level above which the patient can perceive pain and below which they cannot is referred to as a *spinal level* and is characteristic of spinal cord disease, although not universally present; the lesion can localize at or above the spinal level found on examination. If the dorsal columns are affected, Romberg sign may be present.

Depending on the tracts of the spinal cord affected by a disease process, different patterns of clinical symptoms and signs can be seen (Table 23.1), including the following:

- Total cord syndrome
- Hemicord (Brown-Séquard) syndrome
- Central cord syndrome
- Posterior cord (dorsal column) syndrome
- Posterolateral cord syndrome
- Anterior cord syndrome
- Anterior horn syndrome

Identification of one of these patterns helps not only to localize the patient's syndrome to and within the spinal cord but also begins to refine the differential diagnosis. However, it should be noted that particular etiologies of myelopathy may cause more than one type of syndrome. For example, cervical spondylotic myelopathy can cause central cord syndrome or posterior column syndrome.

Total Cord Syndrome

This is the most severe form of spinal cord injury and causes dysfunction in all modalities below the level of the lesion. Patients experience bilateral paralysis, sphincter dysfunction, and loss of sensation in all modalities below the level of the lesion. Any form of severe spinal cord injury can cause this syndrome, including spinal cord trauma, spinal cord hemorrhage, and severe inflammatory conditions (transverse myelitis).

TABLE 23.1	Spinal Cord Syndromes		
Syndrome	Lateral corticospinal tract involvement	Dorsal column involvement	Spinothalamic tract involvement
Total cord syndrome	✓ (bilateral)	✓ (bilateral)	✓ (bilateral)
Hemicord syndrome	✓ (ipsilateral)	✓ (ipsilateral)—variably affected	✓ (contralateral symptoms)
Central cord syndrome	✓ (arm > leg)		✓ (hands progressing to cape-like distribution)
Posterior cord (dorsal column) syndrome		✓ (unilateral or bilateral)	
Posterolateral cord syndrome	✓ (unilateral or bilateral)	✓ (unilateral or bilateral)	
Anterior cord syndrome	✓ (typically bilateral)		✓ (typically bilateral)

Hemicord Syndrome (Brown-Séquard Syndrome)

Hemicord syndrome results from injury to one side of the spinal cord. This causes ipsilateral weakness and ipsilateral loss of vibration and joint position sense below the level of the lesion but contralateral loss of temperature/pain sensation below the level of the lesion. Partial forms of the syndrome can also occur in which there is relative preservation of vibration and joint position sense. Dissociated sensory loss with one side of the body impaired in pain/temperature sensation but with preserved vibration and proprioception and the opposite pattern on the contralateral side of the body can only occur with unilateral spinal cord lesions. This syndrome can be seen with any cause of partial cord injuries but is especially common with penetrating trauma and in multiple sclerosis (due to demyelinating lesions affecting only part of the spinal cord).

Central Cord Syndrome

In central cord syndrome, the central region of the spinal cord is involved, predominantly affecting the crossing fibers destined for the spinothalamic tracts (which mediate pinprick/temperature sensation). This causes isolated loss of pain and temperature sensation, most commonly beginning in the upper extremities (since this is a common site of central cord pathology such as a syrinx), progressing to a cape-like distribution over the torso as the lesion expands. More extensive central cord lesions can affect the medial portions of the corticospinal tracts and autonomic pathways, causing bowel and bladder dysfunction. Central cord

syndrome can be seen with cervical hyperextension injury (often in an older adult with preexisting cervical spondylotic disease), syringomyelia (expansion of the central canal of the spinal cord as can be seen in association with Chiari malformation), spinal cord neoplasms (eg, ependymoma) or vascular malformations (eg, cavernous malformation), and inflammatory conditions (eg, neuromyelitis optica spectrum disorder and myelin oligodendrocyte glycoprotein [MOG] antibody-associated disorder; in contrast, myelitis in multiple sclerosis tends to affect the more lateral portion of the cord; see Chapter 20).

Posterior Cord (Dorsal Column) Syndrome

Posterior cord (dorsal column) dysfunction causes impaired vibratory and joint position sense below the level of the lesion, leading to numbness, paresthesias, and sensory ataxia. Patients with posterior spinal cord dysfunction may, therefore, present for evaluation of gait dysfunction. When the dorsal column lesion is in the cervical spinal cord, patients can exhibit the Lhermitte sign. Causes of posterior cord syndrome include multiple sclerosis, syphilis (tabes dorsalis, which also involves the dorsal roots), posterior spinal artery infarct, cervical spondylotic disease, and partial cord trauma.

Posterolateral Cord Syndrome

Posterolateral cord syndrome affects both the dorsal columns and the corticospinal tracts, causing a combination of numbness and sensory ataxia with weakness and upper motor neuron signs. Causes include vitamin B_{12} deficiency (resulting in the syndrome known as *subacute combined degeneration* of the spinal cord), copper deficiency, nitrous oxide misuse, cervical spondylotic disease, and HIV-associated vacuolar myelopathy. Vitamin B_{12} deficiency is the most common cause of this syndrome, and so a serum vitamin B_{12} level should always be assessed in patients with posterolateral cord syndrome so this condition can be rapidly diagnosed and treated.

Anterior Cord Syndrome

Anterior cord syndrome affects the anterior two-thirds of the spinal cord, causing dysfunction of the corticospinal tracts and spinothalamic tracts. Patients, therefore, develop weakness and loss of pain/temperature sensation below the level of the lesion with preserved vibratory and joint position sense since the dorsal columns are spared. The most common cause of anterior cord syndrome is anterior spinal artery infarct, which occurs most commonly in the setting of aortic disease or aortic surgery. Although anterior cord syndrome is characteristic of spinal cord infarct, it is not the only pattern of spinal cord infarct, which can also affect other parts of the cord. Therefore, although anterior cord syndrome suggests spinal cord infarct, the lack of this syndrome does not exclude the diagnosis of spinal cord infarct.

Anterior Horn Syndrome

The anterior (ventral) portion of the spinal cord contains the cell bodies of the lower motor neurons (known as the *anterior horn cells*). In anterior horn syndrome, there is selective injury to the lower motor neurons with preservation of sensation and autonomic function. Poliomyelitis was historically the most common cause of the syndrome but is now rare due to near-eradication. The anterior horns can be selectively affected in West Nile virus myelitis, progressive muscular atrophy (a rare lower motor neuron variant of amyotrophic lateral sclerosis), and spinal muscular atrophy (a genetic condition primarily affecting infants and children).

Diagnostic Evaluation of Myelopathy

If a patient is determined to have myelopathy by history and examination, the next step is evaluation for etiology with neuroimaging of the spine. Magnetic resonance imaging (MRI) is the optimal initial imaging modality for the evaluation of myelopathy (Figure 23.2) since it can evaluate for lesions in the spinal cord itself as well as assess for pathology of the spinal column (eg, vertebrae and intravertebral disks). Computed tomography (CT) and plain radiographs provide excellent visualization of the bony elements of the spinal column but cannot assess for subtle spinal cord pathology. CT and plain radiographs are also useful for the evaluation of implanted hardware from prior spine surgery. Plain radiographs can be obtained in different positions (ie, flexion and extension) to assess for dynamic changes in bony alignment when indicated. CT myelography is a specialized procedure in which radiopaque contrast is injected into the intrathecal space, followed by CT scan. This imaging modality is useful for showing abnormalities in the intrathecal space, such as adhesions in the arachnoid space or cerebrospinal fluid leaks, although it is used less frequently in the MRI era.

MRI studies may be ordered for the total spine or for one specific level (ie, cervical, thoracic, or lumbar). Whole spine imaging can be rapidly obtained

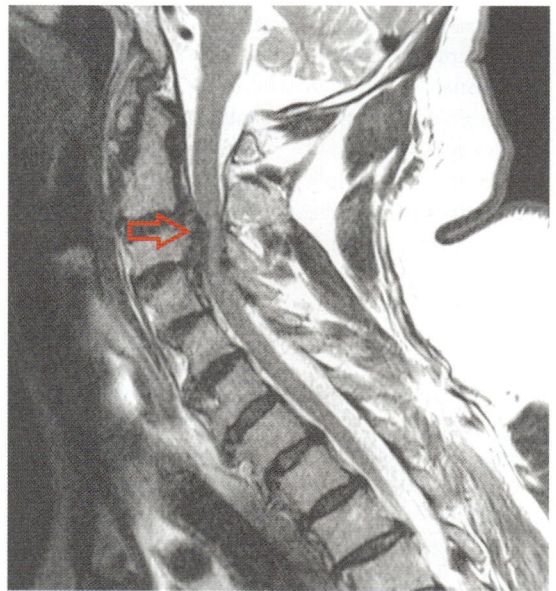

FIGURE 23.2 Cervical spondylotic myelopathy. Sagittal T2 magnetic resonance imaging (MRI) sequence showing severe stenosis of the vertebral canal causing compression of the spinal cord (arrow).

to assess for multifocal structural injury to the spine (eg, after trauma) or in staging of systemic cancer to look for metastases; however, it is not optimal to assess for subtle spinal cord signal change compared to dedicated studies of individual levels of the spine. If the arms are involved in a patient with myelopathy, the cervical spine should be imaged. If the legs alone are involved in a patient with myelopathy, the thoracic spine should be imaged (the spinal cord ends at the L1-L2 level and so a lumbosacral MRI would not be the appropriate study for myelopathy—lesions of the cauda equina in the lumbar spinal canal will cause polyradiculopathy rather than myelopathy). It should be recognized, however, that cervical spinal cord lesions can sometimes primarily affect leg function, so a cervical spine MRI should be obtained if a causative lesion is not seen on thoracic spinal cord imaging of a patient with myelopathic symptoms in the legs alone.

Intravenous contrast is not needed in the evaluation of structural causes of myelopathy. Post-gadolinium contrast studies should be ordered when evaluating for inflammatory, infectious, or neoplastic conditions. Of note, some myelopathies can have normal imaging, such as human T-lymphotropic virus 1 (HTLV-1)-associated myelopathy, metabolic myelopathies (such as vitamin B_{12} and copper deficiency), and genetic conditions such as hereditary spastic paraplegia. Acute spinal cord infarct can also occur with normal neuroimaging.

The imaging and clinical history generally lead to a diagnosis in most patients with common causes of myelopathy, such as structural spinal column disease and neoplasm. If imaging is unremarkable or nonspecific, testing should be guided by the clinical syndrome, time course of disease progression, and clinical context (eg, history of malignancy, immunocompromise, and possible nutritional deficiency). Serum evaluation may include vitamin B_{12} level, HIV testing, and antibody testing (eg, for anti-aquaporin 4 antibodies or MOG antibodies in neuromyelitis optica or MOG antibody-associated disease; see Chapter 20). If there is suspicion for infection, inflammation, or neoplasm, cerebrospinal fluid should be obtained by lumbar puncture to assess cell count, protein, and glucose; obtain microbiologic studies (eg, Gram stain, culture, serology, and polymerase chain reaction

[PCR]); evaluate for neoplasm (eg, cytology and flow cytometry); and assess for autoimmunity (eg, autoantibodies). Table 23.2 summarizes the nonstructural causes of myelopathy.

RADICULOPATHY

Disorders of spinal nerve roots cause the syndrome of radiculopathy. The most common symptom of radiculopathy is radiating electrical pain from the lateral neck into the upper extremity in cervical radiculopathy and from the buttock into the lower extremity with lumbosacral radiculopathy. Some patients may also note numbness or weakness in affected regions.

The most common sites of radiculopathy are the lower cervical and lower lumbar spine, where the spine is most mobile. In the cervical spine, C5 radiculopathy causes pain radiating from the lateral neck into the shoulder, C6 radiculopathy causes pain down the lateral arm and into the thumb, C7 radiculopathy causes pain down the posterior arm and into the middle finger, and C8 radiculopathy causes pain down the medial arm and into the little finger. In the lumbosacral spine, L4 radiculopathy causes pain wrapping around the leg descending along the medial aspect, L5 radiculopathy causes pain shooting down the lateral leg to the dorsal foot, and S1 radiculopathy causes pain going down the buttock to the posterior calf and to the sole of the foot. It should be noted that these patterns can be variable between patients, and the precise location of cervical or lumbar radiculopathy can be suggested—but not definitively determined—by the clinical pattern alone.

On neurologic examination, patients with radiculopathy may have diminished sensation to pinprick in the sensory distribution of the nerve root (known as the *dermatome* of the nerve root). The distribution of sensory loss and the reflex examination can aid in distinction between radiculopathy and a mononeuropathy (ie, dysfunction of a specific named peripheral nerve). C6 radiculopathy can cause diminution or loss of the biceps and brachioradialis reflexes, C7 radiculopathy can cause diminution or loss of the triceps reflex, and S1 radiculopathy can cause diminution or loss of the ankle reflex. If motor components of the nerve roots

TABLE 23.2	**Nonstructural Causes of Myelopathy**
Causes	**Diagnostic clues**
Autoimmune	
Multiple sclerosis	Prior history of episodes of weakness, numbness, or incoordination
Neuromyelitis optica	Positive anti-AQP4 antibody, history of disabling episodes of optic neuritis, myelitis, or refractory nausea/vomiting
MOG antibody–associated disease	Positive anti-MOG antibody, history of multiple episodes of optic neuritis or myelitis, very responsive to corticosteroids
Infectious	
Spinal cord abscess	Rapidly progressive myelopathy with circumscribed collection seen on MRI
HTLV-1-associated myelopathy	Positive serology for HTLV-1, slowly progressive myelopathy most often causing paraparesis
Post- and para-infectious	Myelopathy following a systemic infectious prodrome—cause can be from direct infection (such as in West Nile virus) or immune reaction (such as following *Mycoplasma* infection)
Vascular	
Spinal cord infarct	Rapidly progressive myelopathy (over minutes to hours), noninflammatory cerebrospinal fluid. Imaging can be nonspecific initially. Spinal cord infarct can follow aortic surgery.
Dural arteriovenous fistula	Slow progressive myelopathy with noninflammatory cerebrospinal fluid with imaging evidence of edema in the spinal cord; generally affects older adults
Metabolic/toxic	
Vitamin B_{12} deficiency	Decreased serum level of vitamin B_{12} with elevated methylmalonic acid. Selective impairment of vibratory and joint position sense with spastic weakness. Often accompanied by macrocytic anemia (pernicious anemia), peripheral neuropathy, and cognitive slowing.
Copper deficiency	Decreased serum level of copper. Appears clinically similar to vitamin B_{12} deficiency
Delayed radiation myelopathy	History of exposure to ionizing radiation to the spinal cord months or years prior to onset of syndrome
Genetic	
Hereditary spastic paraplegia	Slow progressive myelopathy of genetic origin progressing usually over years (can have only myelopathy or other neurologic changes such as cognitive impairment). Inheritance pattern can be autosomal dominant, recessive, or X-linked

AQP4, aquaporin 4; HTLV-1, human T-lymphotropic virus 1; MOG, myelin oligodendrocyte glycoprotein; MRI, magnetic resonance imaging.

are involved, weakness may also be seen in affected muscles (in a distribution known as the *myotome* of the nerve root).

The most common cause of radiculopathy is degenerative disease of the spine, including disk herniation, spondylosis (a term referring to various degenerative processes involving bone, disks, and ligaments, often occurring in combination), spondylolisthesis, facet arthropathy, ligamentous hypertrophy, and synovial cysts. The roots may also be affected by malignancy, infection (eg, epidural abscess, infectious radiculitis [eg, due to varicella zoster virus [VZV], cytomegalovirus [CMV], and Lyme]), or inflammatory conditions (eg, inflammatory arthritis, sarcoidosis, primary immune-mediated radiculopathies, and radiculoneuropathies such

as Guillain-Barré syndrome and chronic inflammatory demyelinating polyradiculoneuropathy [CIDP]; see Chapter 24). Further evaluation for these etiologies should be considered in patients with concerning features on history (eg, fever, severe and progressive symptoms, unexplained weight loss, and older age) or past medical history (eg, cancer, intravenous drug use history, immunocompromise, and autoimmune disease).

Diagnostic Evaluation of Radiculopathy

MRI is the preferred modality to evaluate radiculopathy since it allows for visualization of the nerve roots in the vertebral canal and as they exit through the intervertebral foramina. If there are red flags for infection, neoplasm, or inflammation (see preceding text), MRI with contrast should be obtained. For presumed structural degenerative etiologies of radiculopathy, MRI should be considered if there is persistent painful radiculopathy despite physical therapy or if there is progressive weakness, numbness, or bladder/bowel incontinence. In most adults older than age 50, degenerative disease of the spine is present to some degree, and imaging findings may not correlate with clinical symptoms. Therefore, careful correlation between the clinical findings and imaging is essential.

Nerve conduction studies/electromyography (NCS/EMG) can be considered if there is ambiguity between neuropathy and radiculopathy or to determine the degree of contribution from both etiologies when there is dual pathology. However, it should be noted that NCS/EMG is insensitive for detection of purely sensory radiculopathy as the dorsal roots cannot be assessed with this technique. In addition, since NCS/EMG is dependent on the skill of the examiner, this test should not be used as a screening test to decide on the need for imaging. If a patient has multiple radiculopathies (known as *polyradiculopathy*) and no apparent etiology on MRI, CSF analysis should be considered (assessing the same parameters for inflammation, infection, or neoplasm as described earlier for the evaluation of myelopathy).

DIAGNOSIS AND TREATMENT OF DEGENERATIVE SPINE DISEASES

Degenerative disease of the spine refers to conditions such as disk herniation, spondylosis, spondylolisthesis, facet arthropathy, ligamentous hypertrophy, and synovial cysts. Degenerative disease of the spine is one of the most common causes of musculoskeletal neck and back pain, radiculopathy, myelopathy, or a combination of these. Other structural causes of these conditions include vertebral compression fracture in older adults or metastatic bony lesions in patients with cancer. Degenerative disease of the spine is most common in the cervical and lumbar regions, as these are the most mobile regions of the spinal column; degenerative disease of the thoracic spine is uncommon, as the thoracic spine is fixed.

Many patients with degenerative spine disease complain of back pain or neuropathic symptoms. The first step in diagnosis is to categorize the sensory symptoms as axial or appendicular. Axial symptoms involve the spine and proximal limbs (shoulders and thighs) and are associated with musculoskeletal disease of the spine or paraspinal structures. Patients often describe musculoskeletal pain as achy with intermittent superimposed sharp pain. In contrast, appendicular symptoms in the arms and legs are more often associated with structural radiculopathy (foraminal or vertebral canal narrowing leading to nerve root compression) or myelopathy (central canal stenosis causing spinal cord compression). Patients can experience shooting pain (especially with radiculopathy) or more generalized numbness with pins and needles sensations in myelopathy.

The most common cause of acute axial neck pain is cervicalgia or cervical strain. This is characterized by achy pain with sharp exacerbations in the neck and proximal shoulders that is worse with periods of decreased mobility (such as while driving or prolonged phone conversations). Imaging of cervical strain is generally unremarkable (or may show incidental unrelated structural disease). Similarly, axial lumbar spine pain is caused by musculoskeletal causes ranging from ligamentous sources to facet arthropathy to muscle sprain to disk herniation. The quality of the pain is not specific to the cause. On physical examination, the most frequent finding in patients with axial cervical and lumbar spine pain is restricted range of motion. For example, the neck may be restricted in rotation unilaterally, or patients may have difficulty flexing forward because of pain in the lumbar spine.

Compression of spinal nerve roots leads to shooting pain down the arm or the leg, tends to be provoked by specific positions, and can, therefore, be reproduced with physical examination maneuvers, including the Spurling maneuver and shoulder abduction test for cervical radiculopathy and straight leg test for lumbosacral radiculopathy. In the Spurling maneuver, the patient tilts the head toward the symptomatic side and the examiner applies pressure to the top of the head. If the maneuver reproduces the patient's radicular symptoms, this is a positive test result. In the shoulder abduction test, the patient places the hand on the symptomatic side on top of the head with the elbow pointing out (shoulder abducted). Improvement in pain with this maneuver is a positive test result. Both tests have good specificity (estimated at around 80%) but limited sensitivity (estimated at about 50%).

For lumbosacral radiculopathy, the provocative test is called the *straight leg test*. In the ipsilateral straight leg test, the patient is asked to lie supine, and the symptomatic leg is passively lifted (flexed at the hip) to at least 40° to 50°. Reproduction of radicular symptoms is considered a positive test result. In the contralateral straight leg test, the nonsymptomatic leg is passively lifted, with observation for reproduction of radicular symptoms down the other leg. The ipsilateral straight leg test is sensitive but is not very specific (since musculoskeletal low back pain can cause similar findings), whereas the contralateral straight leg test is more specific but less sensitive.

Aside from clinical examination findings broadly indicative of myelopathy, no special physical examination maneuvers distinguish cervical spondylotic myelopathy from other causes of myelopathy. Frequently, however, patients have concurrent cervical radiculopathy in addition to spondylotic myelopathy. The combination of concurrent myelopathic signs in the legs (eg, hyperreflexia and Babinski signs) and radiculopathy in the arms is strongly suggestive of cervical spondylosis. Of note, bladder/bowel dysfunction is not common early in degenerative myelopathy but can occur with severe stenosis or acute neck hyperextension injury.

Treatment of Radiculopathy Due to Degenerative Disease

Treatment of radiculopathy due to degenerative disease can be divided into nonpharmacologic, pharmacologic, interventional pain, and surgical approaches. Nonpharmacologic measures include posture modification (to avoid long periods of immobility of the neck and back, such as prolonged driving or holding the back in fixed positions in occupations such as plumbing), home-based exercises (including gentle range-of-motion exercises of the neck and back along with shoulder rolls to improve paraspinal muscle stiffness often associated with radiculopathy), and physical therapy. Patients do not necessarily need office-based physical therapy for initial treatment of radiculopathy.

For pain relief, patients benefit from nonsteroidal anti-inflammatory drugs as initial therapy. For patients who cannot tolerate or have contraindications to nonsteroidal anti-inflammatory medications, acetaminophen may be used. For severe pain, a short course of oral corticosteroids can be considered. Medications for neuropathic pain (eg, gabapentin and tricyclic antidepressants) may be beneficial in some patients with radicular pain. Skeletal muscle relaxants (eg, cyclobenzaprine) may improve axial muscle stiffness and spasm but can cause significant drowsiness.

With these conservative measures, the majority of patients have marked improvement in pain within 4 to 6 weeks. Patients with initial mild numbness or weakness from radiculopathy improve within the same time scale. For persistent or progressive weakness or numbness, patients may need surgical intervention and should undergo neuroimaging and be referred to a spine surgeon. For persistent radicular pain, patients should be referred to office-based physical therapy and interventional pain management. Epidural steroid injections may improve control of radicular pain for about 1 to 3 months following injection. Patients may need more than one injection for full benefit. Infrequent but serious complications can occur with epidural injections, including infections and nerve and vascular injury (estimated frequency of <1%). Finally, as is true for many conditions causing chronic pain, patients should be screened and treated for concurrent mood disorders, which can contribute to amplification and sensitization of pain.

Treatment of Spondylotic Myelopathy and Lumbar Canal Stenosis Due to Degenerative Disease

Patients with significant myelopathic symptoms, such as difficulty walking attributable to spondylotic cervical disease causing spinal cord compression, should undergo evaluation for surgery with the goal of preventing further progression of neurologic symptoms and improving the level of disability.

Management of milder myelopathic symptoms, such as mild gait stiffness or sensory symptoms in the hands, is less clear. Patients typically do not have relentless progression of neurologic deficits but instead have periods of clinical stability that can last for years, followed by episodes of deterioration. Patients with high surgical risk or who are hesitant about intervention may be treated with physical therapy to improve strength and balance with close clinical monitoring.

As more patients undergo spine imaging for different indications, many patients with clinically asymptomatic but radiographically severe cervical spinal stenosis are discovered. These patients can be observed clinically and do not necessarily need prophylactic surgery. In natural history studies, most patients do not ultimately need surgery; although it is sometimes stated that patients with incidentally noted cervical canal stenosis could become irreversibly paralyzed if they suffer minor trauma, this is not supported by the literature.[1]

Like symptomatic cervical spondylotic myelopathy, symptomatic lumbar canal stenosis causing neurogenic claudication should prompt surgical consultation. Neurogenic claudication is characterized by neuropathic symptoms, with heaviness and discomfort in the legs provoked by standing or walking and relieved by sitting. Most patients with significant neurogenic claudication do not spontaneously improve over time (in contrast to radiculopathy from acute disk herniation) and often gradually worsen. Patients with disabling neurogenic claudication and severe lumbar canal stenosis should be referred to physical therapy and for surgical consultation. If lumbar canal stenosis causes rapidly progressive weakness in the legs or bowel/bladder dysfunction (cauda equina syndrome), immediate surgical decompression is needed.

SUMMARY

Radiculopathy and myelopathy can be caused by structural and nonstructural conditions. Careful correlation of clinical findings, history, and imaging are key to finding a cause. For structural spinal causes, radicular pain and discomfort have a favorable natural history and should be treated initially with conservative measures. For compressive myelopathy, progressive radiculopathy, or severe lumbar canal stenosis, timely referral for surgical evaluation is key to good neurologic outcome. For non-compressive myelopathy, evaluation for immune-mediated, infectious, vascular, and metabolic causes should be pursued.

EDITORS' KEY POINTS

▶ Disorders of the spinal cord (referred to as *myelopathies*) and nerve roots (referred to as *radiculopathies*) are common in clinical practice.

▶ Myelopathies can cause weakness, numbness, gait imbalance, and impaired bladder and bowel control. Patients with cervical myelopathy may report a sensation of electricity running down the spine when they flex the neck forward (Lhermitte sign).

▶ On examination, patients with chronic myelopathy have upper motor neuron signs (including spasticity, hyperreflexia, clonus, and Babinski signs), decreased sensation below the level of the spinal cord lesion, and bladder/bowel dysfunction. Spasticity of the lower extremities can lead to abnormal gait with circumduction of the legs.

▶ Depending on the affected spinal cord tracts, different patterns of symptoms and signs can be seen, including total (transverse) cord syndrome, hemicord (Brown-Séquard) syndrome, central cord syndrome, posterior cord (dorsal column) syndrome, posterolateral cord syndrome, anterior cord syndrome, and anterior horn syndrome. Each is associated with particular etiologies.

▶ Myelopathy is most commonly due to a structural etiology such as cervical stenosis caused by degenerative disease of the spine (eg, spondylosis and disk herniation). MRI of the spinal cord is the investigation of choice to evaluate for a structural cause of myelopathy.

▶ Nonstructural causes of myelopathy include immune-mediated, infectious, vascular, metabolic/toxic, and genetic conditions. Vitamin B_{12} deficiency and copper deficiency are common reversible causes of myelopathy that affect the dorsal columns and corticospinal tracts, causing impaired balance, decreased vibration/proprioception, and upper motor neuron signs; concurrent neuropathy may be present, leading to a mix of upper and lower motor neuron signs.

▶ Patients with significant myelopathic symptoms and signs due to spinal cord compression should be evaluated for decompressive surgery to prevent further progression of neurologic symptoms and improve the level of disability.

▶ Patients with severe lumbar canal stenosis may develop neurogenic claudication, characterized by worsening pain and fatigue in the legs after walking a certain distance. Such patients often benefit from decompressive surgery.

▶ Radiculopathies typically cause radiating electrical pain from the lateral neck into the upper extremity in cervical radiculopathy and from the buttock into the lower extremity in lumbosacral radiculopathy. Some patients may also note numbness or weakness in affected regions.

▶ Radiculopathies are most commonly caused by degenerative disease of the spine (eg, spondylosis and disk herniation). MRI of the spine should be considered if there is intractable pain, progressive motor deficit, or concern for a nonstructural etiology (eg, infection, immune condition, and malignancy).

▶ Treatment of radiculopathy due to degenerative spine disease includes nonpharmacologic, pharmacologic, interventional pain, and surgical options depending on severity and response.

REFERENCE

1. Bednařík J, Sládková D, Kadaňka Z, et al. Are subjects with spondylotic cervical cord encroachment at increased risk of cervical spinal cord injury after minor trauma? *J Neurol Neurosurg Psychiatry.* 2011;82(7):779-781.

Peripheral Nerve Disorders

Kelly Graham Gwathmey

INTRODUCTION

The peripheral nerves carry sensory fibers transmitting sensation (eg, touch, pain, and proprioception) back to the spinal cord (see Chapter 10), motor fibers transmitting impulses from the spinal cord to the muscles (see Chapter 11), and autonomic fibers transmitting impulses to and from the viscera. Therefore, peripheral nerve disorders can cause sensory changes (eg, numbness, imbalance, and painful paresthesias), weakness, and/or autonomic symptoms (eg, orthostasis, sphincter dysfunction, sexual dysfunction, and impaired sweating). This chapter focuses on peripheral neuropathy and motor neuron disease. Peripheral neuropathy can be classified as polyneuropathy (a condition affecting all peripheral nerves), mononeuropathy (a condition

affecting an individual named peripheral nerve [eg, the median nerve, ulnar nerve, fibular (peroneal nerve)], and mononeuropathy multiplex (a condition affecting multiple individual peripheral nerves). Motor neuron disease refers to conditions specifically affecting the motor nerve cells and motor fibers of the peripheral nerves, central nervous system, or both (eg, amyotrophic lateral sclerosis [ALS]).

OVERVIEW OF POLYNEUROPATHY

Polyneuropathies can be categorized by symptom type (ie, sensory, motor, sensorimotor, and autonomic), fiber type involved (ie, small fiber, large fiber, or both), underlying pathophysiology (ie, axonal vs demyelinating), and etiology (ie, acquired, idiopathic, or hereditary). Determining the characteristics of a polyneuropathy based on the patient's symptoms and signs guides the diagnostic evaluation for etiology.

Small nerve fibers carry pain and temperature sensation, so small fiber neuropathy results in painful paresthesias and diminished pain and temperature sensation on examination. Large nerve fibers carry vibration sensation and proprioception, so large fiber neuropathy causes imbalance with impaired vibration sensation and proprioception on examination. The large fibers also carry the afferent impulses responsible for tendon reflexes, and so reflexes are diminished or absent in large fiber neuropathy but normal in small fiber neuropathy. A length-dependent pattern of symptoms and signs—in which the longest peripheral nerves are damaged first, resulting in sensory or sensorimotor deficits in a "stocking" or "stocking glove" pattern—is the most common pattern of polyneuropathy in practice and signifies axonal pathophysiology. In contrast, demyelinating polyneuropathies impact both long and short nerves in the extremities, resulting in both proximal and distal sensory deficits and weakness at onset.

Clinical Presentation

The most common clinical presentation of polyneuropathy is a chronic, distal symmetric sensory polyneuropathy, resulting from length-dependent impairment of small fibers, large fibers, or both types of sensory fibers. Patients develop gradually progressive distal foot numbness, neuropathic pain, and/or imbalance. This presentation is characteristic of polyneuropathies related to toxic and metabolic causes (ie, diabetes and chemotherapy) and is also seen in idiopathic polyneuropathies. Less common patterns of polyneuropathy include acute or subacute presentation, non-length-dependent or asymmetric presentation, and/or early motor involvement. Such patterns are usually encountered in inflammatory polyneuropathies, many of which are demyelinating.

The presence of neuropathic pain often suggests the peripheral neuropathy is acquired rather than inherited or idiopathic. Patients with neuropathic pain will characterize their pain as burning, radiating, or pins and needles. The pain may be intermittent and paroxysmal or constant. In addition to pain, patients may report nonpainful alteration of sensation such as dysesthesia (unpleasant abnormal sensation) and paresthesia (abnormal tingling sensation that may or may not be unpleasant). Patients may have evoked sensations, such as touch-evoked or cold-evoked pain, in addition to spontaneous pain. On examination, patients may complain of pain from a stimulus that would not otherwise cause pain (allodynia) or heightened pain from a stimulus that provokes pain (hyperalgesia). Importantly, these positive neuropathic symptoms will respond to neuropathic pain treatment, whereas negative symptoms such as loss of sensation or weakness will not.

Considering the vast number of causes of peripheral neuropathies, providers must take a detailed history to assess for underlying systemic conditions (eg, infectious processes, rheumatologic or endocrinologic conditions), toxic exposures, and family history of neuropathy. A comprehensive review of systems and determination of comorbid medical conditions will direct the provider to high-yield diagnostic testing that can often lead to a specific diagnosis.

In examining patients with suspected polyneuropathy, particular attention to the deep tendon reflexes and motor and sensory examination will determine the pattern (ie, length-dependent or non-length-dependent; sensory, motor, or sensorimotor). Each pattern guides a targeted diagnostic evaluation. Additionally, identification of pes cavus (high arches in the feet) and hammer toes, especially in a younger individual, is a common finding in inherited polyneuropathies. Inquiring about, or examination of, family members for similar foot deformities may provide evidence for a genetic etiology.

Diagnostic Evaluation

Most polyneuropathies are due to an underlying systemic condition (eg, diabetes and vitamin B_{12} deficiency), medication (eg, chemotherapy), or are idiopathic. Rarer primary neurologic causes of polyneuropathy include inflammatory neuropathies such as Guillain-Barré syndrome (GBS) and chronic inflammatory demyelinating polyradiculoneuropathy (CIDP; both discussed later) and inherited neuropathies such as Charcot-Marie-Tooth (CMT).

American Academy of Neurology guidelines recommend that the laboratory evaluation for the most common pattern of polyneuropathy—chronic distal symmetric polyneuropathy—consist of fasting blood sugar (or hemoglobin A1c), vitamin B_{12} level with methylmalonic acid (with or without homocysteine level), and serum protein electrophoresis with immunofixation (to evaluate for paraprotein-associated neuropathy).[1] If these tests are unrevealing and the patient's symptoms remain chronic and length-dependent, the patient may have an idiopathic polyneuropathy. In patients with a non-length-dependent, subacute, or otherwise atypical presentation, the evaluation may be expanded to include serum evaluation for inflammatory conditions, infections, rarer toxic or metabolic conditions, or genetic conditions (Table 24.1).

If it is not clear based on the history and examination whether the presentation is more consistent with axonal (ie, involving dysfunction of the peripheral nerve axons) or demyelinating (ie, involving dysfunction of the myelin surrounding the peripheral nerves) pathophysiology, electrophysiologic testing (ie, nerve conduction studies [NCS] and electromyography [EMG)]) can be obtained. NCS only evaluate the large fibers and so electrophysiologic testing is normal in isolated small fiber neuropathy. This diagnosis is generally apparent on history and examination, but, if not, can be confirmed by skin biopsy to assess intraepidermal nerve fiber density or autonomic testing if there is a prominent autonomic component.

If an inflammatory neuropathy is under consideration (eg, GBS or CIDP), cerebrospinal fluid (CSF) analysis can aid in diagnosis by demonstrating albuminocytologic dissociation (elevated protein level with a normal or only mildly elevated white blood cell count).

In rare instances of severe, progressive polyneuropathy not able to be diagnosed by the above testing, nerve biopsy may be considered in cases of suspected

conditions such as amyloidosis, sarcoidosis, vasculitic neuropathy, or lymphomatous infiltration of the nerves.

Treatment

Treatment of polyneuropathy should target the underlying systemic condition if identified and neuropathic pain if present. Addressing the systemic condition (eg, diabetes or nutritional deficiency) often stops symptom progression, although it may not reverse the symptoms. However, in the case of inflammatory neuropathies (eg GBS, CIDP, and vasculitic neuropathies), immunomodulatory and immunosuppressive treatments are indicated and may improve symptoms and result in remission of the polyneuropathy. Neuropathic pain treatments (eg, gabapentin, pregabalin) are partially effective in targeting positive neuropathic symptoms (eg, burning pain and paresthesia) but are ineffective at restoring sensation or improving balance or strength.

Guideline-recommended treatments of painful diabetic neuropathy include tricyclic antidepressants, serotonin norepinephrine reuptake inhibitors (SNRIs), gabapentinoids, and sodium channel blockers (Table 24.2); opioids are not recommended.[2] These guidelines can also guide symptomatic therapy of neuropathic pain in non–diabetic neuropathy where there is less evidence. Most providers will initiate either a gabapentinoid or an SNRI first, taking into account the patient's medical comorbidities and concomitant medications. This initial therapy should be increased gradually toward the maximum dose until relief is achieved or side effects encountered. If poorly tolerated or ineffective, then switching to a different therapeutic class of medication is advised. If partially effective, then addition of a medication from another class is frequently helpful. Common combinations include a gabapentinoid with an SNRI or a tricyclic antidepressant with a gabapentinoid.

Alternative therapies that may be beneficial in some patients include α-lipoic acid and acupuncture.

GUILLAIN-BARRÉ SYNDROME

GBS refers to an acute inflammatory polyradiculoneuropathy (ie, affecting both nerve roots and peripheral nerves) that is commonly triggered by infections and rarely by vaccinations. GBS includes both demyelinating

TABLE 24.1	Laboratory Studies in Patients With Suspected Polyneuropathy
Initial laboratory studies in all patients	Fasting blood sugar or hemoglobin A1c Vitamin B$_{12}$ Serum protein electrophoresis and immunofixation
Second-line laboratory studies in select patients	Antinuclear antibody Sjögren syndrome testing (SSA and SSB antibodies) Cholesterol levels including triglycerides
Laboratory studies in those with atypical clinical presentations and specific risk factors (tailored to clinical context)	Vitamin B$_1$ whole blood Vitamin B$_6$ Vitamin E Folate Copper Zinc HIV Lyme Hepatitis B Hepatitis C Cryoglobulins RF CCP ESR CRP ANCA Serum free light chains Antigliadin antibodies Anti-transglutaminase antibodies

ANCA, antineutrophil cytoplasmic antibodies; CCP, cyclic citrullinated peptide; CRP, C-reactive protein; ESR, erythrocyte sedimentation rate; RF, rheumatoid factor.

TABLE 24.2 **First-Line Neuropathic Pain Medications**

Medication	Class	Side effects	AAN level of recommendation[a]	Comments
Gabapentin	Gabapentinoid	Confusion, sedation, weight gait, peripheral edema	B	Renally metabolized
Pregabalin	Gabapentinoid	Sedation, weight gain, peripheral edema	A	Renally metabolized
Amitriptyline, nortriptyline	Tricyclic antidepressants	Anticholinergic side effects, sedation, weight gain	B	Avoid if cardiac conduction concerns and obtain ECG if titration to high dose is a consideration.
Duloxetine	SNRI	Increased blood pressure, nausea, dizziness, hyperhidrosis	B	Avoid if significant hepatic and renal impairment.
Venlafaxine	SNRI	Increased blood pressure, nausea, dizziness, hyperhidrosis	B	Extended-release formulation better tolerated

AAN, American Academy of Neurology; ECG, electrocardiogram; SNRI, serotonin norepinephrine reuptake inhibitor.
[a]The recommendation level was assigned using a modified Delphi process by a panel of clinicians expert in painful diabetic neuropathy based on systematic review of the literature and expert opinion. Level A corresponds to a recommendation of "must" (very strong recommendations), Level B "should" (strong recommendations), and Level C "may" (weak recommendations).

forms (acute inflammatory demyelinating polyradiculoneuropathy [AIDP]) and axonal forms (acute motor and sensory axonal neuropathy [AMSAN] and acute motor axonal neuropathy [AMAN]). Demyelinating forms are most common in North America and Europe, and axonal forms are more common in Asia.

The most common associated preceding infections include *Campylobacter jejuni*, *Mycoplasma pneumoniae*, Epstein-Barr virus, hepatitis E, influenza A, enterovirus, and cytomegalovirus (CMV); coronavirus disease 2019 (COVID-19) is not thought to trigger GBS based on recent epidemiologic data.[3,4] Though the influenza vaccine is associated with triggering of GBS, the risk of influenza infection causing GBS is significantly higher.[5] Regarding the COVID-19 vaccines, the Janssen Ad26.COV2.S vaccine, which utilizes an adenovirus viral vector, appears to carry a heightened risk of GBS compared to messenger RNA vaccines.[6]

Clinical Presentation

The classic presentation of the demyelinating form of GBS (ie, AIDP) is characterized by limb weakness evolving over days. Other common features include paresthesias, neuropathic pain, and cranial neuropathies (most commonly causing facial weakness). Some patients develop severe dysautonomia with fluctuating blood pressure and heart rate. In severe cases, respiratory muscle weakness develops, requiring intubation and mechanical

ventilation. Weakness reaches its nadir at 2 to 4 weeks. Examination is notable for weakness, sensory loss, and areflexia, although reflexes may be normal at initial presentation. There are a number of other GBS variants, such as pure motor, pure sensory, Miller Fisher syndrome (ataxia, ophthalmoplegia, and areflexia), and pharyngeal-cervical-brachial variant, some of which are associated with particular anti-ganglioside antibodies (Table 24.3).

GBS is typically monophasic and recurs only very rarely. Some patients may have a fluctuating course in the initial months following presentation and treatment. If a patient clinically deteriorates beyond the first 2 months, the possibility of acute-onset CIDP should be considered.

Diagnostic Evaluation

CSF in GBS classically demonstrates albuminocytologic dissociation (elevated protein and normal or only mildly increased white blood cell count); however, if lumbar puncture is performed early in the course of the condition, CSF protein may be normal. If CSF reveals an elevated white blood cell count (particularly above 50 cells/mm^3) in a patient with an acute polyradiculopathy, alternative diagnoses such as HIV, sarcoidosis, Lyme polyradiculitis, and CMV (in patients who are immunocompromised) should be considered.

NCS may be normal early in the course of the illness but typically demonstrates features of neuropathy within

TABLE 24.3	Guillain-Barré Variants	
GBS variant	**Clinical features**	**Associated antibodies**
Miller Fisher syndrome	Ataxia, areflexia, and ophthalmoplegia	GQ1b, GT1a, GD1b
Bickerstaff brainstem encephalitis	Ataxia, ophthalmoplegia, hyperreflexia, impaired consciousness	GQ1b
Pharyngeal-cervical-brachial variant	Facial and pharyngeal weakness that may spread into arms	GQ1b, GT1a, GD1a
Sensory GBS	Symmetric sensory deficits Acute onset No motor involvement	None
Ataxic GBS	Acute cerebellar-like ataxia No ophthalmoplegia	GQ1b
Acute sensory ataxic neuropathy	Acute sensory ataxia No ophthalmoplegia	GD1b
AMSAN	Rapidly progressive severe motor and sensory deficits	GM1, GD1a
AMAN	Rapidly progressive motor deficits Deep tendon reflexes may be present or increased.	GM1, GD1a

AMAN, acute motor axonal neuropathy; AMSAN, acute motor and sensory axonal neuropathy; GBS, Guillain-Barré syndrome.

weeks of onset of the disease. Early in the course of GBS, subtle electrophysiologic abnormalities may be observed (eg, absent H reflexes and F waves suggesting proximal nerve root demyelination). If magnetic resonance imaging (MRI) of the spine is obtained, enlargement and contrast enhancement of nerve roots may be observed.

Treatment

Treatment of GBS consists of both supportive intensive care and immunomodulatory therapy with intravenous immunoglobulin (IVIg) or plasma exchange, both of which are equally efficacious and hasten recovery.[7-9] Plasma exchange is usually avoided in patients with significant dysautonomia. Neither IVIg nor plasma exchange results in immediate improvement following treatment; rather, improved outcomes occur weeks to months after treatment. Importantly, lack of immediate response to treatment is not an indication for retreatment, which carries no additional benefits. Patients with very mild symptoms who are still ambulatory can sometimes be observed and do not necessarily require treatment.

Prognosis

Although patients with GBS may be paralyzed and ventilator-dependent at their nadir, many make a full or nearly full recovery over months. Poor prognosis is associated with older age, need for ventilation, antecedent *C. jejuni* infection, and the axonal subtype.[10]

CHRONIC INFLAMMATORY DEMYELINATING POLYRADICULONEUROPATHY

CIDP is a chronic inflammatory condition that affects both nerve roots and peripheral nerves. In contrast to GBS, all forms are demyelinating in nature, and it most commonly arises spontaneously without infectious trigger or vaccination exposure.

Clinical Presentation

The presentation of "typical" CIDP is characterized by symmetric generalized weakness that evolves over months with associated sensory loss. There are also CIDP variants characterized by the distribution of symptoms and fibers involved, including distal CIDP, multifocal CIDP, motor CIDP, and sensory CIDP. In contrast to GBS, dysautonomia and respiratory impairment are very uncommon. Examination findings depend on the form of CIDP, but in the classical presentation, patients will have proximal and distal symmetric weakness, loss of vibration and proprioceptive sensation, and areflexia.

Diagnostic Evaluation

The diagnosis of CIDP relies on electrodiagnostic studies (NCS/EMG) that demonstrate evidence of acquired demyelination on both sensory and motor NCS. Though rarely needed when electrodiagnostic criteria are fulfilled, CSF demonstrates albuminocytologic dissociation, and MRI of the spine may demonstrate enlarged, contrast-enhancing nerve roots.

Treatment

First-line treatment for CIDP includes long-term treatment with IVIg or corticosteroids (usually oral prednisone). Though plasma exchange is effective, it may be logistically challenging to coordinate in the outpatient setting. Steroid-sparing immunomodulatory agents have little evidence but can be considered in patients who cannot tolerate or who do not respond to other therapies.

Prognosis

CIDP may be monophasic, relapsing/remitting, or chronically progressive. Since many patients go into remission, providers should occasionally attempt to withdraw treatment and monitor patients closely for relapse.

COMMON MONONEUROPATHIES

Mononeuropathy refers to pathology of an individual nerve. The most common etiology of mononeuropathy is local compression. In this section, the most frequently encountered mononeuropathies of the upper extremity (median neuropathy at the wrist and ulnar neuropathy at the elbow) and lower extremity (fibular [peroneal] neuropathy at the fibular head) will be discussed. These and other less common mononeuropathies are listed and compared in Table 24.4.

Median Mononeuropathy at the Wrist (Carpal Tunnel Syndrome)

Median Nerve Anatomy

The median nerve is derived from the C6-T1 nerve roots. In the forearm, it innervates the pronators (quadratus and teres) and several of the wrist and finger flexors (flexor carpi radialis, flexor digitorum superficialis, and flexor digitorum profundus to the second and third digits). Since these muscles are innervated proximal to the carpal tunnel at the wrist, they are not impacted by carpal tunnel syndrome. The carpal tunnel is made up of carpal bones and the transverse

carpal ligament (flexor retinaculum); nine finger flexor tendons and the median nerve pass through it. After traversing the carpal tunnel, the median nerve innervates the muscles of the thenar eminence (flexor pollicis brevis, opponens pollicis, and abductor pollicis brevis) and the first and second lumbricals. The median sensory innervation distal to the carpal tunnel supplies the anterior (palmar) portion of the lateral three digits (thumb, index, and middle fingers) and the lateral portion (thumb side) of the fourth digit (ring finger). The palmar cutaneous branch that supplies sensation to the thenar eminence does not pass through the carpal tunnel.

The most common site of median nerve compression is at the wrist (carpal tunnel syndrome), but rarely the nerve may be compressed in the forearm.

Epidemiology and Risk Factors

Carpal tunnel syndrome refers to median nerve compression at the carpal tunnel and is extremely common. Medical conditions that increase the risk for carpal tunnel syndrome by increasing pressure or decreasing volume in the carpal tunnel include pregnancy, diabetes, menopause, hypothyroidism, arthritis, acromegaly, and obesity. Pregnancy-associated carpal tunnel syndrome tends to resolve following delivery, though persistent symptoms are possible. Hobbies and professions with repetitive wrist movement increase the risk of the condition. Patients with underlying polyneuropathies are at increased risk of developing carpal tunnel syndrome. Bilateral carpal tunnel syndrome without apparent risk factors should raise suspicion for amyloidosis.

Clinical Presentation

This first symptom of carpal tunnel syndrome is most commonly nocturnal painful paresthesias in the median nerve distribution of the hand (ie, the distal volar tips of the thumb, second, third, and lateral half of the fourth fingertips), though not uncommonly, patients report paresthesias affecting all five fingers or radiating proximally into the forearm. These paresthesias commonly awaken the patient from sleep, and shaking the hand alleviates the discomfort. As the condition progresses, paresthesias may occur during waking

TABLE 24.4   Mononeuropathies

	Location of compression	Causes	Conservative management	Surgical management
Median mononeuropathy at the wrist	• Carpal Tunnel	• Repetitive wrist movements • Pregnancy • Arthritis • Amyloidosis	• Nocturnal wrist splints • Physical therapy • Corticosteroid injections	• Open or endoscopic carpal tunnel release
Proximal median mononeuropathy	• Ligament of Struthers • Lacertus fibrosus • Pronator teres • Flexor digitorum superficialis	• Compression by various anatomic structures, cysts, nerve tumors	• Activity modification focusing on relieving pressure on the nerve	• Surgical intervention is advised if non-operative treatment was insufficient
Ulnar mononeuropathy at the elbow	• Ulnar groove • Cubital tunnel	• Leaning on flexed elbows • Trauma • Repeated flexion/extension	• Elbow splint	• Decompression and ulnar nerve transposition
Distal ulnar neuropathy (at the wrist)	• Guyon's canal	• Ganglion cyst • Nerve tumor • Postsurgical scars • Trauma • Athletic activities such as cycling, weightlifting	• Avoid triggers/repetitive compression • Protective splints • Physical therapy	• Surgery indicated in moderate-to-severe cases with significant motor deficits
Radial mononeuropathy	• Radiocapitellar joint • Spiral groove of the humerus • Arcade of Frohse • Tendon of the ECRB • Radial tunnel	• Compression of medial arm against a hard surface for a prolonged period • Humerus fracture	• Usually resolves without intervention after 2-3 mo.	• Surgical intervention is if there is a mass lesion or nerve trauma.
Lateral femoral cutaneous mononeuropathy (meralgia paresthetica)	• Inguinal ligament • Sartorius • Fascia lata	• Obesity • Tight clothing • Trauma • Iatrogenesis during surgery	• Avoid constrictive clothing • Neuropathic pain medications • Nerve blocks	• Surgical decompression is uncommon.
Fibular (peroneal) mononeuropathy at the fibular head	• Fibular head	• Leg crossing (especially with weight loss) • Squatting/kneeling • Popliteal/ganglion cyst • Trauma	• Remove provoking factor. • Ankle-foot orthotic	• Surgery indicated in event of compressive mass.
Distal tibial mononeuropathy (tarsal tunnel syndrome)	• Tarsal tunnel between the flexor retinaculum and medial malleolus	• Trauma • Mass	• Neuropathic pain agents • Corticosteroid injections • CAM (controlled, action, motion) boots	• Surgical intervention is standard if patient has had trauma and mass lesions.

ECRB, extensor carpi radialis brevis.

hours and may be triggered by activities that narrow the carpal tunnel, such as gripping a steering wheel. In severe cases, weakness and atrophy of median-innervated thumb muscles may develop, involving weakness of thumb abduction and opposition and atrophy of the thenar eminence. Tinel and Phalen signs can be elicited through bedside tests that attempt to recreate symptoms.[11] The Tinel sign is positive if the patient develops symptoms associated with percussion of the median nerve at the wrist, and the Phalen sign is positive when symptoms emerge following pressing the wrists together with the hands flexed at the wrists ("reverse prayer position") for a minute. The presence or absence of Tinel and Phalen signs should not be relied upon for diagnosis as the sensitivity and specificity of these findings have been found to vary widely in studies.

Diagnostic Evaluation

In a patient with intermittent hand paresthesias that emerge at night or with repeated use, nocturnal wrist splints (that limit the extent of wrist flexion) can be used to see if symptoms improve. If symptoms persist, or in any patient with significant hand weakness, electrodiagnostic studies (NCS/EMG) should be ordered to confirm a median mononeuropathy at the wrist (eg, by showing significantly slower sensory and/or motor median nerve conduction with normal ulnar nerve conduction across the wrist), determine its severity, and assess for potential mimics (or dual pathology) such as a cervical radiculopathy. On occasion, high-resolution ultrasound can be used as an alternative to electrodiagnostic studies or in conjunction with them. Patients with a median mononeuropathy of moderate severity benefit the most from surgical intervention.

Treatment

For patients with mild symptoms of carpal tunnel syndrome (intermittent paresthesias), treatment consists of nocturnal wrist splints, physical therapy, and ergonomic adjustments to causative manual activities. Daytime splinting is not recommended as it could result in compensatory posturing at the elbow and shoulder, which aggravates nerve compression sites proximal to the carpal tunnel. Following a 6-week trial of a nocturnal wrist splint that immobilizes the wrist in the neutral position, patients with persistent symptoms can be considered for corticosteroid injections. If there are severe persistent sensory symptoms or significant weakness in median-innervated muscles, the patient should be referred to a hand surgery specialist for consideration of surgical intervention.

Ulnar Mononeuropathy at the Elbow

Ulnar Nerve Anatomy

The ulnar nerve is derived from the C8-T1 nerve roots. It travels in the ulnar groove between the medial epicondyle of the humerus and the olecranon of the ulna. Distal to the medial epicondyle, the nerve courses under the cubital tunnel, which is comprised of the two heads of the flexor carpi ulnaris muscle. In the forearm, the ulnar nerve innervates one wrist flexor (flexor carpi ulnaris) and the medial portion of the long finger flexors (flexor digitorum profundus to the fourth and fifth digits). The ulnar nerve then continues into the hand via Guyon's canal at the wrist and innervates the majority of the intrinsic hand muscles (hypothenar muscles [abductor digiti minimi, adductor digiti minimi, and opponens digiti minimi], third and fourth lumbricals, interosseous muscles, and adductor pollicis). The sensory innervation of the ulnar nerve consists of two branches that do not go through Guyon's canal: the dorsal cutaneous branch, which innervates the dorsal skin of the fifth digit and medial fourth digit and dorsal hand proximal to these digits, and the palmar cutaneous branch, which innervates the skin of the medial hand on the palmar side. The superficial branch does pass through Guyon's canal and innervates the palmar surface of the fifth digit and medial fourth digit.

The ulnar nerve may become compressed at the ulnar groove, the cubital tunnel (causing ulnar neuropathy at the elbow), or Guyon's canal (causing ulnar neuropathy at the wrist); ulnar neuropathy at the elbow is the most common site of ulnar nerve compression.

Epidemiology, Pathophysiology, and Risk Factors

The ulnar nerve is vulnerable at the elbow due to compression, traction, and frictional forces that occur with flexion and extension of the elbow. The most common cause of ulnar neuropathy at the elbow is leaning on the flexed elbow leading to repeated compression of the nerve, although elbow trauma and hobbies or professions with repeated elbow flexion/extension (eg, playing the violin) can also lead to ulnar mononeuropathy.

Clinical Presentation

Patients with ulnar neuropathy at the elbow develop numbness and paresthesias of the dorsal and palmar surfaces of the fifth finger, medial half of the fourth finger, and medial palm and dorsum of the hand (pinky side). Symptoms are often triggered by repeated flexion of the elbow. Radiating pain or tingling from the elbow into the hand is a common symptom. With progression, patients may develop weakness and atrophy of the ulnar-innervated intrinsic hand muscles causing frequent dropping of objects and leading the fifth digit to catch when putting the hand in a pocket.

On exam, patients with ulnar neuropathy at the elbow often have a sensory deficit in the fifth and medial fourth digits. In more advanced cases with motor involvement, patients have atrophy of their intrinsic hand muscles, most notably the first dorsal interosseous and the abductor digiti minimi, with associated weakness of finger abduction. A Tinel sign may be present when the examiner lightly taps the ulnar nerve at the elbow, but it is neither sensitive nor specific.

In patients with weakness from an ulnar neuropathy, a Froment sign may be present on exam and is demonstrated by asking a patient to hold a sheet of paper between their thumb and index finger. When the examiner tries to remove the paper, the patient will compensate by using their flexor pollicis longus (in lieu of their weak adductor pollicis) and will pinch the paper with the distal phalanx of their thumb.

Diagnostic Evaluation

A diagnosis of ulnar neuropathy at the elbow can often be made clinically, with electrodiagnostic studies reserved for cases with diagnostic ambiguity (eg, to differentiate between a C8/T1 radiculopathy and a lesion of the lower trunk or medial cord of the brachial plexus) or in cases where surgical intervention is being considered.

In patients with ulnar neuropathy at the elbow, electrodiagnostic studies demonstrate focal slowing of conduction velocity across the elbow segment of the nerve. High-resolution nerve ultrasound is also increasingly utilized as an adjunct to electrodiagnostic studies.

Treatment

Patients with mild sensory symptoms can be treated by padding the elbows, avoiding elbow flexion at night by using a flexible elbow splint or wrapping the elbows with a soft towel at night, and avoiding prolonged elbow flexion. Unlike in carpal tunnel syndrome, corticosteroid injections do not have a clear role in the treatment of ulnar neuropathy at the elbow. Patients with prominent weakness in ulnar-innervated hand muscles or in whom conservative management has failed should be evaluated by a hand surgeon for consideration of decompression or ulnar nerve transposition to an adjacent site where it is less likely to be injured; the latter approach may be associated with higher likelihood of complications such as infection or residual sensory deficit.

Fibular (Peroneal) Mononeuropathy at the Fibular Head

Fibular Nerve Anatomy

The common fibular nerve (formerly known as the peroneal nerve) is formed from the L4, L5, and S1 nerve roots. It travels with the tibial nerve in the posterior thigh; together, the two nerves make up the sciatic nerve. Before branching off the sciatic nerve in the popliteal fossa, the fibular nerve innervates the short head of the biceps femoris (one of the hamstring muscles). The fibular nerve wraps around the fibular head and then divides into the superficial fibular and deep fibular branches. The superficial fibular nerve innervates the peroneus longus and brevis muscles and provides sensation to the anterolateral lower leg and dorsum of the foot. The deep fibular nerve descends in the posterior calf to innervate the tibialis anterior, extensor digitorum longus, extensor hallucis longus, peroneus tertius, and extensor digitorum brevis muscles (muscles that dorsiflex and evert the ankle and extend the toes). The deep fibular nerve contributes to the sural nerve (along with the tibial nerve) and provides sensation to the dorsal web space between the first and second toes. The fibular tunnel is an arch made by the peroneus longus, soleus tendon, and proximal fibula just below and lateral to the knee. The common fibular nerve is prone to compression at this site.

Epidemiology and Risk Factors

Fibular neuropathy at the fibular head can be caused by leg crossing (particularly after weight loss, which makes the nerve more prone to compression at this site), frequent squatting and kneeling, popliteal or ganglion cyst, or trauma.

Clinical Presentation

The predominant symptom of fibular neuropathy is foot drop due to weak ankle dorsiflexion. This can lead to tripping and scuffing the front of the shoe. To avoid this, patients develop a steppage gait in which the foot is lifted higher off the ground and slapped down due to inability to dorsiflex for proper heel strike. On examination, patients have weakness of ankle dorsiflexion and eversion, and toe extension. Plantar flexion, foot inversion, and toe flexion are spared as these are tibial nerve-innervated functions. Patients may also have numbness in the anterolateral lower leg and dorsum of the foot. The primary differential diagnosis for fibular neuropathy–associated foot drop is L5 radiculopathy, which will cause weakness of ankle inversion and hip abduction in addition to ankle dorsiflexion and eversion weakness.

Diagnostic Evaluation

When a fibular mononeuropathy is clearly due to acute compression, electrodiagnostic and imaging studies are generally unnecessary. In patients with persistent motor deficits or in whom alternative diagnoses such as an L5 radiculopathy or sciatic mononeuropathy are considered, electrodiagnostic studies are indicated for localization, and MRI should be considered if radiculopathy is suggested clinically.

On electrodiagnostic studies of fibular nerve compression at the fibular head, focal slowing or conduction block of motor conduction is seen at the fibular head. If there is no clear history of mechanical compression, fibular nerve imaging with high-resolution ultrasound or MRI should be considered to evaluate for a compressive lesion such as a ganglion cyst.

Treatment

Most patients will improve with removal of the provoking factor (eg, not crossing the legs) and physical therapy. Patients should wear an ankle-foot orthosis to improve gait until dorsiflexion strength returns. Surgery is rarely indicated unless the cause is a structural compressive lesion (eg, Baker cyst).

MOTOR NEURON DISEASE

Motor neuron disease refers to disorders that specifically affect motor nerves of the peripheral nervous system (lower motor neurons), the central nervous system (upper motor neurons), or both the upper and the lower motor neurons. This leads to progressive weakness of the limbs, cranial nerve–innervated muscles of the head and neck that affect speech and swallowing (called *bulbar weakness*), and the respiratory muscles. The most common motor neuron disease is ALS. Less common motor neuron diseases are presented in Table 24.5.

Epidemiology and Pathophysiology

ALS has a global incidence of 2 per 100,000 patient-years and a prevalence ranging from 5 to 12 per 100,000, with a lifetime risk of 1 in 400 of developing the disease.[12-16] Men are affected more commonly than women (1.5:1 ratio). The most common age of onset is after age 60, although adults of any age can be affected, and the condition may begin at a younger age in rarer genetic cases (about 10%-15% of ALS cases). The pathophysiology of ALS is not completely understood but is thought to arise from a combination of genetic susceptibility, age-related cellular damage, and environmental exposure.

Clinical Presentation

Weakness in ALS often begins in one limb and then progresses to sequentially involve subsequent limbs. Less commonly, weakness begins symmetrically or in the muscles of the head and neck, causing dysarthria and dysphagia (bulbar-onset ALS). Patients may also notice progressive atrophy and fasciculations (muscle twitching). Note that patients presenting with fasciculations and no weakness or reflex changes rarely turn out to have ALS.

Examination demonstrates a mix of upper motor neuron signs (eg, hyperreflexia) and lower motor neuron signs (eg, absent reflexes, atrophy, and fasciculations), often in the same limb. There are no sensory findings (unless the patient has concurrent neuropathy). As the disease progresses, patients become diffusely weak, ultimately requiring a gastrostomy tube for nutrition due to dysphagia as well as noninvasive ventilation for respiratory support. Patients may also develop pseudobulbar affect, characterized by uncontrollable laughing and crying and increased yawning.

It is increasingly recognized that ALS may have neuropsychiatric manifestations, with some patients developing concurrent frontotemporal dementia, particularly in patients with the most common genetic

TABLE 24.5	ALS variants		
Variant	**Clinical presentation**		**Prognosis**
Primary lateral sclerosis	• Pure upper motor neuron syndrome that is gradually progressive • Patients complain of progressive leg and arm spasticity followed by spastic dysarthria. • Most patients presenting with isolated UMN findings will evolve to develop LMN involvement and ultimately clinical ALS.		PLS has a more favorable prognosis than ALS.
Professive muscular atrophy	• Pure lower motor neuron syndrome • A minority of patients will develop UMN symptoms and ALS.		PMA has a more favorable prognosis than ALS.
Progressive bulbar palsy	• Isolated bulbar syndrome may have both UMN and LMN symptoms. • Patients have marked dysphagia and dysarthria and may have pseudo-bulbar palsy (spastic dysarthria and pseudobulbar affect). • Many will evolve to a more classic ALS phenotype.		
Flail arm variant	• Known as *brachial amyotrophic diplegia* • Bilateral asymmetric LMN weakness and atrophy affect both upper limbs but spare other body regions. • Weakness may spread proximal to distal.		More favorable prognosis than ALS
Flail leg variant	• Bilateral and symmetric LMN weakness of the legs		More favorable prognosis than ALS
Hemiplegic variant	• Mix of UMN and LMN signs isolated to one side of the body • Slowly progressive • Can be associated with aphasia		

The syndromes fall under the umbrella of motor neuron diseases but do not satisfy formal diagnostic criteria as they have primarily upper motor neuron or lower motor neuron involvement or are restricted to a single body region.

ALS, amyotrophic lateral sclerosis; DTRs, deep tendon reflexes; LMN, lower motor neuron; PLS, primary lateral sclerosis; PMS, progressive muscular atrophy; UMN, upper motor neuron.

form of ALS due to a mutation in the *C9orf72* gene. Depression, anxiety, and impaired sleep are also common in ALS.

Diagnostic Evaluation

The diagnosis of ALS is made by the combination of clinical examination and NCS/EMG to demonstrate a pure motor neuropathy and exclude potential mimics such as multifocal motor neuropathy. Other tests that should be routinely performed in patients being evaluated for ALS include brain and spine MRIs (depending on site of onset) and occasionally testing for myasthenia gravis, heavy metals, and vitamin B_{12} and copper levels. The ALS Association's think ALS tool (https://www.als.org/thinkals) provides a rapid screening instrument for ALS that encourages primary care providers to refer patients with suspected ALS (progressive dysarthria, dysphagia, extremity weakness, and respiratory impairment) directly to an ALS provider for assessment to improve early referral to a specialist for treatment and consideration of enrollment in clinical trials. With the U.S. Food and Drug

Administration (FDA) approval of a treatment specific to superoxide dismutase 1 (SOD1) ALS, tofersen, genetic testing in ALS has become standard. The most common mutations found in patients with ALS are *C9orf72*, *TARDBP*, *SOD1*, and *FUS*.

Treatment

There is no cure for ALS, but several medications slow progression and prolong survival by months: riluzole (an oral medication), edaravone (available as an infusion or oral solution), and sodium phenylbutyrate and tauroursodeoxycholic acid (an oral medication). However, ALS is relentlessly progressive, culminating in death from respiratory failure within an average of 3 years after symptom onset, and so important components of treatment include supportive care with symptomatic medications (Table 24.6), multidisciplinary care (eg, physical therapists, occupational therapists, speech language pathologists, respiratory therapists, registered dietitians, social workers, palliative care providers, pulmonologists, genetic counselors, and specialized nursing staff), and palliative care. Shortly after

TABLE 24.6 Symptomatic Management and Supportive Care in ALS

Symptom	Treatment
Sialorrhea	Sublingual atropine, glycopyrrolate, scopolamine patch, botulinum toxin injection to salivary glands, radiation, and amitriptyline
Thick bronchial secretions	Mucolytics (eg, N-acetylcysteine and guaifenesin/pseudoephedrine), cough assist device, hydration
Dysarthria	Assistive devices, voice banking
Dyspnea	Noninvasive ventilation
Laryngospasm	Lorazepam, baclofen
Spasticity	Baclofen, tizanidine, botulinum toxin injections
Pseudobulbar affect	TCAs, SSRIs, dextromethorphan-quinidine
Depression	SSRI, referral to psychiatry
Cramping	Baclofen, mexiletine, magnesium oxide, oxcarbazepine, carbamazepine
Functional decline due to motor weakness	Braces (ankle-foot orthotics), mobility aids (eg, walkers, rolling walkers, power wheelchairs), physical and occupation therapy

ALS, amyotrophic lateral sclerosis; SSRIs, selective serotonin reuptake inhibitors; TCAs, tricyclic antidepressants.

the diagnosis is made, conversations about prognosis should be initiated to begin a discussion of the patient's goals and end-of-life decision-making.

SUMMARY

Clinicians will frequently encounter polyneuropathy and compressive mononeuropathies and should be familiar with the typical symptoms, signs, diagnostic evaluation, and treatment. ALS is a progressive motor neuron disease in which patients benefit from early diagnosis, multidisciplinary care, and disease-modifying therapy and should therefore be referred to a specialized center.

EDITORS' KEY POINTS

▶ The most common presentation of peripheral polyneuropathy is chronic, distal symmetric sensory changes (numbness, tingling, and pain) in the feet. The laboratory evaluation for the etiology of these neuropathies includes tests for diabetes (fasting glucose or hemoglobin A1c), vitamin B_{12} level, and serum protein electrophoresis with immunofixation.

▶ If a polyneuropathy is subacute, non-length-dependent (affecting the upper and lower extremities both proximally and distally from onset), or causes significant weakness, evaluation for less common causes of neuropathy such as CIDP should be performed.

▶ Neuropathic pain can be treated with tricyclic antidepressants (eg, amitriptyline and nortriptyline), SNRIs (eg, duloxetine and venlafaxine), and gabapentinoids (gabapentin and pregabalin); opioids are not recommended.

▶ GBS should be considered in patients with rapidly progressive sensory and/or motor symptoms involving the extremities and cranial nerve–innervated muscles of the eyes and face. Diagnosis is made by the finding of albuminocytologic dissociation on CSF analysis (elevated CSF protein with minimal or no elevation in CSF white blood cell count) and findings on NCS, but both may be normal early in the course of the condition. Treatment is with IVIg or plasma exchange.

▶ Common compressive mononeuropathies include median neuropathy at the wrist (causing carpal tunnel syndrome), ulnar neuropathy at the elbow (causing sensory changes in the medial hand and/or intrinsic hand muscle weakness), and peroneal (fibular) neuropathy at the fibular head (causing foot drop). These conditions can generally be diagnosed clinically and treated with splinting, but NCS and EMG should be considered if the mononeuropathy has no clear etiology, is severe, and/or if surgery is being considered.

▶ ALS is the most common type of motor neuron disease, usually presenting with weakness of one limb progressing to other limbs over months with a combination of both upper motor neuron signs (hyperreflexia and Babinski sign) and lower motor neuron signs (hyporeflexia/areflexia, atrophy, and fasciculations) on examination. Diagnosis is made by NCS/EMG findings. Treatments prolong survival by months, and patients require multidisciplinary supportive care.

REFERENCES

1. England JD, Gronseth GS, Franklin G, et al. Practice parameter: evaluation of distal symmetric polyneuropathy: role of autonomic testing, nerve biopsy, and skin biopsy (an evidence-based review). Report of the American Academy of Neurology, American Association of Neuromuscular and Electrodiagnostic. *Neurology*. 2009;72(2):177-184.
2. Callaghan BC, Price RS, Feldman EL. Distal symmetric polyneuropathy: a review. *JAMA*. 2015;314(20):2172-2181.
3. Keddie S, Pakpoor J, Mousele C, et al. Epidemiological and cohort study finds no association between COVID-19 and Guillain-Barré syndrome. *Brain*. 2021;144(2):682-693.
4. Taga A, Lauria G. COVID-19 and the peripheral nervous system. A 2-year review from the pandemic to the vaccine era. *J Peripher Nerv Syst*. 2022;27(1):4-30.
5. Kwong JC, Vasa PP, Campitelli MA, et al. Risk of Guillain-Barré syndrome after seasonal influenza vaccination and influenza health-care encounters: a self-controlled study. *Lancet Infect Dis*. 2013;13(9):769-776.
6. Hanson KE, Goddard K, Lewis N, et al. Incidence of Guillain-Barré syndrome after COVID-19 vaccination in the vaccine safety datalink. *JAMA Netw Open*. 2022;5(4):e228879.
7. Chevret S, Hughes RA, Annane D. Plasma exchange for Guillain-Barré syndrome. *Cochrane Database Syst Rev*. 2017;2(4):CD001798.
8. Hughes RAC, Swan A V, van Doorn PA. Intravenous immunoglobulin for Guillain-Barré syndrome. *Cochrane Database Syst Rev*. 2014;2014(4):CD002063.
9. Ortiz-Salas P, Velez-Van-Meerbeke A, Galvis-Gomez CA, Rodriguez Q JH. Human immunoglobulin versus plasmapheresis in Guillain-Barre syndrome and myasthenia gravis: a meta-analysis. *J Clin Neuromuscul Dis*. 2016;18(1):1-11.
10. Shahrizaila N, Lehmann HC, Kuwabara S. Guillain-Barré syndrome. *Lancet*. 2021;397(10280):1214-1228.
11. Brüske J, Bednarski M, Grzelec H, Zyluk A. The usefulness of the Phalen test and the Hoffmann-Tinel sign in the diagnosis of carpal tunnel syndrome. *Acta Orthop Belg*. 2002;68(2):141-145.
12. Mehta P, Raymond J, Punjani R, et al. Incidence of amyotrophic lateral sclerosis in the United States, 2014–2016. *Amyotroph Lateral Scler Front Degener*. 2022;23(5-6):378-382.
13. Mehta P, Kaye W, Raymond J, et al. Prevalence of amyotrophic lateral sclerosis—United States, 2015. *MMWR Morb Mortal Wkly Rep*. 2018;67(46):1285-1289.
14. Chiò A, Logroscino G, Traynor BJ, et al. Global epidemiology of amyotrophic lateral sclerosis: a systematic review of the published literature. *Neuroepidemiology*. 2013;41(2):118-130.
15. Logroscino G, Traynor BJ, Hardiman O, et al. Incidence of amyotrophic lateral sclerosis in Europe. *J Neurol Neurosurg Psychiatry*. 2010;81(4):385-390.
16. Robberecht W, Philips T. The changing scene of amyotrophic lateral sclerosis. *Nat Rev Neurosci*. 2013;14:248-264.

CHAPTER 25

Neuromuscular Junction and Muscle Disorders

Joome Suh and Amanda C. Guidon

INTRODUCTION

Diseases of the neuromuscular junction (NMJ) and muscle cause weakness without sensory abnormalities. Important features to elicit on clinical history include area(s) of the body affected by weakness; whether symptoms are static, progressive, or fluctuating; medication history; and a complete family history. When terms such as "weakness" or "numbness" are used by the patient to describe symptoms, further clarification is warranted, as patients may use these terms nonspecifically to describe various symptoms. Asking about task-specific weakness is informative, such as the ability to climb stairs or reach above the head (both requiring proximal strength) or manual dexterity (requiring

distal strength). A discussion of the history and examination in patients with weakness is presented in Chapter 11; disease-specific considerations are discussed in detail here.

DISEASES OF THE NEUROMUSCULAR JUNCTION

The NMJ refers to the synapse between the motor nerve and muscle. Disorders of the NMJ include myasthenia gravis (MG), Lambert-Eaton myasthenic syndrome (LEMS), and botulism; the former two are discussed here.

Myasthenia Gravis

MG is a disorder of the NMJ. MG can be immune-mediated or, much more rarely, hereditary (ie, congenital myasthenic syndrome). In autoimmune MG, antibodies form against structures of the postsynaptic muscle membrane. These antibodies impair muscle depolarization that occurs from the binding of acetylcholine to its receptor. Congenital myasthenic syndromes are due to genetic mutations that cause abnormalities of various presynaptic, synaptic, and postsynaptic structures of the NMJ. These conditions may be considered in children who develop MG or in adults with MG who lack MG-specific antibodies.

MG is characterized by fatigable skeletal muscle weakness, that is, weakness that worsens with repeated use and improves with rest. This should be distinguished from nonspecific "fatigue," "tiredness," or "sleepiness" without muscle weakness. Smooth muscle and sensory functions are not affected by MG. Autoimmune MG often begins with ocular symptoms (such as ptosis or diplopia), but weakness of the extremities and/or muscles of the face, larynx, and/or pharynx develops in most patients within 2 years of onset. Involvement of the respiratory muscles can lead to restrictive ventilatory defects and, when severe, can be fatal if not recognized and urgently treated. Myasthenic weakness limited to extraocular movements causing binocular diplopia, eye closure weakness, and/or ptosis is called *ocular MG*. When myasthenia causes weakness in areas beyond the eyes, it is classified as *generalized MG*.

Many patients experience myasthenic exacerbation during the disease course with worsening symptoms, and a smaller subset experience myasthenic crisis, defined as MG-induced respiratory failure requiring noninvasive or invasive ventilatory support. Severe neck or bulbar weakness (eg, difficulty swallowing food, liquids or secretions, or severe dysarthria) are signs of impending myasthenic crisis. If disease exacerbation is identified early, prompt treatment interventions can lower the patient's risk of progressing to respiratory failure.

Triggers of MG exacerbation and crisis include illness, stress, surgery (including thymectomy to treat MG), heat, and certain medications, but often no trigger is identified. Medications to avoid or use with caution due to the risk of worsening MG include fluoroquinolone, macrolide, and aminoglycoside antibiotics, intravenous (IV) magnesium, β-blockers (particularly at high doses or given as IV), non-depolarizing neuromuscular blocking agents, and botulinum toxin. A full list can be found in the International Consensus Guidance for Management of Myasthenia Gravis.[1]

MG can rarely occur as a complication of immune checkpoint inhibitor therapies for cancer. In some patients, subclinical MG is thought to be unmasked by immune checkpoint inhibitor therapy, whereas in others, immune checkpoint inhibitor therapy induces MG or a myasthenia-like syndrome de novo. In these patients, symptoms typically arise within the first 3 months of starting immune checkpoint inhibitors and can progress rapidly within days. Unlike sporadic MG, many patients have concurrent myositis and/or myocarditis, which may account for the higher mortality observed in immune checkpoint inhibitor–associated MG compared to idiopathic MG.

Symptoms of Myasthenia Gravis

Asymmetric eyelid drooping (ptosis) and binocular double vision (diplopia) are the most common presenting symptoms of MG. Symptoms are often worse in the evening and generally improve with rest. Additional symptoms may include slurred speech (dysarthria), change in voice quality (dysphonia), and difficulty swallowing (dysphagia); these symptoms are referred to as *bulbar* (ie, related to dysfunction of muscles innervated by the lower cranial nerves). When jaw closure weakness is present, patients may report eating more slowly or restricting their diet to soft foods due to fatigue when chewing. Other symptoms of MG include extremity weakness and difficulty holding up the head (ie, head drop) due to weakness of the neck muscles. Proximal weakness involving the shoulder and hip girdles is more common than distal muscle weakness. Distal weakness, if present, typically affects finger extension and ankle dorsiflexion. Patients may describe difficulty with walking, climbing stairs, getting up from a seated position, brushing hair, shaving, and lifting heavy objects. Respiratory muscle weakness manifests as dyspnea on exertion or at rest and, when severe, respiratory failure. Respiratory symptoms due to neuromuscular weakness are typically worse when supine and improved when sitting upright.

Examination

A standard screening neurologic examination may miss more subtle signs of myasthenic weakness. MG-specific maneuvers can elicit characteristic patterns of weakness and fatigability. These maneuvers are important for both diagnosis and following response to treatment.

Many patients unconsciously compensate for ptosis that obscures vision by raising the eyebrows. This is called the frontalis sign because contraction of the frontalis muscles is responsible for raising the eyebrows. The forehead must be relaxed and the eyebrows in a neutral position to assess ptosis accurately. A contracted forehead will underestimate the severity of ptosis. In addition, older adults often have loose and redundant eyelid skin (dermatochalasis), which must be distinguished from ptosis (Figure 25.1). The loose skin "hooding" the eyelid can be gently moved aside by the examiner's thumb so it no longer obscures the upper lid and ptosis can be assessed.

Having the patient hold upward gaze for at least 30 seconds may induce or worsen ptosis by causing fatigue of eyelid muscles (fatigable ptosis). Ptosis may improve after application of an ice pack to the lid(s) for 2 minutes, a highly sensitive and specific sign for MG (Figure 25.2). Diplopia in MG occurs due to misalignment of the eyes from weakness of extraocular muscles, and so it should resolve completely if either eye is covered; however, this is not specific for MG and can be seen with any cause of binocular diplopia (eg, cranial nerve palsy and thyroid eye disease). Although MG can cause ptosis and diplopia, it does not affect the pupils. If the pupillary size, symmetry, or the pupillary light reflex is abnormal, an alternative diagnosis should be sought (eg, Horner syndrome, cranial nerve 3 palsy and botulism).

Bilateral symmetric eye closure weakness (ie, inability to bury the eyelashes with forced eye closure or resist eye opening by the examiner) is present in most patients with MG. Weakness of the lower facial muscles may also be present. This is demonstrated as an air leak or difficulty sealing the lips in an "O" shape when holding the cheeks inflated against the examiner gently squeezing the puffed cheeks. Weakness of tongue-to-cheek (ie, pushing the tongue as hard as possible into the cheek against the examiner's resistance applied to the outside of the cheek) and symmetrically impaired

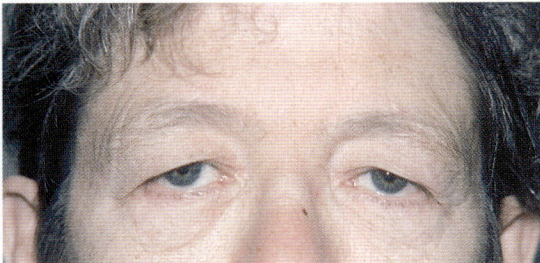

FIGURE 25.2 Ptosis before (A) and after ice-pack test (B), showing improvement. (From Dutton J, Proia A, Tawfik H. *Comprehensive Textbook of Eyelid Disorders and Diseases.* Wolters Kluwer; 2022. Figure 90.3.)

palate elevation may be present. The patient's speech may become more nasal and slurred with prolonged conversation and less commonly hoarser or lower in volume. Proximal worse than distal muscle weakness may be apparent in axial and limb muscles. Neck flexion, elbow flexion and extension, finger extension, and hip flexion are most commonly affected. Neck flexion is best assessed by having the patient lie supine and attempt to elevate the head against resistance with the chin tucked. Neck extension weakness often exists in combination with neck flexion weakness.

Respiratory muscle function can be estimated at the bedside by asking the patient to count as high as possible on a single breath at a rate of about two numbers per second. Inability to count beyond 20 despite maximal effort suggests reduced forced vital capacity (FVC). Respiratory muscle function can be more accurately assessed by measuring negative inspiratory force (NIF) and FVC at the bedside. Oxygen saturation is not a reliable marker

FIGURE 25.1 Dermatochalasis causing "hooding" and creating a false impression of ptosis. This can be gently moved aside to assess for underlying ptosis. (From Penne R. *Oculoplastics.* 3rd ed. Wolters Kluwer; 2018. Figure 5.19a.)

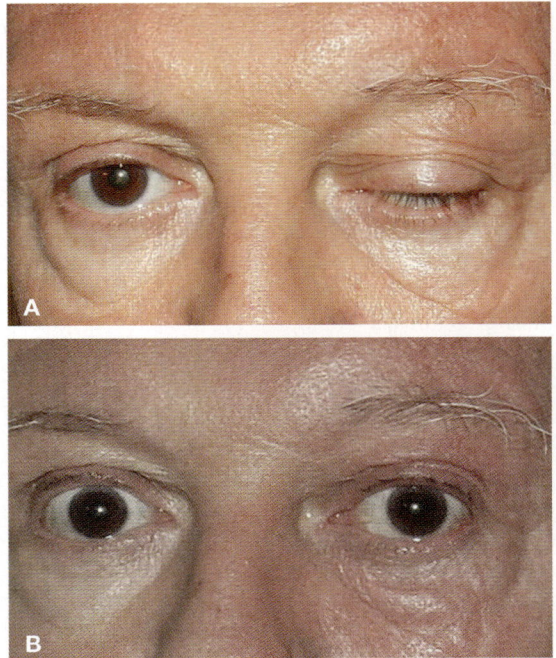

of respiratory impairment in MG since hypercarbia precedes hypoxia. By the time respiratory muscles are affected in MG, weakness is also apparent in other muscle groups. Patients with MG who develop rapidly progressive bulbar weakness and respiratory symptoms over days to weeks should be hospitalized for monitoring and treatment of myasthenic crisis.

Diagnostic Testing for Myasthenia Gravis

An MG diagnosis can be confirmed in most patients with generalized disease by testing for disease-specific serum autoantibodies. Approximately 70% of patients with generalized MG have antibodies against the acetylcholine receptor (AChR), 1% to 10% of patients have antibodies against muscle-specific tyrosine kinase (MuSK), and 1% to 5% of patients have antibodies against lipoprotein-related protein 4 (LRP4).[2] In a small proportion of patients without any of these antibodies, nerve conduction studies (NCSs) with slow repetitive nerve stimulation testing can provide evidence of a disorder of neuromuscular transmission. A decrement in the motor amplitude on repetitive nerve stimulation is supportive, although not specific, for MG. Electromyography (EMG) can be helpful in excluding mimics (eg, myopathy and motor neuron disease). If MG is clinically suspected, it is important to communicate this to the physician performing the NCV/EMG test so that the appropriate electrophysiologic

testing can be performed. However, in purely ocular disease, repetitive nerve stimulation has low sensitivity and AChR antibodies are only present in about 50% of patients.[3] Single-fiber EMG (distinct from routine NCS and EMG) has higher sensitivity, but lower specificity, and is typically only available at medical centers with neuromuscular subspecialists.

In patients newly diagnosed with MG, particularly those with AChR antibodies, chest imaging is needed (computed tomography [CT] or magnetic resonance imaging [MRI]) to evaluate for thymoma. Patients with a thymoma typically require thymectomy.

Treatment of Myasthenia Gravis

Therapies for MG vary in time to onset, dosing frequency, and side effect profile (Table 25.1). Management is tailored to the individual patient. For patients hospitalized with exacerbation or crisis, rescue treatment is with intravenous immunoglobulin (IVIg) or plasma exchange. Corticosteroids may be added or increased in dose. Close monitoring of respiratory function is critical. Supportive care with invasive ventilation and enteral nutrition may be required in some cases until rescue therapy takes effect.

For patients starting treatment in the outpatient setting, pyridostigmine is often the first-line therapy. Pyridostigmine is a symptomatic treatment for MG that works by inhibiting the acetylcholinesterase enzyme

TABLE 25.1   Commonly Used Therapies for Myasthenia Gravis

Treatment name	MG subtype	Route	Mechanism of action	Notable side effects	Notes
Symptomatic therapy					
Pyridostigmine	All	PO (IV should be avoided)	Inhibits acetylcholinesterase at NMJ	Diarrhea, muscle cramps, fasciculations, and increased secretions. Bradycardia (rare, mainly with IV)	Reduced efficacy and increased side effects in MuSK
Rescue therapy					
Intravenous immunoglobulin (IVIg)	All	IV	Unknown, possible neutralization of antibodies	Headache, aseptic meningitis, flu-like symptoms, infusion reaction, TRALI, thrombotic/embolic events (DVT, PE, stroke, and VST), hemolytic anemia, leukopenia, and renal dysfunction	Monitor BMP and CBC with differential at baseline and at clinically appropriate intervals
Plasma exchange	All	IV	Removes antibodies	Hypotension, complications related to central venous access, and coagulopathy	Caution in patients who are anticoagulated; contraindicated in sepsis. Use peripheral IV access when possible.

(continued)

TABLE 25.1	Commonly Used Therapies for Myasthenia Gravis (*continued*)				
Treatment name	**MG subtype**	**Route**	**Mechanism of action**	**Notable side effects**	**Notes**
Oral immunosuppressive therapy					
Corticosteroids	All	PO	Immunosuppression	Hypertension, hyperglycemia, osteoporosis, avascular necrosis, weight gain, fluid retention, cataracts, glaucoma, infection, mood changes, insomnia, and skin thinning	Monitor HbA$_{1c}$, BMP, and other side effects
Azathioprine	All	PO	Inhibits purine synthesis	Idiosyncratic flulike reaction, hepatotoxicity, leukopenia, macrocytic anemia, infection, and malignancy[a]	Monitor CBC with differential and LFT
Mycophenolate mofetil/mycophenolic acid	All	PO	Inhibits synthesis of guanosine nucleotides	Diarrhea, nausea/vomiting, abdominal pain, teratogenic, cytopenia particularly leukopenia, infection, and malignancy[a]	REMS program, monitor CBC with differential
B-cell depleting therapy					
Rituximab	MuSK, all	IV	B-cell depletion	Infection (including TB and HBV reactivation) and infusion reaction	Check for latent TB and HBV prior to starting; if finding is positive, will need concomitant treatment for the infection
Complement inhibitor					
Eculizumab/ravulizumab	AChR	IV	Inhibits complement activation	Meningococcal infection including meningitis	REMS program, requires quadrivalent and serogroup B meningococcal vaccinations
Zilucoplan	AChR	SC	Inhibits complement activation	Meningococcal infection including meningitis, and injection site reaction	REMS program, requires quadrivalent, and serogroup B meningococcal vaccinations
FCRN receptor antagonist					
Efgartigimod[b]	AChR	IV or SC	Inhibits neonatal Fc receptors	Injection site reaction and infection	
Rozanolixizuma[b]	AChR or MuSK	SC	Inhibits neonatal Fc receptors	Injection site reaction and infection	
Thymectomy (see text)					

AChR, acetylcholine receptor; BMP, basic metabolic panel; CBC, complete blood cell count; DVT, deep vein thrombosis; HbA$_{1c}$, hemoglobin A$_{1c}$; HBV, hepatitis B virus; Ig, immunoglobulin; IV, intravenous; LFT, liver function tests; MuSK, muscle-specific tyrosine kinase; NMJ, neuromuscular junction; PE, pulmonary embolism; PLEX, plasma exchange; PO, oral; REMS, risk evaluation and mitigation strategies; SC, subcutaneous; TB, tuberculosis; TRALI, transfusion-related acute lung injury; VST, venous sinus thrombosis.
[a]Mainly skin cancers and lymphoma.
[b]Currently only approved for acetylcholine receptor (AChR) myasthenia gravis (MG), but likely also effective in other subtypes.

from breaking down acetylcholine in the NMJ. In mild ocular disease, this medication may suffice, but most patients require immunomodulatory therapy. Corticosteroids are usually initiated first. Since starting high-dose corticosteroids can sometimes cause paradoxical worsening of symptoms in the first 1 to 2 weeks, corticosteroids are usually started at a low dose and gradually increased until symptomatic control is achieved. Once symptoms are stable, the dose is slowly tapered over months to the minimal effective dose. In patients with moderate to severe generalized disease who require starting corticosteroids at high dose, IVIg or plasma exchange is often used first to prevent the paradoxical worsening of symptoms upon initiating high-dose corticosteroids.

If steroids are insufficient in managing symptoms, symptoms return with tapering steroids, or patients have contraindications to long-term steroid therapy, steroid-sparing agents can be used. The most commonly used oral immunosuppressive therapies are azathioprine or mycophenolate. Given that oral agents typically require 6 to 18 months to take effect, IVIg, plasma exchange, B-cell depletion (rituximab), complement inhibition (eculizumab, ravulizumab or zilucoplan), or neonatal Fc receptor (FcRn) antagonists (efgartigimod or rozanolixizumab) may be required as a bridge (Table 25.1). In MuSK-positive MG, rituximab is highly effective.

Certain medications used in MG require periodic laboratory monitoring and/or vaccinations, as shown in Table 25.1.

Thymectomy is performed in patients with thymoma. Adult patients younger than 50 years of age with AChR antibody–positive, generalized MG without thymoma may also undergo thymectomy, as the procedure is associated with improved long-term clinical outcomes and lower cumulative dose of corticosteroids.[4] Thymectomy may be considered in patients 50 to 65 years old, but there is less evidence to support efficacy in this group. Thymectomy is typically not performed in MuSK or LRP4 antibody–positive patients, exclusively ocular MG, or seronegative patients without thymoma.

In the special case of MG occurring as a complication of immune checkpoint inhibitor therapy, management involves immune checkpoint inhibitor discontinuation, pyridostigmine, and corticosteroids. If patients have severe weakness, concurrent myocarditis or myopathy/myositis, high-dose IV methylprednisolone is first-line therapy. This contrasts with idiopathic MG, where IV steroids are generally avoided due to the risk of worsening. While many patients with MG as a complication of immune checkpoint inhibitor therapy experience rapid improvement over days to weeks on steroids, others may require additional immunomodulatory therapy such as IVIg or plasmapheresis.[5] The decision to restart an immune checkpoint inhibitor is made on a case-by-case basis.

Lambert-Eaton Myasthenic Syndrome

LEMS is a rare disorder of the NMJ caused by antibodies against the voltage-gated calcium channel (VGCC) of the presynaptic nerve terminal, leading to decreased influx of calcium ions into the presynaptic neuron. This results in impaired release of acetylcholine into the NMJ. The disease is paraneoplastic in about 50% of patients; the most commonly associated cancer is small cell lung cancer.[6]

Clinical Symptoms

LEMS is characterized by symmetric proximal weakness, autonomic symptoms, and areflexia or hyporeflexia. Proximal leg muscles are commonly affected, causing difficulty walking, climbing stairs, or getting up from a seated position. Autonomic dysfunction manifests as dry mouth, dry eyes, orthostasis, heat/cold intolerance, constipation, and, in men, erectile dysfunction. Ptosis, diplopia, dysphagia, and dysarthria may be seen but are less common than in MG. Due to proximal weakness, diminished reflexes, and fewer ocular and bulbar symptoms, LEMS may initially be misdiagnosed as myopathy or lumbosacral radiculopathy. However, weakness fluctuates in LEMS, either worsening or improving with prolonged exertion. This variability helps distinguish it from these other disorders.

Examination

The most common examination findings in LEMS are symmetric proximal weakness, especially of the lower extremities, and reduced or absent deep tendon reflexes. Proximal lower extremity weakness may be detected in hip flexion, hip abduction, and hip extension. These muscle groups should be tested with the patient in the supine, lateral decubitus, and prone positions, respectively. This requires the patient to elevate the lower extremities against gravity and makes subtle weakness more apparent on examination. Further observations on examination may include inability of the patient to stand from sitting with the arms crossed so they cannot use the arms to push off from the chair. A waddling gait, characterized by an alternating left and right pelvic tilt with each step, may be present due to hip abductor weakness. Reflexes are typically absent but may become elicitable after brief, maximal contraction of the corresponding muscle, referred to as postexercise facilitation. For example, the biceps reflex may become present after 10 seconds of maximal elbow flexion against resistance by the examiner, and the patellar reflex may become present after 10 seconds of maximal knee extension. Deep tendon reflexes should be tested before manual muscle testing to avoid inadvertent facilitation. Less common findings on examination include ptosis and dysarthria.

Diagnostic Tests

Diagnostic tests include serologic testing and NCS. Serum antibodies may be present against the P/Q-type VGCC. N-type VGCC antibodies may also be present but are not specific for LEMS. On NCS, the main feature that distinguishes LEMS from MG is low-amplitude compound muscle action potentials (CMAPs), which often double to quadruple in amplitude after 10 seconds of voluntary muscle contraction or high-frequency repetitive stimulation. Like MG, LEMS also causes decrement (reduced amplitude) at slow rates of repetitive stimulation. If LEMS is suspected, the clinical suspicion should be communicated when ordering NCS/EMG so that the appropriate protocol is performed. However, most patients with LEMS are initially suspected to have radiculopathy or myopathy, given the pattern of proximal weakness, and the electromyographer is often the first clinician to suspect LEMS based on the characteristic NCS pattern. All patients diagnosed with LEMS should be screened for cancer with body computed tomography (CT) and/or positron emission tomography (PET) imaging. If initial cancer screening is negative, then repeat imaging should be obtained every 6 months for at least 2 years, as LEMS may precede systemic signs of malignancy.[6]

Treatment

In paraneoplastic LEMS, the underlying cancer must be treated. For both paraneoplastic and nonparaneoplastic LEMS, the first-line symptomatic treatment is the potassium channel blocker amifampridine, which works by increasing the release of acetylcholine at the nerve terminal. This medication is contraindicated in patients with a history of seizure as it can lower the seizure threshold. The addition of pyridostigmine may provide further benefit in some patients. In patients who have inadequate symptomatic control despite these medications, corticosteroids, IVIg, or other immunomodulatory therapies may be considered.

DISORDERS OF MUSCLE (MYOPATHY)

Disorders of muscle are referred to as myopathies. Myopathies are commonly characterized by symmetric weakness predominantly in proximal muscles. However, distal, facial, or trunk muscles can be involved. Muscle pain (myalgia) may be present but is not universal. Some patients with myopathy present with full strength, but have exercise intolerance, stiffness, or recurrent episodes of rhabdomyolysis or myoglobinuria. Sensory deficits are absent unless there is concomitant neuropathy. Some myopathies are complicated by involvement of other organ systems (eg, cardiomyopathy).

Proximal limb weakness can cause difficulty walking, climbing stairs, standing up from sitting, raising the arms, lifting groceries, or brushing the teeth or hair. Distal limb weakness can cause foot drop or decreased manual dexterity.

Evaluation for the cause of myopathy includes laboratory studies, NCS/EMG, muscle imaging, muscle biopsy, and/or genetic testing. Elevated creatine kinase (CK) is common in myopathy but not universally present. Aldolase, aspartate transaminase (AST), and alanine transaminase (ALT), although commonly referred to as liver enzymes, are also found in muscle and can be elevated in myopathy. Aldolase can rarely be elevated in myopathy in the absence of CK elevation. When aldolase, AST, and ALT are elevated, γ-glutamyl transferase (GGT) differentiates between skeletal muscle and liver injury, as GGT is not found in muscle.

EMG in myopathy can demonstrate early recruitment of motor units with decreased amplitude and/or duration and, in some cases, abnormal spontaneous activity suggesting muscle membrane irritability, but these findings are nonspecific with respect to the etiology of myopathy. Notably, muscle enzymes and NCS/EMG can be normal in certain myopathies, so normal results do not necessarily exclude a diagnosis of myopathy. MRI may show muscle edema and/or atrophy in specific patterns of involvement related to certain muscle diseases. However, MRI findings can be nonspecific, and abnormalities may be present in both neurogenic and myopathic disorders.

The etiologies of myopathy include toxic (eg, statin), inflammatory (eg, dermatomyositis), genetic (eg, muscular dystrophy), infectious (eg, trichinosis),

TABLE 25.2   Laboratory Testing in the Evaluation of Myopathy

Laboratory test (from serum unless otherwise noted)	Causes of myopathy
CK and aldolase	Nonspecific
Electrolytes: potassium, phosphate, magnesium, and calcium	Hypo/hyperkalemia, hypophosphatemia, hypermagnesemia, and hypo/hypercalcemia
TSH and free T4	Hypothyroidism and hyperthyroidism
Creatinine, GFR, calcium, phosphate, PTH, and vitamin D	Primary and secondary hyperparathyroidism and osteomalacia
24-h urinary free cortisol, late-night salivary cortisol, and dexamethasone suppression test	Cushing syndrome
Serum and urine protein electrophoresis, immunofixation, and free light chains	AL amyloidosis
Carnitine, acylcarnitine profile, and urine organic acids	Metabolic myopathy (lipid storage disease)
Lactate, amino acids, carnitine, acylcarnitine profile, and urine organic acids	Mitochondrial myopathy
Antibody to 5NTc1A	Inclusion body myositis
Antibodies to ANA, Sm, dsDNA, SSA, SSB, RNP, Ku, PM-Scl, and RA	Overlap myositis
[a]Antibodies to Jo-1, PL-7, PL-12, EJ, OJ, KS, Zo, and Ha	Anti-synthetase syndrome
[a]Antibodies to SAE, TIF1-γ, NXP-2, MDA-5, and Mi-2	Dermatomyositis
Antibodies to HMGCR and SRP	Immune-mediated necrotizing myopathy

ANA, anti-nuclear antibody; CK, creatine kinase; dsDNA, double-stranded DNA; GFR, glomerular filtration rate; HMGCR, 3-hydroxy-3-methylglutaryl-coenzyme A reductase; In gray, idiopathic inflammatory myopathies; PM-Scl, polymyositis-scleroderma; PTH, parathyroid hormone; RA, rheumatoid arthritis; RNP, ribonucleoprotein; Sm, Smith; SRP, signal recognition particle; SSA, Sjögren syndrome A; SSB, Sjögren syndrome B; TSH, thyroid-stimulating hormone.
[a]Antibodies are often included in myositis panel.

and associated underlying systemic diseases (eg, thyroid disease). Initial evaluation in suspected myopathy should include past medical history, medication history, family history, social history, neurologic examination, CK and aldolase, and additional testing based on these, as outlined in Table 25.2. NCS/EMG, muscle biopsy, and/or genetic testing may be necessary in some cases.

Toxic Myopathy

Medications that can cause myopathy include statins, corticosteroids, zidovudine, amiodarone, chloroquine/hydroxychloroquine, and colchicine. Alcohol can cause a toxic myopathy from chronic alcohol use disorder or rhabdomyolysis after a binge. Toxic myopathies are typically characterized by progressive proximal weakness, elevated CK, and myopathic abnormalities on EMG. Examples of toxins and associated CK and NCS/EMG findings are shown in Table 25.3. Clinical and NCS/EMG evidence of neuropathy may also be seen if the offending agent can also cause concomitant neuropathy (eg, amiodarone, chloroquine/hydroxychloroquine, colchicine,

and alcohol). In toxic myopathy, when the offending agent is eliminated, symptoms and CK gradually improve over weeks to months.

Statin use can cause muscle conditions ranging from mild asymptomatic CK elevation and myalgia without myopathy (ie, normal strength and normal CK) to rhabdomyolysis to toxic myopathy to immune-mediated necrotizing myopathy, which can cause severe progressive weakness despite statin cessation as discussed in the "Inflammatory Myopathy" section below.

The risk of statin myopathy is associated with drug- and patient-related factors, including older age, female sex, low body mass index, certain comorbidities (eg, renal or hepatic disease, diabetes, and hypothyroidism), higher statin dose, concurrent use of a fibrate medication, and use of a statin metabolized by CYP3A4 (eg, atorvastatin, simvastatin, and lovastatin) concurrently with other drugs that inhibit CYP3A4. In patients with mild CK elevation below 5 times the upper limit of normal, the decision to discontinue the statin, lower the dose, or continue the statin with symptom monitoring is based on symptom tolerability. Alternative causes (eg, hypothyroidism) should also be considered.

TABLE 25.3	CK and NCS/EMG Patterns in Toxic and Endocrine Myopathy	
Etiology	**CK**	**NCS/EMG features**
Steroids	Normal (NI)	NI
Statins	↑	Irritable myopathy
Chloroquine/ hydroxychloroquine	NI or ↑	Irritable myopathy ± polyneuropathy
Amiodarone	NI or ↑	Irritable myopathy ± polyneuropathy
Colchicine	↑	Irritable myopathy ± polyneuropathy
Zidovudine	↑	Myopathy
Alcohol (acute)	↑	Usually not obtained
Alcohol (chronic)	NI or ↑	NI or myopathy ± polyneuropathy
Immune checkpoint inhibitors	NI or ↑	NI or irritable myopathy +/- polyneuropathy +/- myasthenia gravis
Hypothyroidism	NI or ↑	NI or myopathy ± polyneuropathy
Hyperthyroidism	NI	NI or myopathy ± polyneuropathy
Hyperparathyroidism and osteomalacia	NI	NI or myopathy
Cushing syndrome/disease	NI	NI
AL amyloid	NI or ↑	Myopathy ± polyneuropathy

CK, creatine kinase; EMG, electromyography; NCS, nerve conduction study; NI, normal.

In patients with weakness, intolerable symptoms, or CK elevation above 5 times the upper limit of normal, the statin should be discontinued. Once symptoms resolve and the CK level normalizes, usually over weeks to months, reinitiation of the same statin at a lower dose or initiation of a different type of statin can be considered.[7] The treatment of statin-induced immune-mediated necrotizing myopathy is more complex and discussed in the "Inflammatory Myopathy" section below.

Steroid myopathy usually occurs in patients who have been taking a minimum of prednisone 30 mg daily or its equivalent for several weeks or longer.[8] CK and EMG are normal, and, as such, it is a diagnosis of exclusion. Steroid myopathy is relatively uncommon and is likely overdiagnosed.

Myopathy Associated With Systemic Disease

Several endocrine conditions are associated with myopathy. Untreated hypothyroidism or hyperthyroidism can cause muscle weakness, myalgia, and cramps. CK is typically elevated in hypothyroid-associated myopathy and can be asymptomatic. In hyperthyroid-associated myopathy, CK is usually normal. EMG may show myopathic abnormalities in either condition. Symptoms gradually improve with treatment of underlying thyroid disease. Thyrotoxicosis can rarely be associated with hypokalemic periodic paralysis in which acute muscle weakness develops in the setting of hypokalemia. Treatment entails correction of potassium and treatment of underlying thyroid disease. Myopathy may also be seen in parathyroid disease and Cushing syndrome. Table 25.3 shows CK and NCS/EMG patterns that can be observed in myopathies associated with these conditions.

Electrolyte abnormalities (most commonly of potassium, calcium, phosphate, or magnesium) can cause weakness that generally resolves with correction of the underlying electrolyte abnormalities.

Critical illness myopathy is an acute myopathy that develops in critically ill patients and is characterized by proximal worse than distal muscle weakness. Failure to be weaned from mechanical ventilation is the usual setting in which the condition is first suspected. Patients typically have spared eye movements but may be otherwise severely and diffusely weak. Risk factors include multiorgan failure, sepsis, hyperglycemia, use of steroids, use of paralytic agents while the patient is intubated, and duration of intensive care.

In patients with critical illness myopathy, CK is normal or elevated, and NCS/EMG often shows myopathic features, although it may be limited by the patient's reduced voluntary participation in the needle EMG examination. NCS/EMG can be helpful in distinguishing critical illness myopathy from other conditions (eg, MG, Guillain-Barré syndrome, and motor neuron disease) that can cause severe weakness in a patient in an intensive care unit. Muscle biopsy is typically unnecessary for diagnosis of critical illness myopathy unless atypical features are present. Patients may have concurrent critical illness polyneuropathy. Critical illness myopathy improves over weeks to months after resolution of the critical illness with rehabilitation, whereas comorbid critical illness polyneuropathy is associated with worse prognosis and may result in permanent disability.

Myopathies Due to Genetic Mutations

Hereditary myopathies encompass a large, heterogeneous group of muscle diseases that arise secondary to genetic mutations. They can be broadly categorized into muscular dystrophies, myotonic dystrophies, congenital myopathies, metabolic myopathies, and mitochondrial myopathies (Table 25.4). Many patients with hereditary myopathies have a family history of myopathy, although some develop a germline mutation and may lack a family history. Inheritance pattern is variable. Progression of weakness evolves over years. Hereditary myopathies can differ in the age of onset (ranging from the neonatal period to late adulthood), distribution of weakness, associated features (eg, cardiomyopathy), inheritance pattern, and pathologic features. Notably, some myopathies are not associated with weakness but with other muscular features such as exercise intolerance, cramps, or recurrent rhabdomyolysis/myoglobinuria (eg, certain metabolic myopathies). Other hereditary myopathies are associated with a specific clinical feature

TABLE 25.4   Categories of Hereditary Myopathies

Category	Inheritance pattern	Symptom onset	Muscular manifestations[a]	Associated features[b]	Examples
Muscular dystrophy	X-linked recessive AD AR	Infancy to adulthood	Proximal > distal weakness	Cardiac disease, hypoventilation, skeletal deformities (scoliosis), and learning disabilities	Duchenne, Becker, limb girdle, and facioscapulohumeral
Myotonic dystrophy	AD	Childhood to adulthood	Myotonia (inability to relax muscles); Distal > proximal weakness (type 1) or proximal > distal weakness (type 2)	Cardiac disease, hypoventilation, cataracts, cognitive impairment, insulin resistance, and reduced male fertility	Myotonic dystrophy types 1 and 2
Congenital myopathy	X-linked recessive AD AR	Infancy to childhood and occasionally to adulthood	Proximal > distal weakness	Malignant hyperthermia (with a mutation in *RYR1*)	Central core, multi/minicore, nemaline rod, and centronuclear
Metabolic myopathy	AR X-linked recessive	Infancy to young adulthood	Proximal > distal weakness or no weakness but with exercise intolerance, recurrent rhabdomyolysis/myoglobinuria, cramps, and myalgia	Cardiac disease and hepatic disease	Pompe and McArdle
Mitochondrial myopathy	Maternal AD AR X-linked recessive	Infancy to adulthood	Variable; non-fatigable ptosis/ophthalmoplegia and exercise intolerance	Cardiac disease, vision/hearing impairment, seizures, and cognitive impairment	CPEO, MELAS, and MERRF

AD, autosomal dominant; AR, autosomal recessive; CPEO, chronic progressive external ophthalmoplegia; MELAS, mitochondrial encephalomyopathy, lactic acidosis, and stroke-like episodes; MERRF, myoclonic epilepsy with ragged red fibers.
[a]The most common skeletal muscle manifestations of each category are shown.
[b]Features that can be associated with certain types of myopathies within each category. Not all myopathies within a category have these associated features.

called myotonia, which is defined as impaired muscle relaxation. Increased CK and myopathic EMG can be observed in many hereditary myopathies, but these can be normal, and definitive diagnosis is made by genetic testing or muscle biopsy.

Treatment is largely supportive with physical, occupational, and/or speech-language therapy, with the notable exceptions of steroids for Duchenne muscular dystrophy and enzyme replacement therapy for Pompe disease. Patients with hereditary myopathies may require orthoses, ambulatory aids, and, in some cases, ultimately, a wheelchair. In addition, specific conditions may require regular screening for systemic comorbidities (eg, cardiac conduction defect in patients with myotonic dystrophy). Comanagement with additional specialties, such as cardiology for conditions that cause cardiomyopathy or conduction defects, and pulmonology for patients with respiratory muscle weakness, may be necessary. Certain hereditary myopathies, such as myopathy associated with *RYR1* mutations, require special attention when anesthesia is needed for a procedure or surgery, as they are associated with an elevated risk of malignant hyperthermia.

Inflammatory Myopathy

Inflammatory myopathy (myositis) can occur as a sporadic immune-mediated condition (eg, dermatomyositis, inclusion body myositis [IBM], and anti-synthetase syndrome) in response to medications (eg, statins and immune checkpoint inhibitors) or in conjunction with cancer. Myositis can also occur in in conjunction with connective tissue disease (eg, systemic lupus erythematosus, Sjögren syndrome, scleroderma, and rheumatoid arthritis), which is referred to as overlap myositis. Patients with myositis typically present with subacute-onset proximal weakness that may be accompanied by myalgia, although this is not universally present. IBM is distinguished from other inflammatory myopathies by its slow progression over years and unique pattern of weakness predominantly affecting the distal upper extremities and proximal lower extremities (see subsequent text).

EMG in patients with myositis may show early recruitment of motor units with decreased amplitude and/or duration, and abnormal spontaneous activity in the form of fibrillation potentials and/or positive sharp waves (indicative of muscle membrane irritability).

MRI may show edema, hyperintensity, and/or atrophy of affected muscles. Table 25.2 shows laboratory tests that are helpful in the evaluation of noninfectious inflammatory myopathy. Muscle biopsy may be necessary in some cases for diagnosis. Treatment of inflammatory myopathy is with steroids or steroid-sparing immunotherapy. IBM, which does not respond to these treatments, is a notable exception. In addition, patients with inflammatory myopathy may require regular screening for the development of interstitial lung disease or other associated comorbidities (see subsequent text).

Dermatomyositis

Dermatomyositis causes subacute onset of proximal worse than distal weakness and characteristic skin manifestations, such as a purple rash on the eyelids (heliotrope rash), chest (V-neck sign) or upper back (shawl sign); papules on the knuckles, interphalangeal joints, elbows or knees (Gottron papules); periungual erythema; and telangiectasia. Interstitial lung disease may be present. In some patients, a dermatomyositis rash may be present without myositis (dermatomyositis *sine* myositis) or vice versa (dermatomyositis *sine* dermatitis). CK is usually elevated but may be normal. Aldolase can be elevated even when CK is normal. Some patients have dermatomyositis-specific antibodies that correlate with particular clinical features (eg, TIF1-γ dermatomyositis has a stronger association with cancer). Dermatomyositis is associated with malignancy, so thorough cancer screening with PET-CT should be performed in all patients diagnosed with dermatomyositis.

Anti-Synthetase Syndrome

Anti-synthetase syndrome refers to a group of inflammatory myopathies associated with anti-tRNA synthetase antibodies (Jo1, PL-7, PL-12, EJ, OJ, KS, Zo, and Ha) that can cause subacute proximal worse than distal weakness with elevated CK. Interstitial lung disease is more common in anti-synthetase syndrome than in dermatomyositis. Additional features of anti-synthetase syndrome are fever, inflammatory arthritis, mechanic's hands, and Raynaud phenomenon.

Polymyositis

Polymyositis presents similarly to dermatomyositis but without associated skin findings or associated autoantibodies. Patients with polymyositis should also be screened for malignancy with PET-CT.

Inclusion Body Myositis

IBM is the most common acquired inflammatory myopathy in adults older than 50 years of age,[9] and differs in several ways from the other conditions discussed earlier: it is more indolent, can present asymmetrically, and causes a unique pattern of weakness predominantly involving the finger flexors and quadriceps, often accompanied by dysphagia (Figure 25.3). CK may be normal or elevated. A significant proportion of patients have antibodies to cytosolic 5′-nucleotidase 1A (NT5c1A). Conventional immunomodulatory therapies used in other inflammatory myopathies are ineffective in IBM, and treatment is supportive.

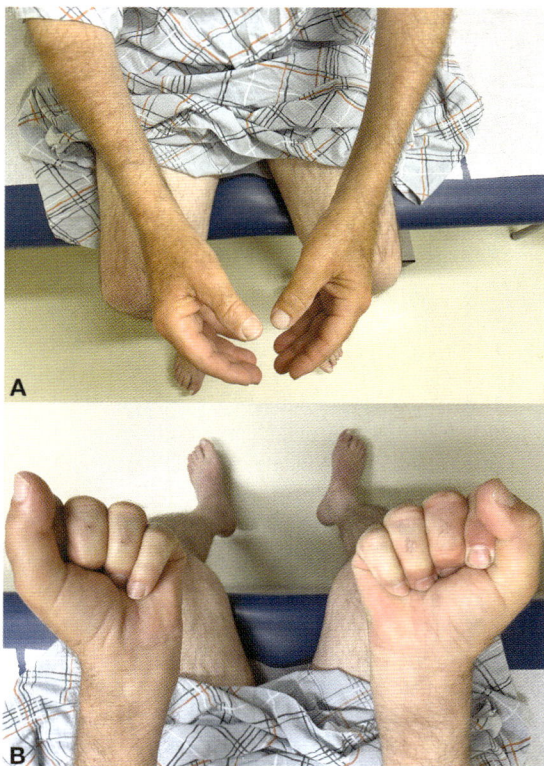

FIGURE 25.3 Bilateral forearm atrophy (A) and asymmetric finger flexion weakness (B), most severely affecting the left thumb, left pinky, and right index finger in this patient with inclusion body myositis. (Picture from author/Dr. Suh; permission has been obtained from the patient.)

Immune-Mediated Necrotizing Myopathy

Immune-mediated necrotizing myopathy (also known as necrotizing autoimmune myopathy) is an autoimmune myopathy that can be triggered by statin exposure, may be paraneoplastic, or can occur sporadically. CK is generally extremely high, and weakness can be severe. Patients may have antibodies to HMG-CoA (3-hydroxy-3-methylglutaryl coenzyme A) reductase or signal recognition particle. Patients who develop this condition should be screened for cancer. In cases triggered by statin use, the statin should be discontinued. These patients should not be rechallenged with another statin. PCSK9 inhibitors may be considered for management of hyperlipidemia in such patients. Immunotherapy is typically required to improve muscle strength.

Immune Checkpoint Inhibitor–Associated Myositis

Immune checkpoint inhibitors for the treatment of cancer can cause various neurologic complications, including myositis (which may be accompanied by MG and/or myocarditis). Onset of weakness is generally acute to subacute (over days to weeks), occurring within months of treatment initiation. Weakness is usually proximal and symmetric, but patients may have focal involvement (eg, orbital myositis). CK is usually elevated but can be normal. Cardiac evaluation for myocarditis is recommended in patients with immune checkpoint inhibitor–associated myositis even if the patient does not have cardiac symptoms since myositis and myocarditis frequently co-occur. The American Society of Clinical Oncology recommends treatment with corticosteroids[5] and at least temporary discontinuation of the immune checkpoint inhibitor unless myositis is mild. Although most cases respond favorably to steroids, patients with insufficient response or relapse during steroid taper may require additional immunosuppressive therapies. A decision to permanently discontinue, resume, or switch to a different immune checkpoint inhibitor therapy after the resolution of complications is made on a case-by-case basis.

Infectious Myositis

Infectious myositis can be caused by bacteria, viruses, parasites, and, rarely, fungi.

Bacterial Myositis

Bacterial infections can cause myositis or pyomyositis (intramuscular infection with abscess formation). Bacteria can reach the muscles by spread from an adjacent infected site, penetrating trauma, bacteremia, or in the setting of muscle ischemia. *Staphylococcus aureus* is the most common bacteria that spreads via the hematogenous route, but others include *Streptococcus pyogenes*, other *Streptococcus* species, gram-negative bacilli, and anaerobes. Risk factors for bacterial myositis and pyomyositis include immunocompromise, IV drug use, and muscle trauma. Bacterial myositis and pyomyositis should be suspected in a patient with focal muscle pain and edema with associated fever, leukocytosis, and elevated inflammatory markers. An abscess in the iliopsoas muscle (a common location for pyomyositis) is not typically associated with visible or palpable swelling but causes back or flank pain that worsens with hip extension; diagnosis is made by CT of the pelvis. CK is usually normal in bacterial myositis and pyomyositis. Antibiotics are the mainstay of therapy and surgical drainage may be required in cases with a purulent collection.

Viral Myositis

Viral myositis typically presents with diffuse weakness, although proximal muscles may be more affected. A notable exception is benign acute childhood myositis, which occurs in school-age children with influenza A/B infection and primarily affects the calves. Other viruses associated with myositis include enterovirus, hepatitis B/C, HIV, human T-cell lymphotropic virus type 1 (HTLV-1), and SARS-CoV-2. CK is often markedly elevated, and rhabdomyolysis may occur. Most cases associated with respiratory viruses are transient and resolve spontaneously, but those associated with retroviruses may be chronic.

Parasitic Myositis

Myositis can occur with various parasitic infections, including *Trichinella* species (trichinosis), *Taenia solium* (cysticercosis), and *Toxoplasma gondii* (primary or reactivation toxoplasmosis). These infections are usually acquired through accidental ingestion of the parasite in raw or undercooked meat (for *Trichinella*), contaminated water or food (for *Taenia solium*), or both (for *Toxoplasma*). *Toxoplasma* infection can additionally occur via accidental ingestion of eggs in cat feces. Parasitic myositis may be subclinical or associated with diffuse or multifocal myalgia, muscle edema, and weakness. Trichinella commonly causes periorbital edema, eosinophilia, myalgia, and febrile myositis with elevated CK. For parasitic myositis, serologic tests, imaging, and muscle biopsy help establish the diagnosis. Treatment includes antiparasitic drugs, often with concurrent corticosteroids.

SUMMARY

NMJ disorders are characterized by fluctuating muscle weakness without sensory abnormalities. Ocular and bulbar weakness are particularly common in MG. Myopathies are characterized by weakness (most commonly proximal) in the absence of sensory abnormalities. Diagnosis of myopathy is suggested by elevated CK, abnormal EMG, and abnormal muscle MRI, although these can be normal. Etiologies of myopathy include medications (eg, statins), inflammatory conditions, systemic conditions, genetic mutations, and infection. Therefore, evaluation should include detailed medical, family, and social history, as well as medication history, with evaluation directed toward the most likely etiologies based on the rate of progression, pattern of weakness, and medical context.

EDITORS' KEY POINTS

▶ Diseases of the NMJ (eg, MG, LEMS, and botulism) and diseases of the muscle (referred to as myopathies) cause weakness without sensory abnormalities.

▶ MG causes fatigable muscle weakness, usually beginning with ocular symptoms (ptosis or diplopia) that may occur alone (ocular MG) or may include— or evolve to include—weakness of the extremities, face, larynx, and pharynx (generalized MG).

▶ Myasthenic crisis can result in respiratory failure requiring noninvasive or invasive ventilatory support. In addition to supportive care, treatment is with IVIG or plasma exchange.

▶ The diagnosis of MG is made by serum autoantibodies (against the AChR or associated structures) and NCS showing a decremental response to slow repetitive nerve stimulation. Patients with MG should be evaluated for thymoma with CT or MRI of the chest.

▶ Therapies for MG include acetylcholinesterase inhibitors (pyridostigmine), corticosteroids, immunomodulatory treatment, and thymectomy (in patients with thymoma or in adult patients without thymoma younger than 50 years old with AChR antibody–positive, generalized MG).

▶ LEMS is a rare disorder of the NMJ caused by antibodies against the VGCC of the presynaptic nerve terminal. LEMS is paraneoplastic in about 50% of patients, most commonly associated with small cell lung cancer. Symptoms of LEMS include symmetric proximal weakness, autonomic symptoms, and hyporeflexia.

▶ Myopathies typically cause symmetric weakness in proximal muscles (causing difficulty reaching above the head and standing from a chair). However, some myopathies can also affect distal, facial, or trunk muscles.

▶ Causes of myopathy include medications (eg, statins, corticosteroids, and immune checkpoint inhibitors), inflammatory conditions (eg, dermatomyositis and IBM), genetic diseases (eg, muscular dystrophy), infections (eg, trichinosis), and underlying systemic diseases (eg, thyroid disease and rheumatologic disease).

▶ Evaluation for the cause of myopathy includes laboratory studies (eg, CK, aldolase, and autoantibody panel), EMG, muscle MRI, muscle biopsy, and genetic testing. Elevated serum CK is common in myopathy but not universally present.

▶ Medications that can cause myopathy include statins, corticosteroids, zidovudine, amiodarone, chloroquine/hydroxychloroquine, and colchicine. Alcohol can cause a toxic myopathy from chronic alcohol use disorder or rhabdomyolysis after excessive intake.

▶ Critical illness myopathy is an acute myopathy that develops in critically ill patients and is characterized by proximal worse than distal muscle weakness. Failure to be weaned from mechanical ventilation is the usual setting in which the condition is first suspected.

▶ Genetic myopathies include the muscular dystrophies, congenital myopathies, metabolic myopathies, and mitochondrial myopathies. Many

patients with genetic myopathies have a family history, although not all.

▶ Inflammatory myopathy (myositis) can occur as a sporadic immune-mediated condition (eg, dermatomyositis, IBM, and anti-synthetase syndrome), in response to medications (eg, statins and immune checkpoint inhibitors), or in association with cancer.

▶ IBM is the most common acquired inflammatory myopathy in adults older than 50 years of age, can present indolently and asymmetrically, and causes a pattern of weakness predominantly involving the finger flexors and quadriceps, often accompanied by dysphagia.

▶ Immune-mediated necrotizing myopathy is an autoimmune myopathy that can be triggered by statin exposure, may be paraneoplastic, or can occur sporadically. CK is generally extremely high, and weakness can be severe. Patients may have antibodies to HMG-CoA reductase or signal recognition particle. In cases triggered by statin use, the statin should be discontinued, and immunotherapy is typically required.

REFERENCES

1. Narayanaswami P, Sanders DB, Wolfe G, et al. International Consensus Guidance for management of myasthenia gravis: 2020 update. *Neurology*. 2021;96(3):114-122.

2. Gilhus NE, Skeie GO, Romi F, Lazaridis K, Zisimopoulou P, Tzartos S. Myasthenia gravis—autoantibody characteristics and their implications for therapy. *Nat Rev Neurol*. 2016;12(5):259-268.

3. O'Hare M, Doughty C. Update on ocular myasthenia gravis. *Semin Neurol*. 2019;39(6):749-760.

4. Wolfe GI, Kaminski HJ, Aban IB, et al. Long-term effect of thymectomy plus prednisone versus prednisone alone in patients with non-thymomatous myasthenia gravis: 2-year extension of the MGTX randomised trial. *Lancet Neurol*. 2019;18(3):259-268.

5. Schneider BJ, Naidoo J, Santomasso BD, et al. Management of immune-related adverse events in patients treated with immune checkpoint inhibitor therapy: ASCO guideline update. *J Clin Oncol*. 2021;39(36):4073-4126.

6. Titulaer MJ, Lang B, Verschuuren JJ. Lambert-Eaton myasthenic syndrome: from clinical characteristics to therapeutic strategies. *Lancet Neurol*. 2011;10(12):1098-1107.

7. Abd TT, Jacobson TA. Statin-induced myopathy: a review and update. *Expert Opin Drug Saf*. 2011;10(3):373-387.

8. Doughty CT, Amato AA. Toxic myopathies. *Continuum (Minneap Minn)*. 2019;25(6):1712-1731.

9. Needham M, Mastaglia FL. Inclusion body myositis: current pathogenetic concepts and diagnostic and therapeutic approaches. *Lancet Neurol*. 2007;6(7):620-631.

Cancer and the Nervous System

Joshua A. Budhu

INTRODUCTION

Cancer can affect the nervous system in various ways: Tumors can arise from or metastasize to nervous system structures, cancer therapies can cause nervous system toxicity, and cancers may cause paraneoplastic syndromes affecting the nervous system. This chapter reviews the diagnosis and treatment of these conditions.

PRIMARY NERVOUS SYSTEM TUMORS

Primary central nervous system (CNS) tumors are less common compared to CNS metastases.[1] Primary CNS tumors are broadly classified by cell of origin; for example, meningiomas arise from the cells of the meninges (the coverings of the brain), gliomas arise from glial cells (nonneuronal cells involved in nervous system homeostasis), and ependymomas arise from the ependyma (lining of ventricles). Here,

the most common CNS tumors—meningioma, glioma, and primary CNS lymphoma—are discussed. While grading of systemic cancers often incorporates metastasis to lymph nodes and other organs, primary CNS tumors generally do not metastasize, and grading is therefore based on cellular and molecular characteristics related to aggressiveness of the tumor and recurrence risk. For example, there is no staging for gliomas, and they are divided from grades 1 to 4 based on an integrated histomolecular diagnosis.

Meningioma

Meningiomas arise from the meninges (the coverings of the brain and spinal cord). They are the most common primary brain tumor, making up about 40% of newly diagnosed brain tumors.[1] Meningiomas most commonly develop over the superior or lateral surface of the brain but can also occur inferior to the brain (at the skull base) or in the spine. Meningiomas are categorized as grades 1, 2, or 3 based on histologic and molecular characteristics. The majority of meningiomas are grade 1, which are very slow growing. Grades 2 and 3 are more aggressive but rare. Although most meningiomas arise spontaneously, risk factors for development of meningioma include previous ionizing radiation to the brain (eg, radiation therapy for a prior cancer) and genetic syndromes such as NF2-related schwannomatosis.

Symptoms of meningioma include headache, seizure, and focal neurologic deficits due to compression of nervous system structures. Many meningiomas

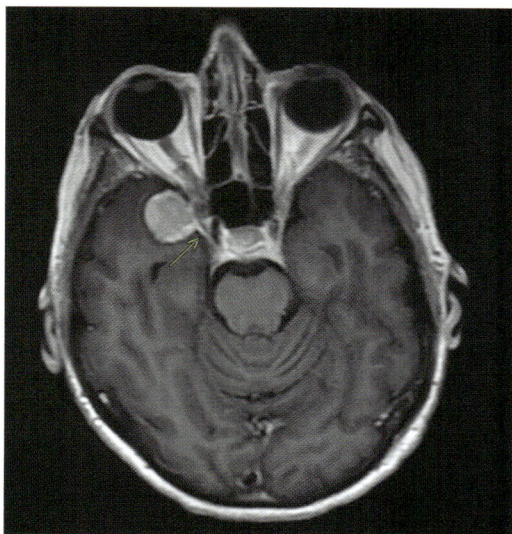

FIGURE 26.1 Axial postcontrast T1-weighted magnetic resonance imaging (MRI) showing a right middle cranial fossa meningioma with an associated dural tail (arrow). The meningioma is extra-axial (ie, outside the brain parenchyma), well circumscribed, and homogeneously enhancing. The dural tail is the result of dural thickening and enhancement.

are asymptomatic, found incidentally during computed tomography (CT) or magnetic resonance imaging (MRI) performed for another purpose. On CT images, meningiomas usually appear isodense or hyperdense and on MRI, meningiomas appear T2 hyperintense with homogeneous enhancement on postcontrast images and often have a characteristic dural tail (Figure 26.1).

Treatment of Meningioma

Incidentally found meningiomas can usually be observed with serial imaging (such as follow-up MRIs annually) unless they are growing rapidly or close to eloquent areas of the brain. Symptomatic meningiomas (eg, causing seizures or focal deficits) should be resected when possible. Treatment decisions are made on an individualized basis; for example, an older patient with a growing meningioma may opt for surveillance, while a younger patient with a growing meningioma may consider early surgery.

The recurrence rate after resection is extremely low for grade 1 tumors but higher for grades 2 and 3 tumors. Therefore, adjuvant radiation to the resection cavity/residual meningioma is recommended for all grade 3 tumors and some grade 2 tumors. In rare, very aggressive grade 3 tumors, chemotherapy may be considered.

Glioma

Gliomas are tumors that arise from glial cells, a nonneuronal cell type found throughout the nervous system that plays various roles in nervous system homeostasis. These tumors are classified depending on histologic characteristics and molecular markers into three tumor types: (1) astrocytoma, isocitrate dehydrogenase (IDH) mutant (ranging from grades 2 to 4); (2) oligodendroglioma, IDH mutant and 1p/19q co-deleted (ranging from grades 2 to 3); and (3) glioblastoma, IDH wild type (grade 4). Grading of these tumors reflects their aggressiveness, and glioblastomas are the most aggressive.

The clinical presentation of gliomas depends on the size and location of the tumor. Patients may present with headache, focal deficits, and/or seizures. Slowly growing tumors may take years to cause symptoms. Glioblastomas, the most common malignant brain tumors, are highly aggressive and often present with focal deficits such as aphasia, weakness, neuropsychiatric symptoms, or sensory changes.

In general, lower-grade gliomas occur in younger patients and higher-grade gliomas present in older patients; however, this is not always the case. Environmental risk factors include exposure to ionizing radiation such as previous radiotherapy to the brain for a childhood cancer. Currently, there is no clear association of radiofrequency fields (cellphone usage) with an increased risk of glioma.

On MRI, lower grade tumors demonstrate T2 hyperintensity with little to no contrast enhancement (Figure 26. 2). IDH mutant tumors may demonstrate the T2-FLAIR (fluid-attenuated inversion recovery) mismatch sign, in which there is T2 hyperintensity of the tumor on T2 sequences but hypointensity on

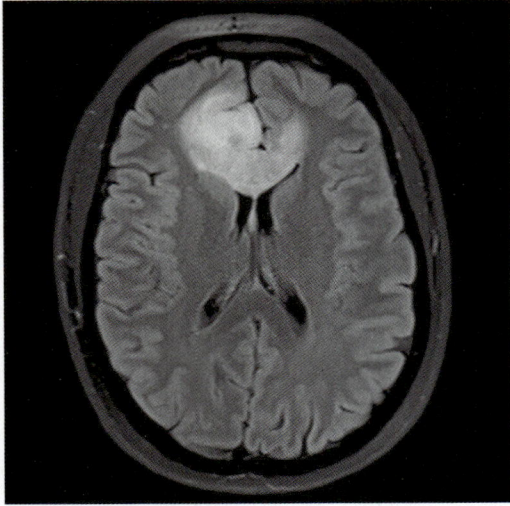

FIGURE 26.2 Grade 2 IDH mutant astrocytoma on an axial fluid-attenuated inversion recovery (FLAIR) magnetic resonance imaging (MRI). Note the indistinct borders indicating this is an infiltrative tumor. This lesion did not exhibit contrast enhancement.

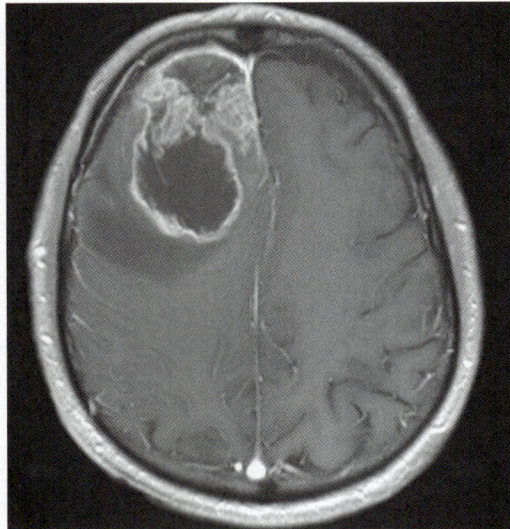

FIGURE 26.3 Right frontal glioblastoma on axial postcontrast T1-weighted magnetic resonance imaging (MRI). There is a large, right frontal, heterogeneously enhancing mass, with central hypointensity indicative of necrosis, along with vasogenic edema and midline shift.

FLAIR sequences.[2] Glioblastomas and higher grade tumors have heterogeneous contrast enhancement, necrosis, and associated vasogenic edema (Figure 26.3).

Treatment of Glioma

If possible, surgical resection is recommended for all gliomas. If a gross total resection can be achieved and pathology shows low-risk features and is consistent with a grade 1 or 2 tumor, it may be reasonable to monitor with close surveillance. For grade 2 gliomas with a subtotal resection or higher-risk features, radiation followed by chemotherapy is the mainstay of treatment. Grade 2 tumors that require adjuvant treatment can be treated with either PCV (procarbazine, CCNU, and vincristine) or temozolomide.

IDH inhibitors, such as vorasidenib, have shown promising response rates in patients with IDH mutant low-grade gliomas.[3] Preliminary data also suggest that these targeted therapies are better tolerated than previously used chemotherapy agents. IDH inhibitors can improve progression-free survival and will likely become standard of care for grades 2 and 3 gliomas.[3]

Grades 3 and 4 tumors, including glioblastoma, are treated with radiation and concurrent temozolomide in a 6-week course, followed by 6 to 12 adjuvant 28-day cycles of temozolomide.[4]

There is no standard of care for recurrence or progression of glioblastoma. CCNU, an oral alkylating nitrosourea, is often used. Bevacizumab, an anti-vascular endothelial growth factor (VEGF) monoclonal antibody, is US Food and Drug Administration (FDA) approved and helps with symptoms and quality of life by decreasing tumor edema, but it has not been associated with a survival benefit. Given the paucity of treatment options, clinical trials are recommended for eligible patients, both for initial treatment and treatment of recurrence.

The prognosis of gliomas depends on the grade of the tumor. Patients with lower-grade gliomas with good prognostic indicators such as younger age of onset (age 40 or younger), favorable molecular features, and near-total or gross total surgical resection can routinely live 15 years or more. However, even with molecular data, prognosis can be difficult to predict. Patients with grade 3 astrocytomas and oligodendrogliomas generally live about 5 years after diagnosis, depending on treatment. Patients with glioblastomas, depending on molecular features and location, have median survival between 12 and 18 months after diagnosis, even with maximal therapy.

Apart from direct anti-tumor treatment, supportive care is very important in the management of patients with gliomas. Patients can have neuropsychiatric symptoms, both from the tumor itself and from side effects of therapy, including anti-seizure medications (ASMs) and corticosteroids used to treat symptomatic edema. Deep venous thrombosis and pulmonary embolism are common in patients with glioblastoma; anticoagulation is generally safe for these patients unless they have significant intratumoral hemorrhage or thrombocytopenia.

Central Nervous System Lymphoma

Primary CNS lymphoma is a rare non-Hodgkin lymphoma. Ninety percent of cases of primary CNS lymphoma are diffuse large B-cell lymphomas. Primary CNS lymphoma can occur in both patients who are immunocompetent and patients who are immunocompromised; in the setting of immune compromise, the tumor is usually associated with the Epstein-Barr virus (EBV).

Symptoms of primary CNS lymphoma include focal neurologic deficits, signs of raised intracranial pressure (headache, nausea, vomiting, and double vision), and neuropsychiatric symptoms; symptoms often emerge and progress over weeks to months. Unlike systemic lymphomas, most patients do not have any constitutional B symptoms (eg, fever and night sweats).

In patients who are immunocompetent, brain MRI usually reveals one or more T2 hyperintense, homogeneously enhancing lesions with diffusion restriction (Figure 26.4). In patients who are immunocompromised, tumors exhibit ring enhancement and are more commonly multifocal.

Unlike other primary CNS tumors, evaluation for systemic involvement is a key part of the evaluation for primary CNS lymphoma. This includes MRI of the brain and spine, positron emission tomography (PET)-CT to evaluate for systemic involvement, lumbar puncture, ophthalmologic evaluation, HIV testing, and testicular ultrasound for male patients.

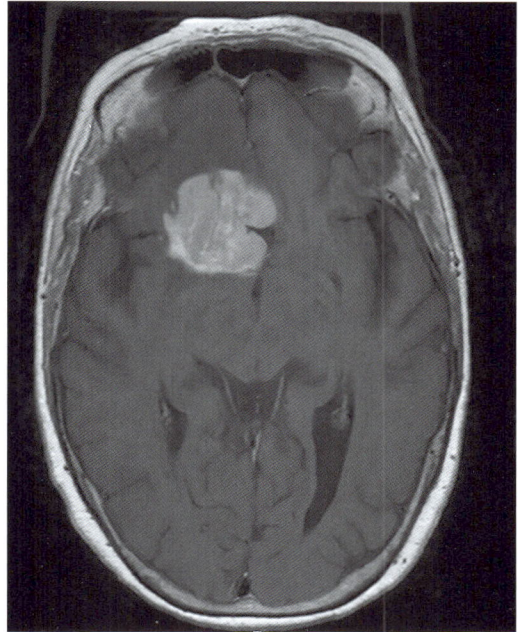

FIGURE 26.4 Axial postcontrast T1-weighted magnetic resonance imaging (MRI) of a diffuse large B-cell primary central nervous system (CNS) lymphoma. There is a solitary lesion with homogeneous contrast enhancement and some associated vasogenic edema in the inferior right frontal lobe.

If testicular involvement is found, an orchiectomy can be performed. If there is evidence of systemic involvement, the disease is considered secondary CNS lymphoma (rather than primary CNS lymphoma), and treatment will involve a combination of systemic and CNS penetrant agents.

Steroids are cytotoxic to lymphoma and should be avoided before biopsy, as they can produce inconclusive pathology results.

Treatment of Primary Central Nervous System Lymphoma

Treatment involves two stages: induction with the goal of achieving remission of disease and consolidation to prevent relapse or recurrence. Induction regimens vary depending on institution but always include high-dose methotrexate. Additional treatment agents include combinations of rituximab, temozolomide, procarbazine, vincristine, carmustine, etoposide, cytarabine, and thiotepa. Consolidation therapy regimens include high-dose chemotherapy followed by stem cell transplant, Bruton tyrosine kinase (BTK) inhibitors, and immunomodulatory drugs such as lenalidomide. There are ongoing trials studying chimeric antigen receptor T-cell (CAR-T) therapies. Radiotherapy can be used as a bridge in patients with extensive tumor burden, but the response is generally not durable.

The treatment of primary CNS lymphoma in patients who are immunocompromised also involves addressing the underlying cause of immunocompromise, such as starting antiretroviral therapy in patients with HIV or discontinuing immunosuppressive agents.

METASTASES TO THE NERVOUS SYSTEM

Metastases to the brain and spine are much more common than primary CNS tumors. The tumors that most commonly metastasize to the brain are lung cancer, breast cancer, melanoma, colorectal cancer, and renal cell cancer. Prostate cancer rarely metastasizes to the CNS but may metastasize to the spine, skull, or dura, leading to brain or spinal cord compression. Leptomeningeal metastases are metastases to the arachnoid and pia mater (the leptomeninges). Previously, the spread of cancer to the nervous system portended a very poor outcome, but recent advancements in targeted therapies and radiation have improved survival and quality of life for patients with CNS metastases.

CNS metastases can present with a variety of symptoms depending on the location and number of metastases. Brain metastases can cause headache, seizures, focal neurologic deficits, and neuropsychiatric symptoms. Spine metastases can cause back pain, weakness, and sensory changes in the extremities due to compression of the spinal cord or cauda equina. Most symptoms related to CNS metastases present subacutely, but sudden-onset symptoms may be seen with hemorrhage into a brain metastasis (most common with melanoma, choriocarcinoma, thyroid cancer, and renal cell cancer) or spinal cord compression due to collapse of a vertebra weakened by metastasis. Leptomeningeal metastases can present with signs of increased intracranial pressure (eg, headache, nausea, and vomiting), focal neurologic deficits including cranial neuropathies and cerebellar dysfunction,

encephalopathy, radiculopathy, and cauda equina syndrome. Leptomeningeal metastases may also cause transient increases in intracranial pressure that can occur when changing position and are characterized by changes in level of consciousness or stereotyped movements.

Brain metastases typically appear on MRI as small, multiple, discrete ring-enhancing lesions with a propensity for the gray-white junction (Figures 26.5 and 26.6). However, metastases can occur in any part of the brain and may be solitary and/or large. Leptomeningeal metastatic disease is usually characterized by wispy enhancement of the sulci, cerebellar folia, and enhancement surrounding the nerve roots of the cauda equina; in addition, bulky nodular deposits may develop. Patients with suspected leptomeningeal metastases should have a lumbar puncture for pathologic confirmation with cytology and flow cytometry (for hematologic malignancies). The most common cerebrospinal fluid (CSF) profile in leptomeningeal metastatic disease is a lymphocytic pleocytosis and increased protein; glucose level may be normal or decreased.

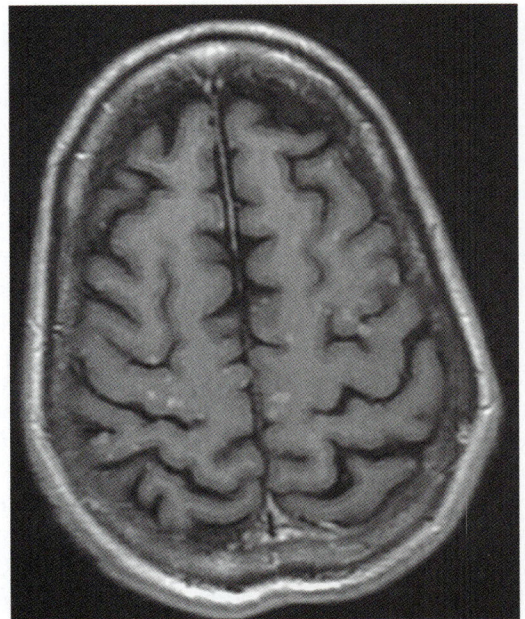

FIGURE 26.5 Axial postcontrast T1-weighted magnetic resonance imaging (MRI) of a patient with innumerable small, asymptomatic brain metastases from non-small cell lung cancer.

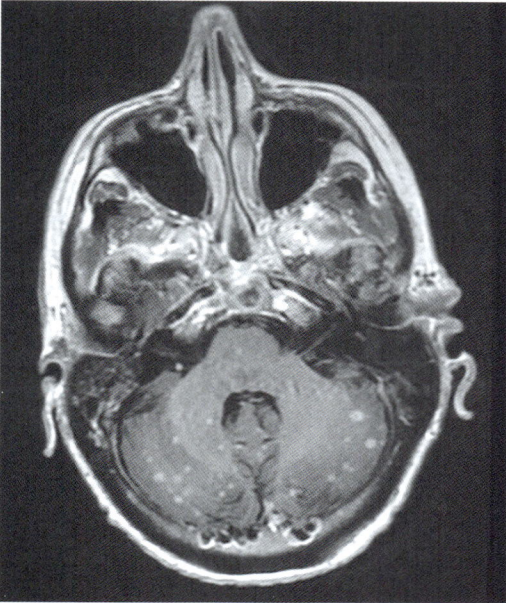

FIGURE 26.6 Axial postcontrast T1-weighted magnetic resonance imaging (MRI) of a patient with innumerable small, asymptomatic brain metastases from non-small cell lung cancer.

In patients with known systemic cancer and a classic appearance of metastases on MRI, further diagnostic testing of the brain lesion(s) is generally unnecessary. However, if the primary tumor is unknown and not determined by biopsy of a lesion discovered by CT and/or PET of the body, age-appropriate cancer screening, and detailed skin examination, brain biopsy may be necessary to diagnose the systemic cancer.

Treatment of Central Nervous System Metastases

Large, symptomatic brain metastases are treated with surgical resection with postoperative radiation, whether solitary or a single large symptomatic metastasis among multiple metastases. Stereotactic radiosurgery, which provides a focused amount of radiation in limited fractions, can be used when there are fewer than 10 metastases less than 3 cm in size, whereas intensity-modulated radiation therapy or whole-brain radiation is used for larger metastases and/or a greater number of metastases.[5] In patients with leptomeningeal metastases, radiotherapy often includes the entire craniospinal axis. Craniospinal irradiation targets a large area and can have side effects, especially on the bone marrow. If available, proton therapy can mitigate some of these side effects.

Specific chemotherapy and/or immunotherapy with CNS penetration is used for certain cancers such as lung, breast, and melanoma. Intrathecal chemotherapy is sometimes used for leptomeningeal metastases but may not be effective in bulky disease.[6] If there are signs or symptoms of increased intracranial pressure, then CSF diversion with a ventriculoperitoneal shunt may be considered.

Anticoagulation in Patients With Brain Metastases

Similar to glioblastomas, it is generally safe to use anticoagulation for treatment of venous or arterial thromboembolism in patients with brain metastases. Relative contraindications include intratumoral blood products (more common in cancers such as melanoma) or thrombocytopenia that may lead to a bleeding event. Each patient should be evaluated for appropriateness of anticoagulation. For example, patients who are slightly thrombocytopenic ($<150,000/\mu L$) and are receiving platelet-depleting chemotherapy will need to be closely monitored and potentially require dose adjustment of chemotherapy. Historically, enoxaparin has been the preferred anticoagulant, but recent data has validated the use of direct oral anticoagulants (DOACs).[7,8]

Management of Seizures in Patients With Brain Tumors

Patients undergoing surgery for both primary brain tumors and brain metastases are often placed on prophylactic antiseizures medications (ASMs) during the perioperative period. If a patient does not have a history of seizures, then the ASMs can be weaned off postoperatively. Given the side effects of ASMs, including neuropsychiatric symptoms, it is not routine practice to place patients with brain tumors who have not seized on prophylactic ASMs when they are not undergoing a procedure.

In patients who develop a seizure secondary to a brain tumor, levetiracetam is the preferred initial agent because of ease of titration, mild side effect profile (compared to other ASMs), and lack of interaction with other agents. There are no contraindications to other ASMs, but clinicians should be aware of drug-drug interactions, especially with strong inducers of the cytochrome P450 system such as phenytoin, phenobarbital, and carbamazepine. These medications may also render patients ineligible for clinical trials due to drug-drug interactions.

NEUROLOGIC COMPLICATIONS OF CANCER THERAPY

Radiation Therapy

Radiation therapy can cause side effects during treatment, in the immediate posttreatment period, and chronically. During treatment, patients often develop fatigue, impaired memory, and word-finding difficulty. These side effects are more common with whole-brain radiation therapy as compared to stereotactic radiosurgery.

Weeks to months after fractionated radiotherapy, there can be radiation-induced inflammatory changes and tissue injury at the site of radiation in the brain. This is termed pseudoprogression and can be difficult to discern from viable tumor growth as it may cause worsening symptoms and imaging findings. Advanced imaging techniques, such as perfusion imaging, PET-CT, or PET-MRI, and biopsy/resection of the lesion are used to distinguish pseudoprogression from tumor growth. Management depends on symptoms; if pseudoprogression is large and symptomatic, then steroids and resection are considered.

Radiation necrosis can develop months or years after radiation treatment. Like pseudoprogression, radiation necrosis can appear similar to progressive disease on neuroimaging but can be distinguished with advanced neuroimaging techniques such as perfusion imaging and nuclear medicine studies such as PET-CT and PET-MRI. Symptoms depend on the size and location of radiation necrosis and can cause headaches, focal neurologic symptoms, seizures, and neuropsychiatric symptoms. The condition may resolve spontaneously but can be treated with dexamethasone, bevacizumab, and, in severe cases, surgery (Figures 26.7 and 26.8).

Radiation therapy to the brain can also cause a dementing syndrome years after treatment, associated with diffuse symmetric white matter changes on

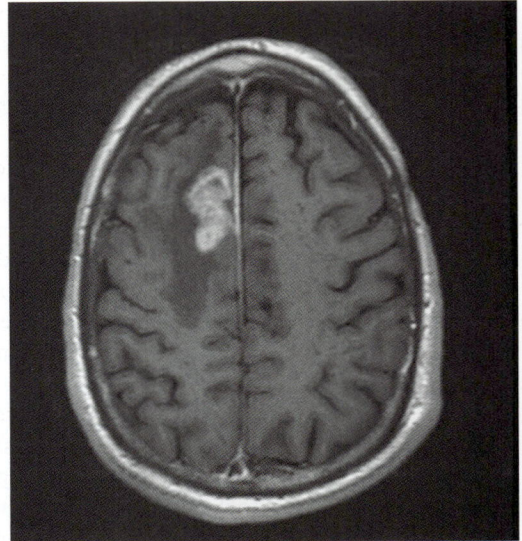

FIGURE 26.7 Axial postcontrast T1-weighted magnetic resonance imaging (MRI) showing radiation necrosis in the right frontal lobe.

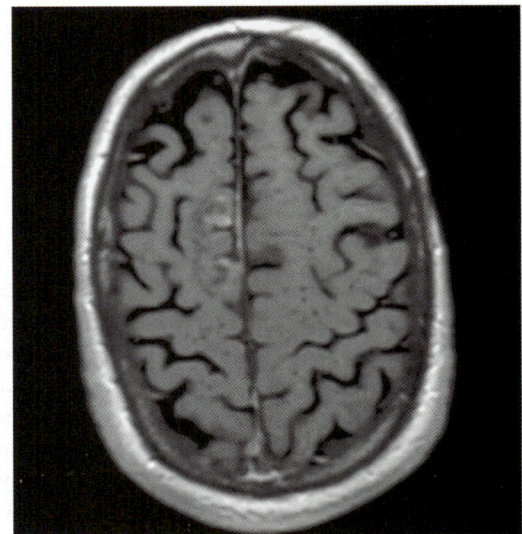

FIGURE 26.8 Same patient (Figure 26.7) after treatment with bevacizumab, with decrease in enhancement and edema.

MRI; patients who received concurrent methotrexate may be at higher risk. The use of hippocampal-sparing radiation therapy protocols has decreased the risk of long-term cognitive impairment after brain radiation.

Radiation myelopathy (ie, spinal cord dysfunction as a consequence of radiation) can also occur months to years after treatment. This was more common in the past with older techniques such as mantle field radiation. Newer forms of radiation delivery are less likely to cause radiation myelopathy; however, radiation sensitizing chemotherapy agents (eg, gemcitabine) can increase the risk.

Radiation can also impair CSF resorption, causing normal pressure hydrocephalus, leading to gait difficulties, cognitive impairment, and urinary symptoms. Patients with a history of brain radiation who present with these symptoms and hydrocephalus on neuroimaging should be evaluated for CSF diversion with ventriculoperitoneal shunt.

Radiation to the head and neck can cause a vasculopathy that can lead to strokes.

Stroke-like migraine attacks after radiation therapy (SMART) syndrome present with acute focal neurologic deficits, seizures, and/or headache years after radiation therapy with unilateral gyral enhancement and T2 hyperintensity on brain MRI with no evidence of tumor recurrence or stroke. This condition usually resolves spontaneously but may recur.

Neurologic Complications of Systemic Chemotherapy

Chemotherapy-Induced Peripheral Neuropathy

The most common neurologic complication of cancer treatment is chemotherapy-induced peripheral neuropathy, which can be caused by a wide variety of medications, including platinum-based agents, taxanes, vinca alkaloids, bortezomib, thalidomide, brentuximab, and lorlatinib. Oxaliplatin can also cause an acute-onset neuropathy with paresthesia and sensitivity to temperature that may require dose reduction or cessation. The vinca alkaloids can also cause an autonomic neuropathy that affects the gastrointestinal and genitourinary systems.

Clinical symptoms include numbness and tingling of the hands and feet. Some patients develop sharp, stabbing pain, and/or sensory ataxia, predisposing them to falls. Chemotherapy-induced peripheral neuropathy is typically dose dependent; more doses of the offending agent will cause worsening symptoms. The diagnosis is usually made clinically given the temporal relationship to chemo therapy, but a nerve conduction study and electromyogram (NCS/EMG) may be used to confirm the diagnosis.

There are no current recommended agents for preventing chemotherapy-induced peripheral neuropathy.[9] Patients often improve after the cessation of chemotherapy and many make a full recovery, though symptoms may persist in some patients. There are multiple treatments that can be used for symptomatic treatment of painful chemotherapy-induced peripheral neuropathy. Duloxetine has the most evidence for use. Other agents that are typically used for neuropathic pain include gabapentin, pregabalin, tricyclic antidepressants, and serotonin-norepinephrine reuptake inhibitors. Topical agents such as capsaicin cream, baclofen, and ketamine may provide relief. Additional strategies include acupuncture, scrambler therapy (a device that provides electric stimulation to the skin at the site of the neuropathy, "scrambling" the pain signals that are transmitted to the brain), and transcutaneous electrical nerve stimulation (TENS) unit.

Posterior Reversible Encephalopathy Syndrome

Posterior reversible encephalopathy syndrome (PRES) is a clinicoradiologic syndrome characterized by encephalopathy, visual changes, headaches, focal deficits, and T2 hyperintensities on brain MRI that usually predominantly affect the posterior white matter. The presentation can vary from mild symptoms that spontaneously resolve to a fulminant course that can cause residual neurologic deficits. The condition can be caused by hypertensive emergency, eclampsia, immunosuppressant medications, and a wide variety of anti-neoplastic treatments, including rituximab, gemcitabine, vincristine, vinblastine, cytarabine, etoposide, bortezomib, cyclophosphamide, methotrexate, cisplatin, oxaliplatin, carboplatin, sunitinib, sorafenib, capecitabine, and 5-fluorouracil (5-FU), among others. The treatment of PRES related to anti-neoplastic treatment is usually supportive and involves removing the offending agent.

Depending on the severity of PRES, rechallenge with the offending chemotherapy agent can be considered, particularly if there were additional factors such as high blood pressure or other medications that could have caused PRES.

Additional Neurologic Complications of Chemotherapy

Acute ataxia and cerebellar symptoms at the time of administration can be seen with 5-FU and cytarabine arabinoside. Methotrexate can cause a wide variety of neurologic syndromes, including acute encephalopathy, chronic leukoencephalopathy (white matter disease) causing cognitive changes, and, in the case of intrathecal methotrexate, spinal cord toxicity. Methotrexate can also cause a stroke-like syndrome that is characterized by transient confusion, seizures, and focal neurologic deficits.

Ifosfamide is an alkylating agent that can produce an acute encephalopathy with confusion, hallucinations, cerebellar dysfunction, and coma. This is usually reversible; methylene blue is sometimes used as a rescue agent.[10] Busulfan is an alkylating agent that is often used in conditioning regimens for stem cell transplants and can increase the risk of seizures.[11,12] Anthracycline antibiotics such as daunorubicin, doxorubicin, and mitoxantrone can cause cardiomyopathy, leading to an increased risk of lft ventricular thrombus formation and cardio embolic stroke. L-asparagine can cause encephalopathy that may be related to ammonia production,[13] as well as clotting factor deficiencies that can result in both ischemic and hemorrhagic neurologic complications, including venous sinus thrombosis.[14]

Biologic Agents and Targeted Therapies

Since the mid-1990s, many biologic agents and targeted agents have been developed for anti-neoplastic treatment. This reflects the evolution of cancer care from nonspecific cytotoxic therapies to nuanced targets and additional approaches such as immunotherapy. In some cases, targeted therapy has become first-line therapy; in other cases, these treatments represent adjunct or second-line treatment. Many can cause neurologic side effects.

Monoclonal Antibodies

Rituximab is a CD20 monoclonal antibody used to treat lymphomas that can rarely cause progressive multifocal leukoencephalopathy (PML).[15] This is a leukoencephalopathy that is caused by the reactivation of the JC virus and has a subacute presentation with personality changes, focal neurologic deficits, visual changes, and headaches. Immunotherapy is an emerging treatment approach for PML.[16,17]

Bevacizumab is a monoclonal antibody targeted against VEGF that can increase the risk of thrombotic events and bleeding.[15,18] It can also very rarely cause coagulation necrosis of the brain due to chronic hypoxia when used for CNS indications, which is grounds for discontinuation.[19] Trastuzumab, an anti-HER2 humanized monoclonal antibody used for the treatment of breast cancer, can often cause headaches after infusion. Recently, there have been combinations of trastuzumab with antibody drug targets, such as the combination with emtansine (TDM-1) or deruxtecan (T-Dxd). There is increasing evidence that these agents may have CNS penetration and can potentially worsen radiation necrosis.[20,21]

Tyrosine Kinase Inhibitors

Lorlatinib, which is a third-generation ALK inhibitor, can cause peripheral neuropathy, neuropsychiatric syndromes, auditory hallucinations, and cognitive impairment.[22] BRAF and MEK inhibitors, which have good CNS penetration, can cause headache and blurry vision. Tyrosine kinase inhibitors (eg, imatinib and dasatinib) used for chronic myelogenous leukemia can cause headaches, and, in rare cases, dasatinib can cause an optic neuropathy.[23] VEGF inhibitors (eg, sunitinib and sorafenib) can also cause PRES, similar to bevacizumab. The IDH inhibitor ivosidenib has been associated with Guillain-Barré syndrome. Ibrutinib and acalabrutinib (BTK inhibitors used in B-cell malignancies, such as diffuse large B-cell lymphoma [including primary CNS lymphoma]) have been linked with opportunistic fungal infections, such as invasive CNS aspergillosis.[24] Bortezomib, used for multiple myeloma, has a high incidence of peripheral neuropathy. Lenalidomide, also used for the treatment of multiple myeloma, can increase the risk of thrombotic events including stroke.

Immunotherapies Including Chimeric Antigen Receptor (CAR) T Cell Therapy

Immunotherapies have shown great promise in certain cancers, such as metastatic melanoma.[25] Immunotherapies range from immune checkpoint inhibition, cancer vaccines, immune effector cells including tumor-infiltrating lymphocytes and CAR-T, and oncolytic virus therapies.

Immune checkpoint inhibitors enhance T-cell-mediated immune responses against cancer cells. The most commonly targeted proteins include programmed death 1 (PD-1; eg, pembrolizumab and nivolumab), programmed death ligand 1 (PD-L1; atezolizumab and durvalumab), and cytotoxic T-lymphocyte antigen-4 (CTLA-4; ipilimumab). These therapies can trigger systemic autoimmune responses affecting the CNS (eg, autoimmune encephalitis and aseptic meningitis) or peripheral nervous system (eg, myasthenia gravis, Guillain-Barré syndrome, myositis, peripheral neuropathies, and cranial neuropathies). Treatment of neurologic complications of immune checkpoint inhibitors involves glucocorticoids, with consideration of intravenous immune globulin (IVIg) or plasmapheresis in severe or refractory cases. If the adverse effect is severe (ie, grade 3 or 4 toxicities such as autoimmune encephalitis or myasthenia gravis), it warrants permanent discontinuation of the offending medication.

Bispecific T-cell engagers, such as blinatumomab, which target both CD19 and CD3 on precursor B-cell acute lymphoblastic leukemia (ALL) tumor cells and CD3 on cytotoxic T cells, frequently cause neurotoxicity, including tremor, dizziness, and encephalopathy. These toxicities usually occur within days of administration, are typically transient and reversible, and respond to glucocorticoids.

CAR-T is FDA-approved for both leukemias and lymphomas, with ongoing investigations in multiple other cancers including CNS cancers. The majority of patients experience neurotoxicity after infusion, ranging from mild confusion and tremor to seizures and cerebral edema. Symptoms usually occur within the first 10 days of infusion, although they can be delayed up to 28 days of infusion. Treatment is with glucocorticoids along with anti-interleukin agents such as tocilizumab, anakinra, and siltuximab. Most patients recover completely.

PARANEOPLASTIC SYNDROMES

Paraneoplastic syndromes are autoimmune disorders that can affect any level of the nervous system. In the CNS, cerebellar degeneration and autoimmune encephalitis are common paraneoplastic syndromes, whereas in the PNS, peripheral neuropathy, myasthenia gravis (most commonly associated with thymoma), and Lambert-Eaton myasthenic syndrome (most commonly associated with small cell lung cancer) are prototypical paraneoplastic syndromes.

Paraneoplastic disorders can precede the diagnosis of an underlying malignancy. The presentation is subacute and occurs over weeks to months. Initial symptoms can be vague but often develop into a discrete syndrome. The subacute onset of a new neurologic syndrome, especially a prototypical paraneoplastic syndrome such as Lambert-Eaton myasthenic syndrome or cerebellar degeneration, should prompt evaluation for systemic malignancy.

The initial diagnostic evaluation for a possible paraneoplastic syndrome depends on the symptoms. For cases affecting the brain or brainstem, such as suspected autoimmune encephalitis or paraneoplastic cerebellar degeneration, a contrast-enhanced brain MRI and lumbar puncture are recommended. In cases of encephalitis, the MRI may show areas of inflammation that preferentially affect the limbic system (eg, medial temporal lobes). CSF can show a pleocytosis with elevation of protein. Paraneoplastic antibody panels can be sent from both CSF and serum; however, these may take days to weeks to return. The decision to initiate treatment should not be delayed while awaiting antibody results in a patient with a progressively worsening classic syndrome.

Additional ancillary testing depends on the type of syndrome. NCS/EMG can be used to make the diagnosis of myasthenia gravis, Lambert-Eaton myasthenic syndrome, or other types of paraneoplastic PNS syndromes. PET-CT imaging is used to search for the underlying cancer.

Immunomodulatory therapies such as steroids, IVIg, and plasmapheresis are mainstays of treatment of paraneoplastic neurologic syndromes.[26] Sometimes longer-term immunosuppression may be required.

Definitive treatment of a paraneoplastic syndrome is treatment of the underlying cancer. In cases of complete responses or remissions, either due to systemic therapy or resection of the underlying cancer, the paraneoplastic syndrome may completely subside. In cases with either a highly probable or confirmed paraneoplastic syndrome and no identified primary malignancy, serial screening for a primary malignancy for 2 years with PET-CT is recommended.

SUMMARY

The nervous system can be affected by cancer in many ways: primary tumors of the nervous system, metastases to CNS structures, side effects of treatment, and paraneoplastic syndromes. Treatment of these entities is rapidly evolving, requiring close collaboration between neurologists and oncologists to provide patients with optimal care.

EDITORS' KEY POINTS

▶ Metastases to the nervous system are more common than primary brain tumors (eg, meningioma, glioma, and primary CNS lymphoma).

▶ Incidental asymptomatic meningiomas discovered on routine neuroimaging can generally be followed up with serial annual neuroimaging to evaluate for growth. Large and/or symptomatic meningiomas are treated with surgery.

▶ Gliomas are treated with a combination of maximal surgical resection, radiation, and chemotherapy, depending on the genetic profile of the tumor.

▶ Primary CNS lymphoma can occur in both immunocompetent and immunocompromised patients.

▶ Large symptomatic brain metastases are treated with surgery. Multifocal small metastases may be treated with radiation therapy.

▶ The most common neurologic toxicity of chemotherapy is peripheral neuropathy. Symptoms resolve in many patients after chemotherapy concludes, although they may persist in some patients. Patients who develop this complication are generally treated symptomatically for neuropathic pain.

▶ Immunotherapies for cancer can cause immune-mediated neurologic syndromes, including encephalitis, myelitis, Guillain-Barré syndrome, myasthenia gravis, and myositis. Treatment of these complications is with steroids and may require discontinuation of immunotherapy in severe cases.

▶ Paraneoplastic neurologic syndromes include cerebellar degeneration, encephalitis, and Lambert-Eaton myasthenic syndrome. Paraneoplastic syndromes may precede the diagnosis of the underlying cancer.

REFERENCES

1. Ostrom QT, Cioffi G, Waite K, Kruchko C, Barnholtz-Sloan JS. CBTRUS statistical report: primary brain and other central nervous system tumors diagnosed in the United States in 2014–2018. *Neuro Oncol.* 2021;23(Supplement_3):iii1-iii105. doi:10.1093/neuonc/noab200

2. Deguchi S, Oishi T, Mitsuya K, et al. Clinicopathological analysis of T2-FLAIR mismatch sign in lower-grade gliomas. *Sci Rep.* 2020;10(1):10113. doi:10.1038/s41598-020-67244-7

3. Mellinghoff IK, van den Bent MJ, Blumenthal DT, et al. Vorasidenib in IDH1- or IDH2-mutant low-grade glioma. *N Engl J Med.* 2023;389(7):589-601. doi:10.1056/NEJMoa2304194

4. Stupp R, Mason WP, van den Bent MJ, et al. Radiotherapy plus concomitant and adjuvant temozolomide for glioblastoma. *N Engl J Med.* 2005;352(10):987-996. doi:10.1056/NEJMoa043330

5. Vogelbaum MA, Brown PD, Messersmith H, et al. Treatment for brain metastases: ASCO-SNO-ASTRO guideline. *J Clin Oncol.* 2022;40(5):492-516. doi:10.1200/JCO.21.02314

6. Wang N, Bertalan MS, Brastianos PK. Leptomeningeal metastasis from systemic cancer: review and update on management. *Cancer.* 2018;124(1):21-35. doi:10.1002/cncr.30911

7. Schrag D, Uno H, Rosovsky R, et al. Direct oral anticoagulants vs low-molecular-weight heparin and recurrent VTE in patients with cancer: a randomized clinical trial. *JAMA.* 2023;329(22):1924-1933. doi:10.1001/jama.2023.7843

8. Giustozzi M, Proietti G, Becattini C, Roila F, Agnelli G, Mandalà M. ICH in primary or metastatic brain cancer patients with or without anticoagulant treatment: a systematic

review and meta-analysis. *Blood Adv.* 2022;6(16):4873-4883. doi:10.1182/bloodadvances.2022008086

9. Loprinzi CL, Lacchetti C, Bleeker J, et al. Prevention and management of chemotherapy-induced peripheral neuropathy in survivors of adult cancers: ASCO guideline update. *J Clin Oncol.* 2020;38(28):3325-3348. doi:10.1200/JCO.20.01399

10. Howell JE, Szabatura AH, Seung AH, Nesbit SA. Characterization of the occurrence of ifosfamide-induced neurotoxicity with concomitant aprepitant. *J Oncol Pharm Pract.* 2008;14(3):157-162.

11. Ciurea SO, Andersson BS. Busulfan in hematopoietic stem cell transplantation. *Biol Blood Marrow Transplant.* 2009;15(5):523-536. doi:10.1016/j.bbmt.2008.12.489

12. Soni S, Skeens M, Termuhlen AM, Bajwa RPS, Gross TG, Pai V. Levetiracetam for busulfan-induced seizure prophylaxis in children undergoing hematopoietic stem cell transplantation. *Pediatr Blood Cancer.* 2012;59(4):762-764. doi:10.1002/pbc

13. Leonard JV, Kay JD. Acute encephalopathy and hyperammonaemia complicating treatment of acute lymphoblastic leukaemia with asparaginase. *Lancet.* 1986;1(8473):162-163. doi:10.1016/S0140-6736(86)92304-4

14. Kieslich M, Porto L, Lanfermann H, Jacobi G, Schwabe D, Böhles H. Cerebrovascular complications of L-asparaginase in the therapy of acute lymphoblastic leukemia. *J Pediatr Hematol Oncol.* 2003;25(6):484-487. doi:10.1097/00043426-200306000-00011

15. Keene DL, Legare C, Taylor E, Gallivan J, Cawthorn GM, Vu D. Monoclonal antibodies and progressive multifocal leukoencephalopathy. *Can J Neurol Sci.* 2011;38(4):565-571. doi:10.1017/S0317167100012105

16. Muftuoglu M, Olson A, Marin D, et al. Allogeneic BK virus–specific T cells for progressive multifocal leukoencephalopathy. *N Engl J Med.* 2018;379(15):1443-1451. doi:10.1056/nejmoa1801540

17. Cortese I, Muranski P, Enose-Akahata Y, et al. Pembrolizumab treatment for progressive multifocal leukoencephalopathy.

N Engl J Med. 2019;380(17):1597-1605. doi:10.1056/nejmoa1815039

18. Zukas AM, Schiff D. Neurological complications of new chemotherapy agents. *Neuro Oncol.* 2018;20(1):24-36. doi:10.1093/neuonc/nox115

19. Agarwal A, Desai A, Gupta V, Vibhute P. Bevacizumab-induced coagulative necrosis with restricted diffusion. *Radiol Imaging Cancer.* 2022;4(5):e220089. doi:10.1148/rycan.220089

20. Park C, Buckley E, Van Swearingen AE, et al. Effect of type and timing of systemic therapy on risk of radiation necrosis in patients with HER2+ breast cancer brain metastases. *J Clin Oncol.* 2021;39(15_suppl):e14002-e14002. doi:10.1200/JCO.2021.39.15_suppl.e14002

21. Carlson JA, Nooruddin Z, Rusthoven C, et al. Trastuzumab emtansine and stereotactic radiosurgery: an unexpected increase in clinically significant brain edema. *Neuro Oncol.* 2014;16(7):1006-1009. doi:10.1093/neuonc/not329

22. Solomon BJ, Besse B, Bauer TM, et al. Lorlatinib in patients with ALK-positive non-small-cell lung cancer: results from a global phase 2 study. *Lancet Oncol.* 2018;19(12):1654-1667. doi:10.1016/S1470-2045(18)30649-1

23. Monge KS, Gálvez-Ruiz A, Alvárez-Carrón A, Quijada C, Matheu A. Optic neuropathy secondary to dasatinib in the treatment of a chronic myeloid leukemia case. *Saudi J Ophthalmol.* 2015;29(3):227-231. doi:10.1016/j.sjopt.2014.12.004

24. Lionakis MS, Dunleavy K, Roschewski M, et al. Inhibition of B cell receptor signaling by ibrutinib in primary CNS lymphoma. *Cancer Cell.* 2017;31(6):833-843.e5. doi:10.1016/j.cell.2017.04.012

25. Carlino MS, Larkin J, Long G V. Immune checkpoint inhibitors in melanoma. *Lancet.* 2021;398(10304):1002-1014. doi:10.1016/S0140-6736(21)01206-X

26. Graus F, Vogrig A, Muñiz-Castrillo S, et al. Updated diagnostic criteria for paraneoplastic neurologic syndromes. *Neurol Neuroimmunol Neuroinflamm.* 2021;8(4):e1014. doi:10.1212/NXI.0000000000001014

Neurologic Complications of Systemic Disease

Ethan Hoang and Joseph E. Safdieh

INTRODUCTION

Neurologic complications of systemic illness are common. Neurologic conditions may be the presenting feature of systemic diseases or may emerge during the course of a systemic condition or its treatment. This chapter provides an overview of the neurologic manifestations of systemic diseases, organized by organ system.

CARDIAC DISORDERS

Cardiac disorders are frequently associated with neurologic complications. The brain receives a relatively large percentage of cardiac output and is highly reliant on regular and consistent blood flow to maintain normal function. The most common neurologic manifestation of cardiac disease is cardioembolic stroke, especially in patients with atrial fibrillation, which is covered in Chapter 16. This section focuses on the neurologic complications of endocarditis and common cardiac procedures.

Endocarditis

Patients with endocarditis have inflammation of the endocardial lining, typically involving the cardiac valves. Neurologic complications of endocarditis are largely related to septic emboli from the heart, which can lead to ischemic stroke, hemorrhagic stroke, mycotic aneurysm, and cerebral abscess. These complications typically manifest with the development of focal or multifocal neurologic deficits, seizures, or, in the case of a shower of small emboli, as an acute confusional state that can be mistaken for delirium. The associated bacteremia may also lead to seeding of the meninges causing meningitis. Some patients with endocarditis may develop headache, altered mental status, and/or generalized weakness as constitutional symptoms without focal lesions. The risk of neurologic complications decreases with appropriate antimicrobial and/or surgical treatment of endocarditis.

Stroke due to septic embolization has a relatively high rate of hemorrhagic conversion as compared to noninfectious stroke etiologies. Due to the high potential for hemorrhage, intravenous (IV) thrombolysis should be avoided in cases of acute ischemic stroke in the setting of endocarditis. Although mechanical thrombectomy may be an option for large vessel occlusion caused by septic embolization, there is very limited data on the benefit and safety of catheter-based acute stroke procedures in this population, and the decision to proceed with mechanical thrombectomy should only be made after careful discussion between the neurologist, neuroendovascular physician, and patient regarding potential risks and benefits. For secondary stroke prevention, anticoagulant and antiplatelet

medications pose a significant risk for hemorrhagic transformation and should be avoided in most patients with stroke due to septic embolization. The best approach to primary and secondary stroke prevention in patients with endocarditis is antimicrobial therapy and, if indicated, valve surgery. In select cases where anticoagulation is absolutely necessary (eg, mechanical valve), IV heparin can be used with careful dose titration based on monitoring of serum partial thromboplastin time (PTT) as well as frequent serial neurologic examinations to look for any worsening, which would indicate the need for immediate imaging.

Mycotic cerebral aneurysms are caused by infection of the blood vessel wall, which can lead to vessel wall breakdown. They occur in a minority of patients with endocarditis but can lead to significant morbidity due to hemorrhagic complications. Unlike traditional berry aneurysms that tend to be located along the circle of Willis, mycotic aneurysms tend to be distal and may be multiple. Screening for mycotic aneurysms is not routinely recommended for all patients with endocarditis but should be obtained in patients with intracerebral hemorrhage in the setting of endocarditis. Computed tomography angiography (CTA) and magnetic resonance angiography (MRA) will detect most mycotic aneurysms, but due to the distal location and small size of the aneurysms, they can be missed on noninvasive imaging modalities. Digital subtraction cerebral angiography is the gold standard and should be performed if a high suspicion exists for mycotic aneurysms despite negative noninvasive testing.

Most mycotic aneurysms resolve with appropriate antimicrobial therapy and usually do not require specific intervention. Surgical or endovascular treatment of mycotic aneurysms is challenging and generally only considered in the setting of aneurysmal rupture. Surgical or endovascular intervention in the setting of unruptured aneurysm prior to cardiac surgery depends on the size and location of the mycotic aneurysm; currently, no established guidelines exist. The management of rarer complications of endocarditis such as cerebral or epidural abscess, meningitis, and seizures is similar to when these develop in other contexts.

Although many patients with endocarditis can be managed successfully with antibiotics, some patients will require surgical valve repair or replacement. Indications for surgery generally include severe heart failure, severe valve dysfunction, large mobile vegetations, and recurrent septic embolization or prolonged sepsis despite appropriate antimicrobial therapy. Surgical treatment of endocarditis is often urgent or emergent, and the intracranial bleeding risks are high in patients with stroke or mycotic aneurysm. This risk is driven by the requirement for intraoperative anticoagulation as well as the risk of intraoperative hypotension. This leads to challenging clinical decisions related to balancing the potential risks of perioperative neurologic complications with the potential cardiovascular risks of surgical delay. The American Heart Association guidelines recommend early valvular surgery (when indicated) if a patient is found to have small ischemic strokes or subclinical strokes noted incidentally on neuroimaging, but recommend delay of surgery for at least 4 weeks in the setting of large ischemic stroke or intracerebral hemorrhage.[1]

Cardiac Procedures and Surgeries

Neurologic Complications of Cardiac Catheterization

Cardiac catheterization can be complicated by embolic stroke caused by dislodging of aortic plaque by the catheter tip or thrombus formation on the catheter tip. Patients who develop focal neurologic symptoms, seizures, or do not return to baseline in the expected timeline following the procedure should undergo urgent neuroimaging with CT, though this may be insensitive for small embolic strokes that would only be visible on MRI.

Contrast-induced encephalopathy is an uncommon clinical entity that can occur during or immediately after cardiac catheterization. It manifests as confusion, seizures, and/or focal neurologic deficits. The mechanism is thought to be related to blood-brain barrier disruption, hyperosmolarity, and neurotoxicity from the contrast medium. Patients with renal failure and history of stroke are at increased risk. MRI should be obtained to evaluate for stroke. Deficits are usually transient and resolve over days with supportive care and hydration.

Neurologic Complications of Cardiac Surgery

Cardiac surgery carries a risk of ischemic stroke due to embolization from the aortic arch during cross-clamping/unclamping or intraoperative hypotension. IV thrombolysis is contraindicated immediately after open-heart surgery, but mechanical thrombectomy can be considered for proximal cerebral artery occlusion. Although postoperative delirium can occur after cardiac surgery, providers should have a high index of suspicion for stroke, as multiple small embolic strokes can cause a global encephalopathy without clear focal deficits and may not be apparent on CT.

Cognitive decline after cardiac surgery can be classified into two types: short term and long term. Short-term cognitive decline can last up to 6 weeks and occur in up to half of patients, while long-term cognitive decline occurs 6 months after surgery and occurs in up to 30% of patients. The diagnosis can be made by bedside cognitive testing, although formal neuropsychological testing may be required to detect more subtle cognitive changes.

Neurologic "Clearance" for Cardiac Procedures

Often, neurologists are asked to "clear" patients for cardiac surgery. While neurologists cannot "clear" patients for surgery, they can assist with identifying any underlying neurologic disorder that could influence surgical risk or anesthesia considerations, participating in discussion of potential neurologic risks (eg, stroke risk) and how to mitigate them, and performing and documenting a complete neurologic examination that can be used as a baseline if there are any postprocedural changes in neurologic status.

PULMONARY DISORDERS

Neurologic Complications of Endotracheal Intubation

Neurologic complications of endotracheal intubation are uncommon. During intubation, airway manipulation can lead to stretching of cranial nerve branches in the laryngeal region or injury to the ascending pharyngeal branch of the carotid artery supplying those nerves. Impacted nerves may include the recurrent laryngeal nerve or hypoglossal nerve. In rare cases, both nerves can be affected on the same side, a condition known as Tapia syndrome. Patients can also develop isolated unilateral or bilateral vocal cord paralysis, leading to dysphonia.

Patients with acute cervical injury or known severe cervical spine disease should be intubated with caution, avoiding hyperextension of the neck due to the risk of spinal cord damage. Fiberoptic intubation is preferred in this group of patients.

Neurologic Complications of Hypercapnia

Hypercapnia can present with neurologic symptoms including lethargy, confusion, and headache. While hypercapnia most commonly occurs due to pulmonary disease, neurologic causes of hypoventilation include neuromuscular conditions with diaphragmatic weakness (eg, Guillain-Barré syndrome, myasthenia gravis), obstructive sleep apnea, and, rarely, brainstem lesions.

RENAL AND ELECTROLYTE DISORDERS

Renal disorders can cause neurologic dysfunction due to the accumulation of uncleared toxins (uremic encephalopathy, uremic neuropathy) or electrolyte disorders. In addition, renal replacement therapy with dialysis can have several neurologic complications, including dialysis disequilibrium syndrome and ischemic monomelic neuropathy.

Renal Failure

Central Nervous System Manifestations of Renal Failure

Uremic encephalopathy presents with altered mental status ranging from confusion to coma. Abnormal involuntary movements such as asterixis (brief loss of muscle tone best observed with the arms outstretched and wrists extended) and myoclonus may be seen, but these are nonspecific and can also occur in other toxic-metabolic encephalopathies. The differential diagnosis of encephalopathy in patients with renal insufficiency includes hypertensive encephalopathy/posterior reversible encephalopathy syndrome (PRES), dialysis

disequilibrium syndrome (see later), fluid and electrolyte disturbances (see later), and toxic effects of renally cleared medications (eg, cefepime). In uremic encephalopathy, brain imaging is typically normal. Electroencephalogram (EEG) may demonstrate nonspecific patterns such as diffuse slowing and triphasic waves, which can be seen in other causes of encephalopathy. Mental status generally improves to baseline with improvement in renal function due to the treatment of the underlying cause and/or dialysis, if indicated.

Dialysis disequilibrium syndrome is characterized by neurologic symptoms occurring during the first session of dialysis or when resuming dialysis after one or more missed sessions. Symptoms range from mild (eg, fatigue, headache, nausea/vomiting, confusion) to severe (eg, seizures, coma). The pathophysiology is thought to be related to osmotic shifts causing cerebral edema. Most cases are mild and resolve with modification of the dialysis parameters. If there are severe and persistent symptoms, hyperosmolar treatment may be needed, and the patient should be evaluated for other potential causes of neurologic symptoms (eg, electrolyte abnormalities, structural lesions).

Peripheral Nervous System Manifestations of Renal Failure

Renal disease is also a risk factor for various types of peripheral neuropathies. Neuropathy is also a significant contributor to ulceration and amputations, especially if patients have comorbid peripheral vascular disease. Symptoms often present in the distal lower extremities with numbness, tingling, and/or weakness. Patients on hemodialysis with arteriovenous fistulas may develop ischemic monomelic neuropathy, which causes sudden onset of pain, numbness, and/or weakness in the limb in which the fistula has been placed due to ischemic insult affecting one or more nerves of the affected extremity.

Electrolyte Disorders

The nervous system requires electrolyte homeostasis to allow for strict control over concentration gradients across cellular compartments. When these relationships are disturbed, neurologic signs and symptoms can occur as demonstrated by Table 27.1. Central

TABLE 27.1	Neurologic Manifestations of Electrolyte Disorders				
Electrolyte	Disorder	Mental status changes	Seizures	Weakness	Paresthesias
Sodium	Hyponatremia	✓	✓	✓	
	Hypernatremia	✓	✓	✓	
Potassium	Hypokalemia			✓	✓
	Hyperkalemia			✓	✓
Calcium	Hypocalcemia	✓	✓		✓
	Hypercalcemia	✓	✓	✓	
Magnesium	Hypomagnesemia		✓		
	Hypermagnesemia	✓		✓	
Phosphorus	Hypophosphatemia	✓		✓	
	Hyperphosphatemia	✓		✓	

nervous system (CNS) manifestations of electrolyte disturbances most commonly include seizures and encephalopathy and are typically associated with derangements in sodium or calcium levels. Peripheral nervous system (PNS) manifestations include weakness, cramps, numbness, and tingling and are typically associated with derangements in potassium, magnesium, phosphate, and calcium.

Sodium

Hyponatremia

Encephalopathy and seizures are the most common neurologic manifestations of hyponatremia. Although neurologic manifestations of hyponatremia generally only occur with serum sodium levels lower than 120 mmol/L, the absolute sodium level is not a good predictor of whether a patient will be symptomatic. The rapid development of even mild hyponatremia in patients who are usually eunatremic can cause seizures and encephalopathy. Hyponatremia should be corrected slowly (8-10 mmol/L/day) with normal saline (0.9%), since more rapid correction may lead to osmotic demyelination syndrome, which can affect the pons (central pontine myelinolysis), causing quadriparesis/quadriplegia, locked-in syndrome, or death, or may affect the cerebral hemispheres (extrapontine myelinolysis), causing movement disorders such as parkinsonism.

Hypernatremia

Hypernatremia (serum sodium level >145 mmol/L) can cause weakness, hyperreflexia, tremor, myoclonus, or encephalopathy. Extremely high levels (>160 mmol/L) can lead to coma. Slow correction of hypernatremia (0.5 mmol/L/h or 10 mmol/L/day) is preferred since rapid correction of a hypertonic state may lead to cerebral edema, seizures, coma, or death.

Potassium

Hypokalemia

Aberrations in serum potassium levels predominantly affect the neuromuscular system. Generalized proximal more than distal weakness can occur with potassium levels <2.5 mmol/L. Hypokalemic periodic paralysis is a rare genetic condition that should be considered in patients presenting with transient flaccid weakness in muscles of the extremities with serum potassium levels <3 mmol/L. Attacks may last hours to days and tend to be provoked by vigorous exercise or a carbohydrate-rich meal.

Hyperkalemia

Hyperkalemia is often asymptomatic but can rarely manifest neurologically with muscle weakness and hyporeflexia in the legs that ascends to the trunk and is associated with burning paresthesias. Hyperkalemic periodic paralysis is a genetic disorder that can manifest with episodic muscle weakness in the setting of hyperkalemia.

Calcium
Hypocalcemia

Although hypocalcemia (serum calcium <8.5 mg/dL) is often asymptomatic, it can cause PNS and CNS manifestations. PNS manifestations include extremity and perioral numbness and tingling. Neuromuscular irritability in hypocalcemia can be demonstrated by observing facial twitching when tapping on the facial nerve (Chvostek sign) or observing involuntary hand contracture when inflating a blood pressure cuff (Trousseau sign). In rare cases, hypocalcemia can cause tetany and respiratory compromise. CNS manifestations are uncommon but may include seizures.

Hypercalcemia

Patients with hypercalcemia (serum calcium >10 mg/dL) are often asymptomatic, but levels >14 mg/dL can cause drowsiness, neuropsychiatric symptoms, seizures, and coma.

Phosphate
Hypophosphatemia

Hypophosphatemia is defined as serum levels <2.5 mg/dL. Peripheral neurologic symptoms of hypophosphatemia begin when the level falls below 1 mg/dL. Signs can include areflexia with diaphragmatic weakness. CNS deficits may appear when phosphate levels are less than 0.5 mg/dL and can include altered mentation with seizures, tremors, ataxia, and/or nystagmus.

Hyperphosphatemia

Hyperphosphatemia (serum phosphate levels >4.5 mg/dL) can be associated with clinical features like those of hypocalcemia (see prior section).

Magnesium
Hypomagnesemia

Hypomagnesemia leads to increased neuromuscular excitability. Weakness, muscle cramps, fasciculations, tremor, and hyperreflexia can be seen with serum magnesium levels <1.25 mg/dL. Seizures are a rare manifestation.

Hypermagnesemia

Hypermagnesemia is defined as serum magnesium >2.6 mg/dL, but CNS complications generally only occur with magnesium >5 mg/dL and can include lethargy, confusion, weakness, and generalized hyporeflexia.

GASTROINTESTINAL DISORDERS
Vitamin Deficiencies
Vitamin B$_1$ (Thiamine) Deficiency

Vitamin B$_1$ (thiamine) deficiency can cause the syndromes of Wernicke encephalopathy and dry beriberi. Wernicke encephalopathy classically presents with ataxia, confusion, and ocular abnormalities, such as oculomotor palsies or nystagmus, but patients rarely present with the complete triad. Confusion is the most common manifestation at the time of diagnosis. Although the condition is classically associated with alcohol use disorder, thiamine deficiency can also be caused by any cause of malnutrition or malabsorption, such as hyperemesis gravidarum and gastric bypass. Brain MRI may demonstrate abnormalities in midline structures, including the mammillary bodies, thalamus, and the dorsal midbrain. Delayed thiamine repletion may result in a progression to Korsakoff syndrome, a dementia characterized by amnesia and confabulation. Serum thiamine levels are not reliable; although serum erythrocyte transketolase activity coefficient is a more reliable marker of thiamine activity, the test is rarely useful in clinical practice as results are often delayed, and treatment with thiamine should be immediate when Wernicke encephalopathy is clinically suspected.

Thiamine deficiency can also cause dry beriberi, resulting in a progressive sensorimotor peripheral neuropathy. Thiamine repletion can lead to a slow recovery over months.

Vitamin B$_3$ (Niacin) Deficiency

Vitamin B$_3$ (niacin) deficiency can cause a triad of symptoms, including dermatitis, dementia, and diarrhea (pellagra). Neurologic symptoms can range from lethargy and mild confusion to coma. The full triad is rarely seen at presentation. Diagnosis is made by serum niacin level. High-risk populations include patients with malnutrition (eg, alcohol use disorder, gastrointestinal [GI] tract disease, malignancy). Niacin administration can lead to symptom improvement.

Vitamin B₆ (Pyridoxine) Deficiency

Vitamin B₆ (pyridoxine) deficiency can cause peripheral neuropathy, usually characterized by painful distal paresthesias. Although pyridoxine is readily available in the diet, those at high risk for deficiency include patients with chronic alcohol use disorder, patients on hemodialysis, and patients using certain medications (eg, isoniazid, phenelzine, hydralazine, or penicillamine). Repletion of pyridoxine or stopping the offending agent can lead to symptom stabilization and improvement.

Vitamin B₉ (Folate) and Vitamin B₁₂ (Cyanocobalamin) Deficiency

Vitamin B₉ (folic acid) and vitamin B₁₂ (cyanocobalamin) deficiencies cause similar symptoms, though vitamin B₁₂ deficiency is more common due to fortification of grains with folate. Risk factors for vitamin B₁₂ deficiency include pernicious anemia, malabsorption, metformin use, gastric bypass surgery, and a vegan diet. Vitamin B₁₂ deficiency can cause subacute combined degeneration of the spinal cord, a length-dependent sensory or sensorimotor neuropathy, or a combination of the two (myeloneuropathy). Subacute combined degeneration of the spinal cord affects the dorsal columns (causing proprioceptive loss leading to sensory ataxia and diminished or absent vibration sense on examination) and the corticospinal tracts (causing upper motor neuron signs such as hyperreflexia and Babinski signs). Patients with myeloneuropathy have both spinal cord and peripheral nerve dysfunction and may have a mix of upper and lower motor neuron signs on examination.

In cases of suspected vitamin B₁₂ deficiency with borderline serum vitamin B₁₂ levels, an elevated serum methylmalonic acid supports the diagnosis of true vitamin B₁₂ deficiency. The complete blood count (CBC) is often normal if folate level is normal, since folate can mask the hematologic abnormalities seen in vitamin B₁₂ deficiency, but neurologic manifestations can still occur. MRI of the spine can show T2 hyperintensity of the posterior and lateral columns of the spinal cord, predominantly in the cervical and thoracic cord. If detected early, many patients improve with B₁₂ repletion.

Copper Deficiency

Copper deficiency can mimic the subacute combined degeneration or myeloneuropathy caused by vitamin B₁₂ deficiency and should be considered in patients with a clinical syndrome suggesting vitamin B₁₂ deficiency with normal serum B₁₂ levels. Patients usually present with sensory ataxia due to dorsal column dysfunction. Similar to vitamin B₁₂ deficiency, MRI of patients with copper deficiency can demonstrate abnormal spinal cord signal in the dorsal columns. Causes of copper deficiency include gastric bypass, zinc supplementation, and the use of zinc-containing denture cream. Low serum copper levels are diagnostic. Zinc levels should be checked and the source of zinc excess should be addressed in addition to replenishing copper levels. Copper supplementation can lead to improved neurologic symptoms.

Vitamin Excess

Vitamin A (Retinoic Acid) Toxicity

Retinoic acid toxicity can be caused by topical or oral vitamin A. Vitamin A toxicity is typically due to increased vitamin A supplementation or exogenous use with topical creams for the skin. Neurologic manifestations can include headaches and blurred vision due to increased intracranial pressure (pseudotumor cerebri; see Chapter 12). Stopping the offending agent can lead to symptom improvement.

Vitamin B₆ (Pyridoxine) Toxicity

Pyridoxine toxicity can cause a sensory ganglionopathy (also called a *sensory neuronopathy*), a condition affecting the dorsal root ganglia. This syndrome presents as sensory ataxia (ataxia of the limbs and gait due to proprioceptive dysfunction), diminished reflexes, and impaired sensation. Pyridoxine toxicity tends to be from excessive supplement use.

Celiac Disease

Neurologic manifestations of celiac disease are uncommon and include cerebellar ataxia and painful small fiber neuropathy. These may occur in the absence of GI symptoms and are diagnosed by the presence of celiac antibodies. Neurologic manifestations of celiac disease typically improve with a gluten-free diet.

Inflammatory Bowel Disease

Neurologic manifestations of inflammatory bowel diseases include peripheral neuropathy and cerebrovascular complications due to hypercoagulability. Peripheral neuropathy is an uncommon neurologic manifestation and may be caused by vitamin deficiency due to malabsorption or may be immune mediated; the former is usually chronic and causes length-dependent sensory changes, whereas the latter may be acute, non-length-dependent, sensorimotor, and painful. The hypercoagulable state of inflammatory bowel disease may lead to ischemic stroke or cerebral venous sinus thrombosis.

Immunomodulatory treatments for inflammatory bowel diseases targeting tumor necrosis factor-α (TNF-α) (etanercept, infliximab, adalimumab) can rarely cause CNS demyelination, with a similar appearance to multiple sclerosis on MRI. These medications can also lead to the development of chronic inflammatory demyelinating polyradiculoneuropathy (CIDP). Discontinuation of the offending medication usually leads to resolution, though corticosteroids may be used to treat the acute symptoms of the demyelinating event.

Whipple Disease

Whipple disease is a multisystem condition caused by the bacterium *Tropheryma whipplei* that predominantly affects the GI tract but can also involve the nervous system, causing dementia, movement disorders, ataxia, and/or seizures. A rare but pathognomonic manifestation is known as *oculomasticatory myorhythmia*, characterized by pendular oscillations of the eyes with synchronous myoclonus of the jaw. Rarely, neurologic manifestations can occur in isolation without GI involvement. Diagnosis is made by detection of *T. whipplei* polymerase chain reaction (PCR) or brain biopsy of lesions demonstrating foamy macrophages. Treatment is with IV antibiotics followed by 1 year of oral antibiotics.

Viral Hepatitis

Hepatitis C is associated with several types of peripheral neuropathy, including distal sensorimotor neuropathy and mononeuropathy multiplex, the latter associated with cryoglobulinemia. Mononeuropathy multiplex signifies a sequential involvement of multiple individual nerves, causing asymmetric and often painful sensory and motor symptoms in the limbs. The etiology is typically due to ischemia of the nerve due to the involvement of the vasa nervorum. Hepatitis C is also associated with an increased risk of stroke.

Liver Failure

Acute Liver Failure

Acute liver failure may cause an acute encephalopathy with diffuse cerebral edema. In severe cases, symptoms may progress to a comatose state and subsequently death if not recognized and treated promptly with agents and interventions aimed at lowering elevated intracranial pressure.

Chronic Liver Failure

Chronic liver failure can lead to several neurologic manifestations, such as hepatic encephalopathy, hepatocerebral degeneration, and hepatic myelopathy.

Hepatic encephalopathy causes neuropsychiatric symptoms ranging from mild confusion to coma. Patients may have asterixis on examination and triphasic waves on EEG, but both are nonspecific and can be seen in other toxic-metabolic conditions. Serum ammonia is often elevated, but the level does not correlate with the degree of encephalopathy. MRI may show bilateral T1 hyperintensities in the basal ganglia without enhancement, though this is not universally present and may be seen in patients with chronic hepatic disease even without encephalopathy. Hepatic encephalopathy is often precipitated by an infection, GI bleed, or medications, and symptoms may improve with the treatment of the underlying etiology and ammonia-lowering therapies such as lactulose and rifaximin.

Acquired hepatocerebral degeneration is a rare complication of chronic liver failure that can be seen in patients with surgical or spontaneous portosystemic shunts. Neurologic symptoms include extrapyramidal signs (parkinsonism), ataxia, and cognitive changes. As in any patient with chronic liver failure, MRI may show hyperintensities in the basal ganglia on noncontrast T1-weighted images.

Hepatic myelopathy is a rare spinal cord complication of chronic liver failure that can be seen in patients with surgical or spontaneous portosystemic shunts. It manifests as chronic paraparesis, usually without sensory or bowel/bladder dysfunction. MRI of the spine is usually normal. Hepatic myelopathy generally does not respond to ammonia-lowering therapies but may improve with liver transplantation.

Wilson Disease

Wilson disease is an autosomal recessive disorder leading to copper accumulation in various organs, including the liver and brain. Patients generally present in early adulthood with movement disorders, such as parkinsonism, tremor, dystonia, and ataxia. Dysarthria and neuropsychiatric symptoms may occur. Kayser-Fleischer rings (gold-colored rings that encircle the iris of the eye due to copper deposition) are almost always present in patients with neurologic symptoms but may require slit-lamp examination to detect, especially in patients with darker irises. Patients often present with neurologic symptoms without overt laboratory evidence of liver failure. A young patient presenting with a movement disorder of unclear etiology should be screened for Wilson disease with serum ceruloplasmin, 24-hour urine copper, and slit-lamp examination for Kayser-Fleischer rings. MRI may demonstrate T2 hyperintense signal in the bilateral thalami, putamen, and midbrain. Ambiguities in laboratory findings and lack of family history may require liver biopsy or genetic testing for definitive diagnosis. Treatment is with copper-chelating agents.

ENDOCRINE DISORDERS

Thyroid Disorders

Hypothyroidism

Hypothyroidism can affect the CNS or PNS. In the CNS, hypothyroidism can cause altered mental status, ranging from mild cognitive impairment to coma (myxedema coma). Thyroid-stimulating hormone

(TSH) levels are, therefore, an important part of the evaluation for potentially reversible causes of altered cognition. Systemic clues to hypothyroidism include fatigue, constipation, weight gain, hair loss, and dry skin. In the PNS, hypothyroidism can cause myopathy (presenting with proximal weakness) and predispose to entrapment neuropathies (such as carpal tunnel syndrome).

Hyperthyroidism

The most common neurologic manifestation of hyperthyroidism is tremor, which typically presents as a high-frequency, low-amplitude postural tremor in the hands. Like hypothyroidism, hyperthyroidism can also cause altered mental status and myopathy, and TSH is part of the evaluation for reversible causes of either presentation. Hyperthyroidism-associated changes in mental status are characterized by hyperactivity, anxiety, agitation, and psychosis. Clues to hyperthyroidism as a cause of altered cognition include systemic symptoms such as palpitations, disturbed sleep, weight loss, heat intolerance, and increased sweating. Thyrotoxic periodic paralysis is a form of hypokalemic periodic paralysis, which usually presents as sudden onset weakness in the proximal muscles. It is a reversible condition that can be treated with rapid repletion of potassium and normalization of thyroid hormones.

Glycemic Disorders

Hypoglycemia

Acute hypoglycemia can cause autonomic symptoms, such as diaphoresis, tachycardia, and nausea. If left untreated, severe hypoglycemia can lead to seizures and/or coma and irreversible CNS injury; therefore, assessment for and prompt management of hypoglycemia is a critical part of the investigation of altered mental status.

Hyperglycemia

Acute hyperglycemia causing a hyperosmolar state can cause altered mental status, seizures, and/or chorea (a movement disorder characterized by spontaneous irregular movements of the extremities). In contrast to many neurologic manifestations of systemic conditions that cause bilateral neurologic dysfunction,

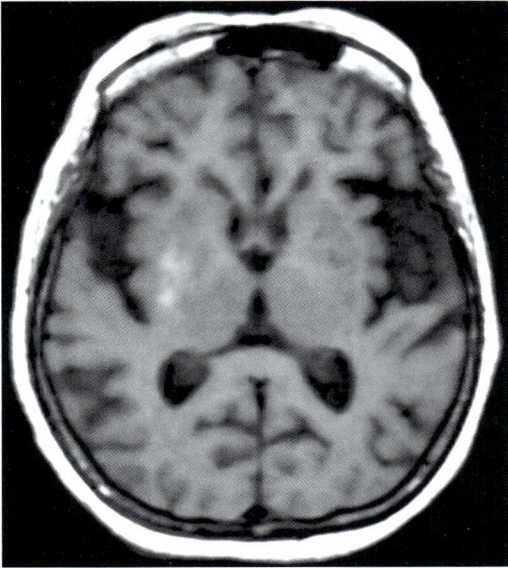

FIGURE 27.1 Axial T1-weighted MRI demonstrating T1 hyperintensity in the right basal ganglia in a patient with left-sided hemichorea due to severe hyperglycemia. (Image provided courtesy of A. John Tsiouris MD.)

seizures and chorea may be unilateral (focal seizures, hemichorea) in hyperglycemia. Hyperglycemic hemichorea can be associated with contralateral T1 hyperintensity in the basal ganglia on MRI (Figure 27.1).

Chronic hyperglycemia in diabetes can lead to a variety of types of peripheral neuropathy, including distal sensory neuropathy, autonomic neuropathy, acute neuropathy, and diabetic lumbosacral radiculoplexus neuropathy (also known as diabetic amyotrophy). Most commonly, diabetic neuropathy presents as distal sensory neuropathy with numbness, tingling, and/or pain in the feet, sometimes accompanied by imbalance. Symptomatic treatment of painful neuropathy is discussed in Chapter 24, but such treatments are ineffective for other symptoms of neuropathy, such as imbalance. Diabetic autonomic neuropathy can lead to gastroparesis, orthostatic hypotension, and sexual dysfunction.

Patients with diabetes are susceptible to the development of a microvascular ocular motor palsy due to occlusion of the blood vessels (vasa nervorum) supplying cranial nerves 3, 4, or 6. Patients present with sudden-onset diplopia and an isolated cranial nerve palsy, often with associated periorbital pain. In the case of a microvascular cranial nerve 3 palsy, the eye is deviated downward and outward and the lid is ptotic, but the pupil is often spared (in contrast to a compressive cause of a cranial nerve 3 palsy, such as from an aneurysm). Most patients recover over months.

Diabetic lumbosacral radiculoplexus neuropathy usually presents as a period of unilateral severe pain of one lower extremity (usually proximal in the thigh) followed by the development of proximal weakness of the affected limb. Symptoms increase over weeks to months and then plateau. Treatment includes physical therapy, pain control, and improved control of diabetes. Steroids or intravenous immune globulin (IVIg) may be considered, but data on treatment are limited.

RHEUMATOLOGIC DISORDERS

Neurologic manifestations of rheumatologic diseases can occur at any time over the course of the illness and may be the presenting features before systemic features of the condition emerge as demonstrated in Table 27.2.

Systemic Lupus Erythematosus

Systemic lupus erythematosus (SLE) can be associated with myriad CNS and PNS manifestations. Some manifestations of neuropsychiatric lupus are nonspecific and often lack neuroimaging correlates but occur at higher frequency than in the general population, such as headache, mood disorders, cognitive dysfunction, psychosis, and seizures. Stroke in SLE should lead to evaluation for antiphospholipid antibodies. The existence of "lupus cerebritis" is considered controversial, and evaluation for alternative etiologies of neurologic manifestations (such as infectious complications of immunomodulatory treatment) should be pursued before attributing new neurologic symptoms to SLE.

If transverse myelitis occurs in a patient with SLE, the patient should be evaluated for neuromyelitis optica (NMO; see Chapter 20) with serum testing for anti-aquaporin 4 antibodies, as NMO and SLE may coexist.

SLE may cause a wide variety of neuropathies, with the most common being sensory polyneuropathy such as painful small fiber neuropathy.

TABLE 27.2   Neurologic Manifestations of Rheumatologic Disorders

Rheumatologic Disorder	CNS				PNS		
	Encephalitis	Strokes	Cranial neuropathy	Myelopathy	Dorsal root ganglionopathy	Peripheral neuropathy	Myopathy
SLE	✓	✓		✓		✓	✓
Sjögren syndrome			✓	✓	✓	✓	
Rheumatoid arthritis				✓		✓	
Systemic vasculitis		✓				✓	
Behçet disease	✓	✓	✓	✓			
Sarcoidosis	✓	✓	✓	✓		✓	✓

CNS, central nervous system; PNS, peripheral nervous system; SLE, systemic lupus erythematosus.

Acute neurologic manifestations of SLE that are thought to be related to active inflammation are generally treated with high-dose steroids.

Sjögren Syndrome

Neurologic manifestations of Sjögren syndrome primarily affect the PNS. The most common neurologic conditions are painful small fiber neuropathy and sensory ganglionopathy (neuronopathy); the latter presents with severe sensory ataxia. Cranial neuropathies may occur, most commonly involving the trigeminal nerve causing numbness or tingling in the face. These conditions may precede the development of classic glandular manifestations and so diagnostic evaluation for Sjögren syndrome should be considered in patients with these clinical syndromes. Rarely, patients with Sjögren syndrome can develop transverse myelitis; similar to SLE, patients may have coexistent NMO and should be tested for serum anti-aquaporin 4 antibodies.

Rheumatoid Arthritis

Neurologic manifestations of rheumatoid arthritis (RA) are most commonly due to inflammatory changes and destruction of synovial joints, leading to compression of nearby structures of the CNS or PNS. The most concerning articular manifestations occur in the cervical spine and can lead to atlantoaxial instability or pannus formation, causing severe spinal cord (or rarely lower brainstem) compression. Articular disease can also lead to focal entrapment neuropathies, such as

carpal tunnel syndrome. Rarer neurologic manifestations of RA include aseptic meningitis and CNS vasculitis. Rheumatoid meningitis presents with headache, cognitive changes, seizure, and/or cranial nerve palsies, with MRI demonstrating enhancement of the dura (pachymeninges). CNS vasculitis causes headache, cognitive changes, and focal deficits due to stroke. Peripheral neuropathies and myositis can also occur in RA. Patients treated for RA with anti-TNF therapies can develop demyelination of the CNS or PNS (discussed above under "Inflammatory Bowel Disease"). Discontinuation of the offending medication usually leads to resolution of the neurologic complications.

Systemic Vasculitis

CNS vasculitis can occur secondary to systemic vasculitis, infections (eg, syphilis, aspergillosis) or can more rarely be primary (ie, isolated to the nervous system with no systemic involvement, called *primary CNS vasculitis*). Rheumatologic conditions that can cause CNS vasculitis include anti-neutrophil cytoplasmic antibody (ANCA)-associated vasculitis syndromes, polyarteritis nodosa, Henoch-Schönlein purpura, Takayasu arteritis, giant cell arteritis (GCA), and RA. Patients with CNS vasculitis typically present with headache, cognitive dysfunction, and focal or multifocal neurologic deficits. MRI may demonstrate areas of infarction along with confluent white matter changes in the subcortical white matter. Angiography may demonstrate multifocal vascular stenoses, although it is frequently normal, since most CNS vasculitides affect small vessels that cannot be visualized radiologically. Cerebrospinal fluid (CSF) demonstrates modest elevations in protein and white cell count, but these findings are nonspecific. If no systemic vasculitis is diagnosed in a patient with presumed CNS vasculitis, brain biopsy is necessary for the diagnosis of primary CNS vasculitis.

GCA is a medium vessel vasculitis initially affecting branches of the external carotid artery. It almost exclusively affects patients over age 50. Classically, patients present with headache, often with pain upon palpation of the temporal arteries. Commonly associated symptoms include jaw claudication, proximal muscle pain due to polymyalgia rheumatica, and constitutional symptoms, such as fevers, chills, and unexplained weight loss. If the disease progresses, it can cause permanent visual loss due to arteritic anterior ischemic optic neuropathy. Erythrocyte sedimentation rate (ESR) and C-reactive protein (CRP) are typically elevated but can be normal in some cases. If there is clinical concern for GCA, patients should be treated urgently with high-dose steroids to avoid permanent visual loss. Biopsy of the affected temporal artery demonstrates the presence of inflammation, giant cells, and disruption of the internal elastic lamina. Steroids are generally tapered very slowly and may need to be maintained if symptoms recur. Tocilizumab or methotrexate are steroid-sparing agents that may be considered in patients needing prolonged immunomodulatory treatment.

Behçet Disease

Behçet disease can cause CNS parenchymal lesions (often with brainstem predominance) and cerebral venous sinus thrombosis. Patients generally have other systemic clues to the diagnosis such as oral or genital ulcers, uveitis, and pathergy (pustule development at the site of needlestick for blood draw).

Sarcoidosis

Neurologic involvement of sarcoidosis occurs in 5% to 10% of patients with sarcoidosis and can sometimes be the presenting or only manifestation. Sarcoidosis can affect any part of the nervous system, but the most common neurologic manifestation of sarcoidosis is cranial neuropathy, most commonly unilateral or bilateral cranial nerve 7 palsy causing lower motor neuron pattern

facial droop (ie, involving both the upper and lower face on the affected side). Other neurologic manifestations include hypothalamic-pituitary involvement, parenchymal brain lesions, aseptic meningitis, optic neuritis, spinal cord lesions, peripheral neuropathy, and myopathy. In patients with suspected neurosarcoidosis and no systemic symptoms, body imaging with CT or positron emission tomography (PET) should be performed to look for an enlarged and accessible lymph node biopsy target. CSF angiotensin-converting enzyme (ACE) level is insensitive and nonspecific. In patients with no evidence of systemic disease, biopsy of affected nervous system tissue may be necessary.

HEMATOLOGIC DISORDERS

Sickle Cell Disease

The most common neurologic complication of sickle cell disease is stroke. Sickle cell disease causes a vasculopathy that predisposes to ischemic stroke, intracerebral hemorrhage, subarachnoid hemorrhage, and moyamoya syndrome (in which a large network of friable blood vessels develops in relation to stenosis of a proximal cerebral artery). Infarcted brain tissue can serve as a nidus for the development of epilepsy. Routine screening using transcranial Doppler to assess flow velocity of the middle cerebral artery can help detect patients at high risk of stroke and need for blood cell transfusion, which is the mainstay of primary and secondary stroke prevention in children with sickle cell disease.

Thrombotic Thrombocytopenic Purpura

Thrombotic thrombocytopenic purpura (TTP) can cause ischemic stroke, intracerebral hemorrhage, or PRES (see below).

Polycythemia Vera

Neurologic complications of polycythemia vera are due to serum hyperviscosity and include ischemic stroke and, rarely, chorea.

Paroxysmal Nocturnal Hemoglobinuria

The most common neurologic manifestation of paroxysmal nocturnal hemoglobinuria is cerebral venous sinus thrombosis, which can present with headache, altered mental status, and/or seizures. Diagnosis is made by CT venogram or MR venogram.

POSTERIOR REVERSIBLE ENCEPHALOPATHY SYNDROME

PRES is a neurologic condition characterized by vasogenic cerebral edema causing neurologic symptoms, such as headache, seizures, change in mental status, or visual disturbances. Vasogenic edema in PRES occurs due to failure of the blood-brain barrier. Brain MRI in PRES demonstrates subcortical vasogenic edema on T2-weighted sequences (Figure 27.2). The edema is usually most apparent in posterior

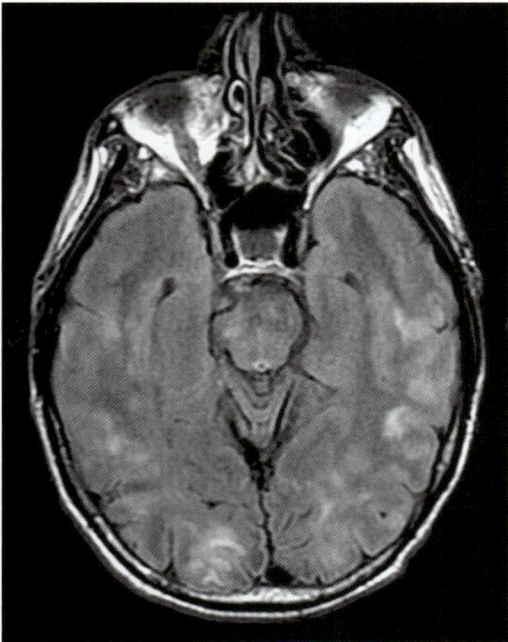

FIGURE 27.2 Axial fluid attenuated inversion recovery (FLAIR) MRI demonstrating posterior-predominant T2 hyperintensities representing vasogenic edema consistent with the diagnosis of PRES. (Image provided courtesy of A. John Tsiouris MD.)

cortical areas such as parieto-occipital and parieto-temporal regions but can also be anterior or more widespread. PRES can be caused by hypertensive crisis, preeclampsia/eclampsia, calcineurin inhibitors (eg, cyclosporine, tacrolimus), organ transplantation, chemotherapy agents (eg, bevacizumab, bortezomib, cytarabine), synthetic marijuana (such as K2 or spice), and sympathomimetic drugs (such as cocaine and amphetamines). Management includes strict blood pressure control, withdrawal of the offending agent, and symptomatic management of headache and seizures, if they occur. As the name implies, the condition is almost always reversible, although some patients can develop stroke.

SUMMARY

Many systemic diseases can cause neurologic complications, and these may be the presenting symptoms of the underlying systemic disease. Therefore, systemic disease should be considered in the differential diagnosis of patients with new neurologic symptoms or signs. In patients with known systemic disease, neurologic manifestations may be related to the underlying condition or its treatment, but could also represent a separate superimposed neurologic disease. Knowledge of common and uncommon neurologic complications of systemic diseases is essential in the diagnosis and treatment of patients with medical illness.

EDITORS' KEY POINTS

▶ Many systemic conditions have neurologic manifestations, which, in some cases, can be the presenting feature of the underlying condition.

▶ Strokes due to septic emboli from endocarditis have a high risk of hemorrhage and, therefore, should not be treated with thrombolysis, antiplatelet agents, or anticoagulation (unless the latter is required for a mechanical heart valve).

▶ Patients with ischemic or hemorrhagic stroke due to endocarditis should be screened for mycotic aneurysms with CT angiography or MR angiography.

▶ Hyponatremia, hypocalcemia, and hypomagnesemia can cause seizures.

► Hypokalemia and hyperkalemia can cause PNS manifestations, such as weakness.

► Bariatric surgery and GI disease predispose patients to vitamin and mineral deficiencies that may present with neurologic manifestations, including vitamin B_1 (thiamine) deficiency causing Wernicke encephalopathy and/or neuropathy (dry beriberi); vitamin B_{12} (cobalamin) deficiency causing neuropathy, subacute combined degeneration of the spinal cord, or both; and copper deficiency, which can cause the same manifestations as vitamin B_{12} deficiency.

► Patients with SLE or Sjögren syndrome who develop myelitis should be evaluated for NMO by sending serum anti-aquaporin 4 antibodies.

► Neurosarcoidosis can affect any level of the nervous system, but cranial neuropathy is the most common manifestation (most commonly unilateral or bilateral CN 7 palsy causing facial weakness).

REFERENCE

1. Baddour LM, Wilson WR, Bayer AS, et al. Infective endocarditis in adults: diagnosis, antimicrobial therapy, and management of complications: a scientific statement for healthcare professionals from the American Heart Association. *Circulation*. 2015;132(15):1435-1486.

Neurology of Pregnancy

Mary A. O'Neal

INTRODUCTION

Pregnancy causes significant physiologic changes in the mother that support the developing fetus, including alterations in hemodynamics (volume expansion, lower blood pressure, and increased cardiac output), hypercoagulability (to reduce the risk of bleeding at delivery), and increased immune tolerance (to avoid rejection of fetal tissue). These changes can have effects on the nervous system, leading to the development of neurologic conditions or exacerbations of underlying neurologic diseases. In addition, changes in metabolism and volume of absorption affect the efficacy of medications, raising particular challenges for dosing of antiseizure medications (ASMs) in pregnant patients with epilepsy. This chapter discusses eclampsia and cerebrovascular complications of pregnancy as well as special considerations in the diagnosis and treatment of headache disorders, epilepsy, multiple sclerosis (MS), and myasthenia gravis in patients who are pregnant.

NEUROLOGIC COMPLICATIONS OF PREGNANCY AND THE POSTPARTUM PERIOD

Preeclampsia/Eclampsia

Preeclampsia is defined as the development of hypertension after 20 weeks of gestation with one or more of the following: proteinuria, thrombocytopenia, elevated creatinine, rising liver transaminases, pulmonary edema, new-onset headache (not accounted for by an alternative diagnosis and not responding to analgesics), or visual symptoms.

The most common neurologic symptoms of preeclampsia are headache, confusion, and visual changes (which can include both positive symptoms, such as blurred vision and flashing lights, and negative symptoms, including hemianopia and cortical blindness). Stroke (both ischemic and hemorrhagic) may also occur.

Eclampsia is defined as seizures in a patient with preeclampsia. Seizures in eclampsia are usually generalized tonic-clonic, but can be focal, often with impaired awareness (manifesting as staring, associated automatisms, and confusion).

Definitive treatment for preeclampsia is delivery as soon as the fetus is at term. While awaiting this time frame for delivery, hypertension should be controlled, and intravenous (IV) magnesium is used to prevent eclampsia. Treatment of seizures in eclampsia is with IV magnesium. If seizures continue despite IV magnesium treatment, other ASMs such as IV levetiracetam or others may be considered.

Posterior Reversible Encephalopathy Syndrome and Reversible Cerebral Vasoconstriction Syndrome

The pathophysiology of preeclampsia is due to endothelial dysfunction and vasoconstriction involving multiple organ systems. In the brain, the posterior cerebral circulation may be particularly vulnerable to these changes due to decreased capacity for autoregulation, which can lead to posterior reversible encephalopathy syndrome (PRES). PRES is characterized on neuroimaging by vasogenic cerebral edema, most commonly in the white matter of the parietal and occipital lobes (see Figure 27.2 in Chapter 27). PRES should be considered in pregnant women who develop unremitting headache and visual symptoms as described earlier. In addition to preeclampsia/eclampsia, PRES can occur in hypertensive urgency and due to immunosuppressive and chemotherapy agents. The radiographic changes of PRES are generally reversible after the underlying cause is treated, but stroke or intracerebral hemorrhage rarely occurs.

Reversible cerebral vasoconstriction syndrome (RCVS) can occur either in conjunction with PRES or independently. The condition presents with recurrent thunderclap headaches (severe headaches with maximal intensity at onset). In addition to preeclampsia/eclampsia, triggers of this condition include marijuana, sympathomimetics, serotonergic agents, and over-the-counter decongestants. In the postpartum setting, bromocriptine used to inhibit lactation and ergometrine for postpartum hemorrhage are potential culprits. Therefore, patients should be asked about use of these agents before the condition is attributed to pregnancy or the postpartum period in which it commonly occurs. The diagnosis of RCVS is made by the finding of vascular irregularities ("beading") on computed tomography angiography (CTA) or magnetic resonance angiography (MRA), sometimes accompanied by small foci of subarachnoid hemorrhage in the cerebral sulci. These findings resolve with the treatment of the underlying trigger. The condition is rarely complicated by ischemic stroke or intracerebral hemorrhage. Treatment of RCVS consists of withdrawal of any offending agents, symptomatic treatment of headache and seizures if present, and, in pregnancy-associated or postpartum cases, IV magnesium.

Stroke in Pregnancy

Strokes in pregnancy are rare (<0.05%), occurring most commonly in the third trimester and postpartum period. The risk of stroke is elevated due to the normal hypercoagulability of pregnancy, as well as bed rest, dehydration, and compression of the iliac veins by a gravid uterus, all of which increase thrombotic risk. Preeclampsia and eclampsia increase the risk for both ischemic and hemorrhagic stroke. In women with arteriovenous malformations (AVMs), rupture risk is increased in the second and third trimesters due to pregnancy-associated changes in intravascular volume and cardiac output.

In pregnant patients who develop acute ischemic stroke and present within the appropriate time window, expert opinion is that IV thrombolysis and thrombectomy should be considered on a case-by-case basis, balancing potential benefit in moderate or severe stroke with the potential risk of uterine bleeding.[1] Secondary prevention depends on the underlying etiology. Aspirin, low-molecular-weight heparin, and unfractionated heparin are considered safe in pregnancy and lactation if indicated. Warfarin is teratogenic and should be avoided during pregnancy but can be used during lactation if needed. Data are limited on clopidogrel and direct oral anticoagulants in pregnant patients and should be avoided.

Cerebral Venous Sinus Thrombosis

The hypercoagulability of pregnancy and the postpartum period predisposes to thrombosis of the cerebral venous sinuses. The primary presenting symptom of cerebral venous sinus thrombosis is headache, which may be progressive over days or sudden in onset (thunderclap). Headache may be accompanied by seizure, blurred or double vision (which may be accompanied by papilledema on examination), and/or focal neurologic deficits if secondary intracerebral hemorrhage or ischemic stroke complicates venous sinus thrombosis.

The diagnosis is made by CT venogram or MR venogram, demonstrating a filling defect in the affected venous sinus(es). Cerebral venous sinus thrombosis is treated with anticoagulation, even in the presence of intracerebral hemorrhage. During pregnancy, IV heparin or low-molecular-weight heparin is considered safe; postpartum, if the woman is breastfeeding, warfarin is recommended since the safety of direct oral anticoagulants in breastfeeding remains uncertain. If pregnancy alone is considered the provoking factor, anticoagulation is generally continued for 3 to 6 months and prophylactic dose low-molecular-weight heparin is recommended during subsequent pregnancies to prevent recurrence. If an underlying thrombophilia is identified, lifelong anticoagulation is generally recommended.

DIAGNOSIS AND TREATMENT OF NEUROLOGIC CONDITIONS IN PREGNANCY

Headache in Pregnancy

In the first trimester of pregnancy, primary headache disorders such as migraine are most common. Later in pregnancy, secondary headaches (ie, those caused by underlying disorders; see Chapter 8) become more frequent, and preeclampsia, RCVS, cerebral venous sinus thrombosis, intracerebral hemorrhage, and idiopathic intracranial hypertension should be considered (Table 28.1). Preeclampsia, RCVS, and cerebral

venous sinus thrombosis can also occur in the postpartum period. Additional considerations in patients with postpartum headache include intracranial hypotension (due to cerebrospinal fluid [CSF] leak from inadvertent dural puncture during epidural anesthesia) and cervical artery dissection (which can occur during labor).

Red flags for headaches that warrant evaluation with neuroimaging include new-onset headache in a patient with no history of headache, change in headache character or frequency in a patient with a known headache disorder, thunderclap headache (maximal severity at onset), headache worse in the morning or awakening the patient from sleep (associated with elevated intracranial pressure), and headache with additional neurologic symptoms. If any of these features are present, the patient should undergo evaluation with neuroimaging. If there is a concern for acute stroke, head CT and CT angiogram of the head and neck should be obtained. Brain MRI without gadolinium is considered safe in pregnancy in all trimesters. MR angiography and venography can both be performed without gadolinium. Gadolinium contrast is generally avoided due to the risks to the developing fetus, but may be considered if the benefits of diagnostic information obtained are thought to merit this risk.[2]

Migraine in Pregnancy

Migraine is a primary headache disorder characterized by severe headache that is usually unilateral, throbbing, and associated with photosensitivity,

TABLE 28.1	Headaches in Pregnancy	
Historical features	**Headache type**	**Neuroimaging**
First trimester	• Likely migraine or tension type	None (except if there are red flags)
Prior similar headache	• Likely migraine or tension type	Not needed
Thunderclap onset	• Subarachnoid hemorrhage • Reversible cerebral vasoconstriction syndrome • Cerebral venous thrombosis	Brain MRI, MRA or CTA of the head/neck, brain MRV or CTV
Postural	• Idiopathic intracranial hypertension • Postdural puncture headache	Brain MRI with gadolinium (only if postpartum)
Hypertension, proteinuria	• Preeclampsia/eclampsia	Brain MRI

CT, computed tomography; CTA, computed tomography angiography; MRA, magnetic resonance angiography; MRI, magnetic resonance imaging.

TABLE 28.2 Preventive Medications for Migraine During Pregnancy

Drug class	Generic name	Level of risk during pregnancy category	Breastfeeding safety
Nutraceuticals	Magnesium oxide Coenzyme Q	B	Safe
Antihistamines	Cyproheptadine	B	Avoid
Tricyclic antidepressants	Amitriptyline	C	Safe
SNRIs	Duloxetine Venlafaxine	C C	Little data
CGRP inhibitors	Erenumab Fremanezumab Galcanezumab	No data	No data
Gepants	Rimegepant Eptinezumab	No data	No data

CGRP, calcitonin gene-related peptide; SNRI, serotonin norepinephrine reuptake inhibitor. Refer to Table 28.3 for explanation of levels of risk.

phonosensitivity, nausea/vomiting, and, in some patients, aura (see Chapter 15). The hormonal changes in pregnancy can lead to new onset of migraines or exacerbation in migraine frequency in patients with preexisting migraines. This occurs most commonly during the first trimester, though most patients will have improvement in migraine by the second trimester. Migraine is associated with an increased risk of preeclampsia.

Given that migraines often improve as pregnancy progresses, and since most preventive medications carry risks for the developing fetus, patients should ideally be tapered off preventive medications prior to conception. If a preventive agent is required due to the frequency and severity of migraines, the safest options in pregnancy are magnesium oxide and coenzyme Q10 (Table 28.2). Valproate and topiramate should be avoided due to the high risk of teratogenicity. For acute abortive treatment, acetaminophen and metoclopramide are the safest options (Table 28.3). Triptans can be considered as a second-line migraine abortive medication unless the patient has hypertension, cardiovascular disease, or stroke.

Idiopathic Intracranial Hypertension

Idiopathic intracranial hypertension (also called pseudotumor cerebri) is caused by a rise in intracranial pressure most commonly seen in the setting of weight

TABLE 28.3 Acute Therapy for Migraine in Pregnancy

Drug class	Examples	Level of risk in pregnancy[a]	Breastfeeding safety
Analgesic	Acetaminophen	B	Safe
Antiemetic	Metoclopramide Prochlorperazine	B C	Probably safe May be safe
Nutraceutical	Magnesium IV	A (D)[b]	Probably safe
NSAID	Ibuprofen Naproxen	B (D in the last trimester due to premature closure of the patent ductus arteriosus)	Safe
Triptan	Sumatriptan Rizatriptan	C	Safe
Ergot	Dihydroergotamine	X	Avoid
Ditan	Lasmiditan	No data, but adverse effects not noted in animals	No data
Gepants	Ubrogepant Rimegepant	No data, but adverse effects not noted in animals	No data

A—Appropriate human studies show no risk; B—Insufficient human studies, but animal research suggests safety or animal studies show risk, but human studies show safety; C—Insufficient human studies, but animal studies show risk or no animal studies and insufficient human studies; D—Human studies show fetal risk, but the drug is important to some women to treat their condition; X-fetal risks are evident, there are no situations where risk/benefit justifies use.
IV, intravenous; NSAID, nonsteroidal anti-inflammatory drug.
[a]Although this risk stratification nomenclature no longer used, it is a reasonable first step to begin thinking about the safety of medications during pregnancy.
[b]IV magnesium in high dose for 5 to 7 days has been reported to cause rickets in the infant. In the doses and time frame used to treat preeclampsia or eclampsia, it is generally safe.

gain. The risk of developing this condition increases in the second trimester of pregnancy, which is the time of maximal weight gain. Patients present with headaches, transient visual obscurations (often provoked by bending forward), and pulsatile tinnitus (a "whooshing" sound in the ears). Papilledema may be observed on fundoscopy. In severe cases, patients may develop visual loss. The diagnosis is made by MRI with MR venogram to exclude a structural lesion or venous sinus thrombosis as the cause of elevated intracranial pressure; nonspecific signs of elevated intracranial pressure on MRI may be observed, such as empty sella, tortuosity of the optic nerves, or posterior flattening of the sclera. Lumbar puncture demonstrates elevated opening pressure (greater than 25 cm CSF) with normal CSF analysis. Patients often feel relief of symptoms after lumbar puncture.

In nonpregnant patients who develop this condition, weight loss is a key aspect of treatment, but this is not feasible in pregnancy, so weight gain appropriate to the stage of pregnancy is the goal. Treatment with acetazolamide is considered safe in pregnancy and breastfeeding. In refractory cases with progressive visual loss, repeat lumbar puncture for CSF drainage, ventriculoperitoneal (VP) shunt, or optic nerve sheath fenestration may be required. There is no contraindication to vaginal delivery.

Post-Dural Puncture Headache

If the dura is inadvertently punctured during epidural anesthesia, a CSF leak can develop, which lowers intracranial pressure. The primary symptom of intracranial hypotension is headache that is worse when standing and resolves when supine. Patients may also describe neck stiffness, nausea, dizziness, tinnitus, and blurred or double vision. Signs of intracranial hypotension on brain MRI include sagging of the brain, dural (pachymeningeal) enhancement, pituitary hyperemia, and subdural hematoma or fluid collection (usually bilateral). If bed rest and caffeine do not lead to symptom resolution, epidural blood patch may be considered.

Epilepsy in Pregnancy

Seizures during pregnancy carry risks for both the mother and the fetus (due to hypoxia that may occur with generalized seizures). Many ASMs carry high risks of teratogenicity as well as neurodevelopmental effects such as lower infant IQ and autism. Even ASMs that are safer in pregnancy may require dose adjustments over the course of pregnancy due to shifts in metabolism and volume of distribution. Therefore, in women with epilepsy, pregnancy should ideally be carefully planned and monitored in close collaboration with a neurologist to ensure a healthy pregnancy, adequate seizure control, and minimal risk to the developing fetus. To reduce the risk of unplanned pregnancy, women with epilepsy should be counseled on contraceptives, noting that high-dose contraceptives may be needed in women on enzyme-inducing ASMs (eg, carbamazepine, phenytoin, phenobarbital) and that hormonal contraceptives may reduce the level of lamotrigine, requiring higher dosage of lamotrigine.

The safest ASMs in pregnancy are levetiracetam and lamotrigine, which carry the lowest risk of major congenital malformations and neurodevelopmental disorders. Valproate, phenobarbital, and topiramate have the highest risk of major congenital malformations and should be avoided in women of childbearing age. The smaller number of patient exposures in registries limits the knowledge of pregnancy safety of less commonly used agents, such as zonisamide, gabapentin, and pregabalin (Table 28.4).

If pregnancy is planned, ASM adjustments are made prior to pregnancy with the goal of using monotherapy with the lowest effective dose of the safest possible medication, since the risk to the fetus increases with higher dosage and polytherapy. If a woman becomes pregnant while already on a high-risk medication such as valproate, phenobarbital, or topiramate, the medication is generally maintained because of the risk of seizure with cross-titration and since the period of highest risk of teratogenicity has generally already passed by the time pregnancy is discovered.

Monthly monitoring of serum ASM levels during pregnancy is critical for dose adjustments since changing maternal weight, volume of distribution, protein binding, and metabolism over the course of pregnancy can decrease the levels of ASMs, increasing the risk for seizures. Postpartum, the dose of the ASM should be quickly returned to the prepregnancy level to avoid drug toxicity. Folate supplementation is

| TABLE 28.4 | Antiseizure Medications (ASMs) During Pregnancy and Lactation |

Drug	Pregnancy safety	Lactation safety[a]	% major congenital malformation risk	Neurodevelopmental risk
Lamotrigine	Considered one of the safest ASMs	Can penetrate breast milk in potentially clinically important amounts—side effects can include apnea, rash, drowsiness, or poor sucking	No increased risk	Lower risk
Levetiracetam	Considered one of the safest ASMs	Can penetrate breast milk in potentially clinically important amounts—side effects can include drowsiness and inadequate weight gain	No increased risk	Lower risk
Gabapentin (limited data)	Next safest tier	Levels in breast milk are low.	1.47	Unknown
Oxcarbazepine	Next safest tier	Levels in breast milk are low.	2.39	Unknown
Topiramate	Moderate risk	Levels in breast milk are low.	4.28	Lower risk
Carbamazepine	Moderate risk	Levels in breast milk are relatively high, but no evidence that breastfeeding produces any infant growth or developmental issues.	4.93	Lower risk
Phenytoin	Avoid if possible	Levels in breast milk are low.	6.26	Lower risk
Phenobarbital	Avoid if possible	Levels in breast milk are variable—can cause sedation.	7.10	Higher risk
Primidone	Avoid if possible	Penetrates breast milk in potentially clinically important amounts—can cause drowsiness, inadequate weight gain, poor nursing.	8.49	Unknown (caution)
Valproate	Least safe	Levels in breast milk are low.	10.93	Higher risk

[a]No adverse effects of ASM exposure via breast milk were observed at age 3 years, and breastfed infants had higher IQs and verbal ability. Women with epilepsy should be encouraged to breastfeed. Weston J, Bromley R, Jackson CF, et al. Monotherapy treatment of epilepsy in pregnancy: congenital malformation outcomes in the child. Cochrane Database Syst Rev 2016;11(11):CD010224. doi:10.1002/14651858.CD010224.pub2

recommended throughout pregnancy as it decreases the risk of neural tube defects.

Breastfeeding is safe and encouraged in women on ASMs, since concentrations of ASMs in breast milk are lower than what the fetus was exposed to in utero. Phenobarbital in breast milk can decrease withdrawal symptoms in infants exposed in utero, but it can also cause drowsiness in some infants, especially if the mother is taking any additional sedating medications; infants should, therefore, be monitored for drowsiness and poor weight gain if the mother is taking phenobarbital while breastfeeding. If a new ASM is started in the postpartum period, the first exposure of the infant will be through breast milk (ie, since there is no prior in utero exposure); with some ASMs that reach significant concentrations in breast milk, this may cause side effects in the infant.

Sleep deprivation and missed medications in the postpartum period can lead to breakthrough seizures in women with epilepsy. Patients and their families should be counseled on the importance of maintaining sleep and medication schedules as well as safety in women with persistent seizures to avoid injury to the fetus (eg, assistance with bathing, changing diapers on high tables). Women with epilepsy are at higher risk for postpartum depression and anxiety, which should be screened for and treated.

Multiple Sclerosis in Pregnancy

MS is a demyelinating disease of the central nervous system that most commonly follows a relapsing-remitting course (see Chapter 20). The relapse rate decreases during pregnancy but increases in the postpartum period. Given the decreased risk of relapse in pregnancy and teratogenicity of many disease-modifying therapies, these treatments are generally stopped and may require a washout period before conception; teriflunomide requires elimination with either cholestyramine or activated charcoal (Table 28.5). However, discontinuation

| TABLE 28.5 | Multiple Sclerosis Disease-Modifying Treatments (DMTs) and Pregnancy | | |

DMT	Pregnancy safety	Compatible with lactation	Washout prior to conception
Interferons	Not used	Yes	No washout
Glatiramer acetate	Safe, can be used	Yes	No washout
Teriflunomide	Not compatible	No	Rapid elimination protocol
Dimethyl fumarate	Not compatible	No	No washout
Fingolimod	Not compatible	No	2 mo
Cladribine	Not compatible	It is rapidly eliminated over 24 h and undetectable at 48 h after a dose. It is suggested that breastfeeding be withheld for at least 48 h after a dose of cladribine.	4 mo
Alemtuzumab	Not compatible	Yes, if needed	4 mo
Ocrelizumab	Not compatible	Yes	2 mo
Natalizumab	See standard practice	Yes, if needed	No washout. Standard practice is to continue throughout pregnancy, timing it to the late first trimester and until gestation week ~32, with infusion every 6-8 wk.

of some agents such as natalizumab and fingolimod can result in rebound relapse. In patients with highly active MS, natalizumab may be safely used in pregnancy up to approximately 32 weeks (but should be avoided after 32 weeks due to the risk of hematologic abnormalities in the newborn). Rituximab use within 6 months of conception may also be safe, though this requires monitoring neonatal B cells.

If an MS relapse occurs during pregnancy, IV corticosteroids can be administered, similar to the treatment of flares in nonpregnant patients.

Breastfeeding is encouraged in patients with MS, both for the health of the child and because exclusive breastfeeding lowers postpartum MS relapse risk. The injectable treatments and monoclonal antibodies for MS are considered safe to use during breastfeeding, though the latter may predispose infants to infection and reduce the efficacy of vaccines. Oral MS agents are not recommended during breastfeeding due to the risk to the infant.

Myasthenia Gravis in Pregnancy

Myasthenia gravis is an autoimmune disease caused by antibodies directed against the neuromuscular junction, causing fatigable weakness of the muscles of the eyes, limbs, and/or head and neck (see Chapter 25).

Mild cases are controlled symptomatically with pyridostigmine, whereas more severe cases require immunomodulatory therapy (eg, prednisone, azathioprine, mycophenolate, methotrexate, eculizumab). Pyridostigmine is considered safe in pregnancy and breastfeeding as are some immunomodulatory treatments (prednisone and azathioprine), whereas others are teratogenic and, therefore, contraindicated (eg, methotrexate and mycophenolate) and should be discontinued prior to conception. Myasthenia exacerbations can be treated with intravenous immunoglobulin (IVIg) or plasma exchange as in nonpregnant patients.

If a woman with myasthenia gravis develops eclampsia, IV magnesium should be avoided as it can trigger a myasthenia exacerbation; levetiracetam can be used for seizures. Calcium channel blockers and β-blockers may also cause worsening of myasthenia, and so hydralazine is generally preferred for the treatment of hypertension in preeclampsia in patients with myasthenia.

The first stage of labor uses smooth muscle, which is not affected in myasthenia. However, skeletal muscle weakness in myasthenia may impede the second stage of labor, requiring forceps or vacuum assistance. There is no contraindication to the use of epidural anesthesia in patients with myasthenia.

Infants of mothers with myasthenia should be closely monitored for 48 hours to evaluate for signs of transient neonatal myasthenia that can result from passive transfer of acetylcholine receptor antibodies to the fetus. If this occurs, the neonate may require respiratory support, IV feeding, monitoring in a neonatal intensive care unit (ICU), and treatment with cholinesterase inhibitors.

SUMMARY

Pregnancy and the postpartum period carry an increased risk of stroke and may cause exacerbations in underlying neurologic conditions, such as migraine. Treatments for neurologic diseases such as epilepsy and MS can have adverse effects on the developing fetus. Therefore, careful planning of pregnancy and close collaboration with a neurologist are important for women with neurologic conditions to ensure a safe and healthy pregnancy and delivery.

EDITORS' KEY POINTS

▶ Preeclampsia/eclampsia can be complicated by seizures (due to eclampsia), PRES, and RCVS.

▶ Seizures caused by eclampsia are treated with IV magnesium.

▶ Stroke risk is increased in pregnancy due to hypercoagulability. If a stroke occurs in pregnancy, aspirin, low-molecular-weight heparin, and unfractionated heparin for secondary stroke prevention are considered safe in pregnancy, but warfarin is not. Data are limited on clopidogrel and direct oral anticoagulants in pregnancy, and these medications should be avoided.

▶ Headache in the first trimester of pregnancy is most commonly due to a primary headache disorder (eg, migraine), whereas secondary headaches become more frequent later in pregnancy (eg, preeclampsia, cerebral venous sinus thrombosis, idiopathic intracranial hypertension). MRI (without gadolinium) is considered safe in pregnancy if indicated to evaluate for an underlying cause of headache.

▶ The safest migraine medications for pregnant patients are acetaminophen and metoclopramide for acute abortive treatment, and magnesium oxide and coenzyme Q10 for preventive treatment. Valproate and topiramate should be avoided due to the risks of teratogenicity.

▶ The safest ASMs in pregnancy are levetiracetam and lamotrigine. Valproate, phenobarbital, and topiramate have the highest risk of teratogenicity. The benefits of breastfeeding in women on ASMs are considered to outweigh the risks.

▶ Disease-modifying treatment of MS is generally stopped prior to conception in patients becoming pregnant; however, certain treatments such as natalizumab and rituximab may be considered in patients with highly active disease. If an MS relapse occurs during pregnancy, IV corticosteroids can be administered as in flares in nonpregnant patients.

REFERENCES

1. Miller EC. Maternal stroke associated with pregnancy. *Continuum (Minneap Minn)*. 2022;28(1):93-121.
2. Committee Opinion No. 723: Guidelines for diagnostic imaging during pregnancy and lactation: correction. *Obstet Gynecol*. 2018;132(3):786.

Sleep Disorders

Martina Vendrame

INTRODUCTION

Sleep is essential for physical and mental health, and sleep disorders, therefore, have a significant impact on an individual's quality of life. Sleep disorders include those causing excess sleepiness (the hypersomnias such as sleep apnea and narcolepsy) and inability to sleep (insomnia) as well as sleep-related events (the parasomnias such as rapid eye movement [REM] sleep behavior disorder and sleep-related movement disorders such as restless legs syndrome [RLS]) and specific disruptions to the normal sleep-wake cycle (circadian rhythm disorders). This chapter discusses the diagnosis and treatment of these conditions as well as strategies for improving sleep hygiene.

BIOLOGY OF SLEEP AND WAKEFULNESS

The sleep cycle is made up of several stages: three non-rapid eye movement (NREM) stages and one REM stage. NREM stage 1 is the lightest stage of sleep, characterized by decreased brain activity and heart rate. NREM stage 2 is slightly deeper and marked by the appearance of particular electroencephalographic (EEG) features (sleep spindles and K-complexes). NREM stage 3 is deep sleep, characterized on EEG by predominant slow wave activity (delta waves). In REM sleep, the brain becomes more active, and eye movements become rapid; dreaming occurs during this stage, and muscle tone is normally absent (this is referred to as *REM atonia*) to prevent acting out of dreams. During the three NREM sleep stages, the body undergoes physical restoration, including muscle growth and repair, whereas the brain consolidates memories and processes emotion in REM sleep.[1]

The sleep stages are regulated by complex interactions between multiple neurotransmitters and neuromodulators in neural connections between the brainstem, hypothalamus, and cerebral cortex. The monoaminergic system (including serotonin, norepinephrine, dopamine, and histamine) promotes wakefulness, whereas the γ-aminobutyric acid (GABA) system promotes sleep. The neuromodulator adenosine participates in the transition from wakefulness to sleep. Understanding these neurotransmitters provides a basis for understanding the treatment of some sleep disorders and how medications may affect wakefulness. For example, antihistamines used in the treatment of allergies cause sedation by inhibiting the wakefulness-promoting histaminergic system, hypnotics used in the treatment of insomnia enhance

GABAergic transmission, and caffeine promotes wakefulness by inhibiting adenosine.

The orexin/hypocretin (*orexin* and *hypocretin* are alternative terms for the same molecule) system plays a crucial role in stabilizing wakefulness and regulating transitions between different stages of sleep. Orexin neurons, located in the lateral hypothalamus, are responsible for promoting arousal and maintaining wakefulness. Orexin receptor antagonists have been used to treat insomnia. Dysfunction in the orexin system has also been associated with certain sleep disorders, such as narcolepsy, in which individuals experience uncontrollable bouts of sleep due to a deficiency in orexin production. Orexin receptor agonists are promising options for the treatment of these disorders.

The circadian cycle is a 24-hour rhythm that regulates numerous physiologic processes, including sleep-wake patterns, hormone release, body temperature, and metabolism. The circadian cycle is influenced by environmental cues, with the most crucial being light exposure. Light stimulates retinal cells that send signals to the suprachiasmatic nucleus in the anterior hypothalamus, the pacemaker of the circadian rhythm. In the absence of light stimuli, the suprachiasmatic nucleus stimulates the pineal gland to produce melatonin, inducing drowsiness and sleep. Conversely, with exposure to bright light in the morning, melatonin production is suppressed, signaling wakefulness. Melatonin supplements are sometimes used to help manage sleep disorders by adjusting the timing of the circadian rhythm.

HYPERSOMNIAS

Disorders of hypersomnolence are characterized by chronic, debilitating daytime sleepiness. Hypersomnolence can be caused by insufficient sleep, sedating medications (eg, antidepressants, antipsychotics, sedatives, antihistamines, muscle relaxants), sleep apnea, medical conditions (eg, hepatic failure, uremia, hypothyroidism), psychiatric disorders (eg, major depression, mania, psychosis), and central disorders of hypersomnolence (eg, narcolepsy and idiopathic hypersomnolence; Table 29.1).

Sleep Apnea

Sleep apnea is a common sleep disorder characterized by frequent apneas (ie, pauses in breathing or shallow breaths) during sleep. Apneic pauses can last from seconds to minutes and can occur multiple times

TABLE 29.1	Comparison of Central Disorders of Hypersomnia		
	Narcolepsy type 1	**Narcolepsy type 2**	**Idiopathic hypersomnia**
Clinical features			
Cataplexy	Yes	No	No
Sleep paralysis	Yes[a]	Occasional	Rare
Hallucinations	Yes[a]	Occasional	Rare
Restless sleep	Yes	Occasional	No
Sleep inertia	Rare	Rare	Yes
Restorative naps	Yes	Occasional	No
Diagnostic testing			
MSLT results	MSL ≤8 min 2 or more SOREMP	MSL ≤8 min 2 or more SOREMP	MSL ≤8 min 1 SOREMP or none
Hypocretin-1 (orexin) CSF levels	≤110 pg/mL or one-third the baseline normal levels	>110 pg/mL or more than one-third the baseline normal levels	usually not measured

CSF, cerebrospinal fluid; MSL, mean sleep latency; MSLT, multiple sleep latency test; SOREMP, sleep onset rapid eye movement period.
[a]Cardinal feature, but not needed for diagnosis.

throughout the night, leading to interrupted sleep and daytime fatigue.

Sleep apnea can be classified as obstructive or central. Obstructive sleep apnea, the most common type, is caused by intermittent obstruction of the upper airway. Central sleep apnea is rare and is caused by a failure of the brain to signal the muscles to breathe due to conditions such as congestive heart failure, narcotic use, recent ascent to high altitude, and brainstem disorders. Brainstem lesions and conditions that can disrupt respiratory control mechanisms and cause central sleep apnea include medullary stroke, neoplastic lesions, infections (eg, encephalitis or meningitis), traumatic brain injury, and neurodegenerative diseases (eg, Parkinson disease and amyotrophic lateral sclerosis). This section focuses on the diagnosis and treatment of obstructive sleep apnea.

Diagnosis of Sleep Apnea

The most common symptoms of sleep apnea include loud snoring, gasping or choking during sleep, unrestful sleep, excessive daytime sleepiness, morning headaches, and impaired concentration and memory. The major risk factors for obstructive sleep apnea are obesity, a narrow airway, older age, male sex, the postmenopausal period in women, abnormalities of bony and soft tissue structure of the head and neck, retrognathia (a condition in which the lower jaw is set further back than the upper jaw), Down syndrome, and large tonsils and adenoids. A simple assessment tool called STOP-BANG uses eight yes/no questions to screen for symptoms of, and risk factors for, sleep apnea:[2]

1. Snoring history
2. Tired during the day
3. Observed to stop breathing while sleep
4. High blood pressure
5. BMI (body mass index) more than 35 kg/m^2
6. Age more than 50 years
7. Neck circumference more than 40 cm
8. Male sex

A STOP-Bang score of 5 or more indicates high risk of having sleep apnea.

Definitive diagnosis of sleep apnea requires a sleep study to evaluate for apnea and hypopnea (a milder apnea). Obstructive apneas are defined as cessation of flow (or at least 90% flow reduction) through the airway for at least 10 seconds while the chest and abdomen are moving, often associated with oxygen desaturation. Hypopneas involve at least a 30% drop in airflow and typically last for at least 10 seconds, but there is some variability in how sleep labs define them. The apnea-hypopnea index (AHI) is the combined average number of apneas and hypopneas that occur per hour of sleep. In adults, an AHI of 5 or higher indicates sleep apnea.

Treatment of Sleep Apnea

Untreated sleep apnea is a risk factor for hypertension, hyperlipidemia, diabetes, cardiac arrhythmias, coronary artery disease, stroke, and dementia. These risks can be significantly reduced with the proper treatment of sleep apnea. Treatment options for sleep apnea include lifestyle changes (weight loss and avoidance of alcohol and sedatives), continuous positive airway pressure (CPAP), oral appliances, and surgery.

CPAP delivers a constant stream of air through a mask worn over the nose or mouth to keep the airway open; it is the most effective treatment for sleep apnea. However, many patients find it difficult to use CPAP due to discomfort with the mask and dry mouth. These challenges should be screened for and mitigated with heated humidifiers, different types of masks, and auto-adjusting pressure settings, which can improve adherence.

Surgical treatments for obstructive sleep apnea are considered when conservative therapies, such as CPAP, have not been effective, or the patient cannot tolerate these treatments. Surgical options aim to address anatomic issues that contribute to airway obstruction during sleep. Hypoglossal nerve stimulation is a newer surgical option that helps keep the upper airway open by causing contraction of the tongue muscles, thus reducing obstructive events. It is important to note that surgical treatments for sleep apnea are typically considered only after a thorough evaluation and proper diagnosis by a sleep specialist.

Primary Hypersomnias: Narcolepsy and Idiopathic Hypersomnia

Central (primary) disorders of hypersomnolence present with daytime sleepiness despite sufficient nocturnal sleep. Before diagnosing a central disorder of hypersomnolence, medical and medication-related causes should be ruled out and a detailed sleep history should be obtained; adolescents and young adults in particular frequently suffer from sleep deprivation. Asking patients to keep a sleep diary can aid in understanding sleep patterns and quantity.

Narcolepsy and idiopathic hypersomnia typically present in adolescence or young adulthood. Patients report inability to stay awake during the day and frequent drowsiness resulting in falling a sleep throughout the day, which causes poor school/work performance.

Narcolepsy is divided into narcolepsy type 1 (previously known as narcolepsy with cataplexy) and narcolepsy type 2 (previously known as narcolepsy without cataplexy).[3] Narcolepsy is associated with two cardinal sleep-related symptoms: hypnogogic hallucinations and sleep paralysis. Hypnagogic hallucinations are vivid, often frightening visual hallucinations that occur when falling asleep. Most patients report seeing large obscure shadows or distorted images of people looking down on them; rarely, a tactile or auditory component may be present. These hallucinations are thought to represent intrusion of REM sleep into wakefulness. Sleep paralysis is a temporary inability to move when either falling asleep or waking up that lasts seconds to minutes but may feel subjectively longer, given that it can be frightening and may be accompanied by hallucinations. Sleep paralysis is thought to be related to the persistence of REM atonia into wakefulness.

Both sleep paralysis and hypnagogic hallucinations are common in patients with narcolepsy type 1 but are not specific for the diagnosis since they can occur in the general population, albeit far less frequently; people with narcolepsy have these symptoms weekly or monthly, whereas episodes in the general population occur yearly or less frequently. These symptoms can be seen occasionally in patients with narcolepsy type 2 and rarely in patients with idiopathic hypersomnia.

Some patients with narcolepsy (particularly narcolepsy type 1) may have difficulty waking up, but this is usually only in patients with profoundly disturbed sleep. Idiopathic hypersomnia, by contrast, is associated with an extreme and debilitating difficulty waking up in the morning (called sleep inertia). In sum, patients with narcolepsy cannot stay awake, while patients with idiopathic hypersomnia cannot wake up. Some patients with idiopathic hypersomnia have such a profound degree of sleep inertia that they may need to take a wake-promoting drug 1 to 2 hours before their desired wake-up time (see below).

Patients with narcolepsy often require 1 to 2 hours of daytime naps throughout the day, after which they typically feel refreshed. Such patients may require work accommodations to allow for napping. In contrast, patients with idiopathic hypersomnia typically do not feel restored after a daytime nap, finding it just as difficult as waking up in the morning.

Cataplexy is a sudden, temporary loss of muscle tone triggered by strong emotions, typically positive emotions such as laughter, joking, or excitement, but rarely in response to negative emotions such as intense anger or frustration. The loss of muscle tone can lead to falls if generalized, or may be more focal, leading to grimacing, tongue protrusion, slurred speech, or speech arrest, but will not impact respiration. Episodes of cataplexy generally last minutes and do not impair consciousness. The presence of cataplexy defines narcolepsy type 1 (previously known as narcolepsy with cataplexy), and its absence defines narcolepsy type 2 (previously known as narcolepsy without cataplexy).

Diagnosis of Central Disorders of Hypersomnolence

The diagnosis of central disorders of hypersomnolence is made with a nighttime sleep study (polysomnogram) followed by a daytime sleep study (multiple sleep latency test). Potentially confounding medications (eg, sedatives, stimulants) should ideally be stopped 2 weeks before the sleep study. The purpose of the polysomnogram is to exclude alternative and comorbid causes of daytime sleepiness, such as sleep apnea or periodic limb movement disorder (PLMD). The purpose of the multiple sleep latency test is to determine the patient's tendency to fall asleep and to enter REM sleep after an adequate nocturnal sleep period of at least 6 hours. Patients are allowed four to five nap opportunities, and mean sleep latency and the number of naps with REM (sleep onset rapid eye movement periods [SOREMPs]) are recorded. The diagnosis of narcolepsy is confirmed when the multiple sleep latency test demonstrates an average sleep latency of ≤8 minutes and/or at least two SOREMPs. If sleep studies are not available, narcolepsy type 1 may be diagnosed by a low cerebrospinal fluid hypocretin (orexin) level (≤110 pg/mL or one-third the normal level).

Idiopathic hypersomnia is a diagnosis of exclusion if the patient does not meet the criteria for narcolepsy according to the multiple sleep latency test and lacks cataplexy.

Treatment of Central Disorders of Hypersomnolence

Treatment of central disorders of hypersomnolence aims to reduce daytime drowsiness through the use of wakefulness-promoting agents.[4] For patients exhibiting mild-to-moderate daytime sleepiness, modafinil is generally the first-line treatment. Armodafinil, a more potent, long-acting enantiomer of racemic modafinil, is also available. Both modafinil and armodafinil can cause headaches, nausea, insomnia, and nervousness, although these side effects may lessen over time. Nervousness and insomnia may also be lessened by administering the medication earlier in the day. Modafinil and armodafinil induce cytochrome P450 (CYP450) enzymes, which may reduce systemic levels of drugs metabolized via CYP3A4/5, including oral contraceptives; thus, alternative measures of contraception should be suggested while the patient is taking modafinil (and for at least 1 month following discontinuation).

Alternatives to modafinil and armodafinil include pitolisant and solriamfetol. Pitolisant is a histamine-3 (H3) receptor antagonist/inverse agonist with an adverse effect profile that is similar to modafinil/armodafinil. However, it has been reported to cause a dose-dependent prolongation of the QT interval. Therefore, it is recommended to monitor the QT interval in patients with renal or hepatic impairment and to avoid the use of pitolisant with drugs that can also increase the QT interval. Similar to modafinil and armodafinil, pitolisant can reduce the efficacy of hormonal contraception via CYP3A4 induction. Solriamfetol is a selective inhibitor of dopamine and norepinephrine reuptake. Its side effects are similar to other wakefulness-promoting agents, but small, dose-dependent increases in mean blood pressure, heart rate, and body weight have been observed; therefore, close monitoring is advised.

For patients with narcolepsy experiencing severe and disabling sleepiness, treatment with sodium oxybate may be considered. Sodium oxybate binds GABA$_B$ receptors and can also stimulate dopamine release. The most frequently reported adverse reactions of sodium oxybate include dizziness, sedation, nausea, and difficulty concentrating. Sleepwalking or sleep-driving have also been reported. Since it is a central nervous system depressant, sodium oxybate can lead to increased sedation and respiratory depression when combined with alcohol or other central nervous system depressants.

Stimulants such as methylphenidate and amphetamines are considered second-line wakefulness-promoting agents due to their potential to cause more sympathomimetic side effects than other agents. Therefore, these are generally only considered when patients are unable to tolerate modafinil and armodafinil, or if those drugs are contraindicated due to interactions with other medications.

If cataplexy occurs frequently and is disabling, selective-serotonin reuptake inhibitors (eg, fluoxetine), serotonin-norepinephrine reuptake inhibitors (eg, venlafaxine), or tricyclic antidepressants (eg, protriptyline) can be used. Sodium oxybate or pitolisant may be considered in refractory cases.

In addition to pharmacologic therapy, patients with hypersomnia disorders should be encouraged to maintain regular sleep patterns, take naps, and practice good sleep hygiene (eg, not eating large meals, drinking alcohol, or using back-lit devices in proximity to bedtime). Patients with these conditions should also be counseled on safe driving practices due to an increased risk of motor vehicle accidents as a result of excessive sleepiness. First, it is essential to emphasize the potential risks associated with untreated hypersomnia and the increased likelihood of accidents. Patients should be advised to avoid driving if they experience excessive daytime sleepiness and encouraged to take short naps before driving if necessary and avoid driving during their peak sleepiness hours. It is critical to empower the patient to recognize their own warning signs of drowsiness while driving and take immediate action, such as pulling over to a safe location and resting if they feel fatigued.

INSOMNIA

Insomnia can be due to difficulty falling asleep (sleep initiation insomnia) or difficulty staying asleep (sleep maintenance insomnia). Insomnia results in daytime somnolence, abnormal sleep onset, and impaired concentration and memory. Causes of insomnia include medical conditions (eg, cardiac conditions causing orthopnea or paroxysmal nocturnal dyspnea), pain, stress, psychiatric conditions (eg, depression, anxiety), medications (eg, stimulants, opiates, certain antidepressants; see Table 29.2), and primary sleep disorders (eg, sleep apnea, RLS). Therefore medical, psychiatric, and sleep conditions should be screened for, the patient's medication list should be carefully reviewed,

TABLE 29.2	Some Medications That Can Cause Insomnia
Medication category	**Examples**
CNS stimulants and wakefulness-promoting agents	Methylphenidate, modafinil
Antidepressants	• Serotonergic (fluoxetine, escitalopram, paroxetine, sertraline venlafaxine, duloxetine, reboxetine) • Activating tricyclic antidepressants (imipramine, desipramine, protriptyline), • Bupropion
Dopaminergic medications	Carbidopa-levodopa and pramipexole
Opioids	Oxycodone, hydrocodone, codeine, morphine, fentanyl, methadone
Cold medicines and decongestants	Phenylephrine, pseudoephedrine
Anticonvulsants	Felbamate, lamotrigine, zonisamide
Bronchodilators and asthma medications	Albuterol, ipratropium, levalbuterol, theophylline
Corticosteroids	Prednisone, methylprednisolone
β-Blockers	Acebutolol, atenolol, bisoprolol, metoprolol, nadolol, propranolol
Angiotensin-converting enzyme inhibitors	Captopril, enalapril, lisinopril

CNS, central nervous system.

and patients should be assessed for stressful events or ongoing stressors.

Diagnosis of Insomnia

A sleep diary kept by the patient can aid in determining the nature of the patient's insomnia. The patient should record time spent in bed, number of nighttime awakenings, quality of sleep, sleep onset latency, and total sleep time over a period of 2 to 4 weeks. Insomnia is classified as short term (less than 3 months) or chronic (greater than 3 months).[3] Short-term insomnia is usually due to specific life events (eg, bereavement, employment difficulties, relationship difficulties) and is generally treated with reassurance, discussion of sleep hygiene, and, if needed, a brief course of hypnotic medications.

Treatment of Insomnia

Chronic insomnia is generally treated with a combination of cognitive behavioral therapy to improve the relationship between the patient and their sleep, education on sleep hygiene (Table 29.3), herbal/nutraceutical remedies, and medications.[5] Herbal/nutraceutical remedies include valerian root, kava-kava, chamomile, lavender, and melatonin, but evidence is limited, and these agents are unregulated, leading to lack of standardization of formulation and dose, as well as unknown interactions with other medications.

TABLE 29.3	General Sleep Hygiene Guidelines

Do not go to bed unless you are sleepy and get out of bed if you are unable to sleep.

Go to sleep and wake up at the same time every day.

Minimize nonsleep activities in bed (eg, watching TV, looking at phone).

Do not nap during the daytime.

Limit heavy meals within the 2-3 hours before sleep.

Get exercise during the day to help you get to sleep faster and sleep longer but do not exercise right before bedtime.

Keep the room temperature cool and dark, and do not watch the alarm clock during the night (keep the clock out of clear view).

Develop a relaxing bedtime routine. Consider taking a warm bath before bedtime.

Pharmaceutical agents that may be considered in patients who do not respond to conservative measures include hypnotics (classified as nonbenzodiazepine [zolpidem, eszopiclone, zaleplon] and benzodiazepine), ramelteon (a melatonin receptor agonist), doxepin (a tricyclic antidepressant with antihistamine properties), and the orexin antagonists (lemborexant, suvorexant, daridorexant; Table 29.4). In general, benzodiazepines should be avoided due to the risk of dependence and effects on cognition in older adults. Nonbenzodiazepine hypnotics may be used in patients with difficulty falling asleep, though shorter acting agents such as zolpidem may wear off, leading to awakening during the nighttime; in such cases, extended-release zolpidem or one of the other nonbenzodiazepine hypnotics can be considered. Nonbenzodiazepine hypnotics are generally avoided in older patients, patients with cognitive disorders, and patients at risk for respiratory depression; in such patients, ramelteon is often used. For patients with difficulty staying asleep, doxepin or long-acting nonbenzodiazepine hypnotics can be

considered as well as orexin antagonists, though these latter agents remain costly. In patients with comorbid depression, antidepressants with sedating properties that may improve insomnia include trazodone, mirtazapine, and amitriptyline. In patients with comorbid anxiety, benzodiazepines may be considered.

PARASOMNIAS

Parasomnias are a group of sleep disorders characterized by abnormal behaviors, movements, emotions, and perceptions that occur during sleep and/or sleep-wake transitions. These phenomena can range from mild to disruptive and may cause distress or impairment to the individual experiencing them. Common examples of parasomnias include sleepwalking, night terrors, sleep-related eating disorder, and REM sleep behavior disorder. Parasomnias often result from a complex interplay of environmental and neurobiologic factors. Proper diagnosis and management are essential to alleviate the impact of parasomnias on an

TABLE 29.4 Medications for Insomnia				
Hypnotic	**Mechanism of action**	**Clinical use**	**Common side effects**	**Half-life (hours)**
Zolpidem	Benzodiazepine receptor agonist	Sleep onset or sleep maintenance insomnia	Sleepwalking, morning drowsiness	Max 4.5
Zolpidem ER	Benzodiazepine receptor agonist	Sleep onset or sleep maintenance insomnia	Sleepwalking, morning drowsiness, fogginess	4
Fast-acting sublingual zolpidem tartrate	Benzodiazepine receptor agonist	Sleep maintenance insomnia	Sleepwalking, morning drowsiness	1-4
Eszopiclone	Benzodiazepine receptor agonist	Sleep onset or sleep maintenance insomnia	Unpleasant "metallic" taste, dry mouth, headache, morning drowsiness	6
Zaleplon	Benzodiazepine receptor agonist	Sleep maintenance insomnia	Drowsiness	1
Doxepin	Histamine H1 receptor antagonist	Sleep maintenance insomnia	Nausea, dizziness	15-30
Ramelteon	Melatonin receptor agonist	Sleep onset insomnia	Fatigue, joint pain	1-5
Lemborexant	Orexin receptor antagonist	Sleep onset or sleep maintenance insomnia	Drowsiness, unusual dreams	17-19
Suvorexant	Orexin receptor antagonist	Sleep onset or sleep maintenance insomnia	Drowsiness, unusual dreams	12
Daridorexant	Orexin receptor antagonist	Sleep onset or sleep maintenance insomnia	Drowsiness, fogginess	8

individual's sleep quality and overall well-being, and mostly to ensure the safety of the patient and those around them during these episodes. This section focuses on the diagnosis and treatment of REM sleep behavior disorder.

Rapid Eye Movement Sleep Behavior Disorder

During normal REM sleep, muscle atonia leads to lack of movement during dreams. In REM sleep behavior disorder, patients lose normal atonia and enact their dreams, leading to violent movements (eg, kicking, punching) during sleep that may injure the patient or bed partner. The patient typically recalls unpleasant dream content (eg, being chased, fighting). REM sleep behavior disorder can be idiopathic or caused by medications, most commonly serotonergic antidepressants and, less commonly, β-blockers, central cholinesterase inhibitors, and monoamine oxidase inhibitors, such as selegiline.

Idiopathic REM sleep behavior disorder is part of the prodrome of α-synuclein–associated neurodegenerative conditions such as Parkinson disease, dementia with Lewy bodies, and multiple system atrophy and carries a high risk of conversion to one of these conditions over time.

Diagnosis of Rapid Eye Movement Sleep Behavior Disorder

REM sleep behavior disorder can generally be diagnosed by history, but, if polysomnography is performed (eg, to assess for sleep apnea), it will demonstrate persistence of muscle tone (ie, lack of atonia) during REM sleep. The main clinical features of REM sleep behavior disorder are presented in Table 29.5. REM sleep behavior disorder should be distinguished from periodic limb movements of sleep, in which patients kick in their sleep due to involuntary flexion of the knee and hip with dorsiflexion of the ankle and toe. Unlike REM sleep behavior disorder, periodic limb movements of sleep occur mostly during NREM sleep, are periodic (approximately every 5-90 seconds), and are unrelated to dreaming.

Other disorders to differentiate from REM sleep behavior disorder include NREM parasomnias

TABLE 29.5 History in Patients With REM Sleep Behavior Disorder

Clinical question	Features suggestive of REM sleep behavior disorder
When do the events occur, during the first or the second part of the night?	Events occur mostly after midnight, when periods of REM sleep are more frequent.
How often are these episodes?	Episodes may present weekly or more rarely, at times they may occur every night. Within one night, they may present once or twice. Episodes reported more than 10× per night should raise the suspicion of epilepsy.
Do you recall the dream associated with these abrupt movements?	Patients with REM sleep behavior disorder recall fragments of the dream associated with the events.
Do you recall having abrupt movements?	Patients with REM sleep behavior disorder are most likely not aware of their abnormal behavior. They may present as totally oblivious to the events and have no memory of the movements.
What is the content of the dream?	Patients may recall some fragments of dream contents. Dreams are related to fighting, fear, and other negative and violent content.
Do you injure yourself or your bed partner?	Patients with REM sleep behavior disorder usually injure themselves or their bedpartner (kicking and punching are the most common actions).
Are the episodes brief (less than a minute or so)?	Episodes are usually brief (often less than a minute).
Are you alert and oriented afterward?	Patients are fully alert and oriented after the episodes.

REM, rapid eye movement.

(confusional arousals, sleepwalking, sleep terrors), nightmares, and sleep-related frontal lobe epilepsy. NREM parasomnias typically begin in childhood, whereas REM sleep behavior disorder generally begins in adulthood. NREM parasomnias consist of prolonged, complex, nonviolent behaviors of which patients have no recollection, and from which they are difficult to awaken. They, therefore, contrast with REM sleep behavior disorder in which behaviors are violent and patients generally recall violent dreams, though often do not report panic or anxiety as is the case in nightmares.

Sleep-related hypermotor epilepsy (previously called nocturnal frontal lobe epilepsy) is a familial or sporadic condition that results in seizures, causing complex motor behaviors during sleep such as thrashing, kicking, and articulate vocalizations. Patients typically develop events in childhood or adolescence and are fully unaware during the events and unaware that the events have occurred.

Treatment of Rapid Eye Movement Sleep Behavior Disorder

Patients with REM sleep behavior disorder should be advised to sleep with the mattress on the floor and pad any surfaces near the bed to avoid injury. Bed partners may need to sleep separately to avoid partner injury. Medications that can cause or worsen REM sleep behavior disorder should be discontinued if possible, and patients should avoid potential withdrawal from alcohol, benzodiazepines, or barbiturates.

Medications used to treat REM sleep behavior disorder include melatonin or clonazepam at bedtime. Melatonin is safer and better tolerated but should be used with caution in patients with hepatic impairment, and levels can be impacted by CYP1A inhibitors (eg, fluoroquinolones, estrogen-based hormonal therapies) and inducers (first-generation antiseizure medications, rifampin).[6]

SLEEP-RELATED MOVEMENT DISORDERS

Sleep-related movement disorders are a group of sleep disorders characterized by abnormal movements at bedtime and/or during sleep. These movements can disrupt sleep or sleep onset and may lead to excessive daytime sleepiness and impaired overall sleep quality. The most common sleep-related movement disorders include periodic limb movement disorder (PLMD) and restless leg syndrome (RLS). PLMD involves repetitive and involuntary leg movements during sleep. These movements can be brief, jerky, and occur in a rhythmic pattern, often leading to brief arousals from sleep. While patients with PLMD may not be consciously aware of these movements, the movements can significantly disrupt their sleep and result in daytime sleepiness. This section focuses on the diagnosis and treatment of RLS.

Restless Legs Syndrome

In RLS, patients report an uncomfortable feeling in the legs (eg, "creepy-crawly" sensation) that typically occurs during periods of inactivity, worsens when the patient is trying to fall asleep, and improves when the patient walks or stretches the legs.

Diagnosis of Restless Legs Syndrome

The diagnosis of RLS is purely clinical, and it must be distinguished from nocturnal cramping and PLMD (see earlier). In RLS, there are no involuntary movements of the limbs as in PLMD, though the two conditions frequently co-occur.

RLS can be idiopathic or can occur secondary to medical conditions (eg, iron deficiency, chronic kidney disease), neurologic conditions (eg, polyneuropathy, spinal cord disease), pregnancy, and medications (eg, antidepressants, antipsychotics, antiemetics, antihypertensives, and antiseizure medications; Table 29.6). Therefore, patients should undergo a detailed medical history, medication review, and neurologic examination to assess for any underlying provoking factors. Laboratory evaluation should include ferritin, complete blood cell count, and renal function. If serum ferritin is less than 75 ng/mL, a trial of oral iron therapy should be initiated before considering symptomatic treatment. Response to oral iron is not immediate, and relief of restless legs symptoms may require several months of treatment. In patients with malabsorption or intolerance of oral iron preparations, intravenous (IV) iron may be considered.

TABLE 29.6	Medications That Can Exacerbate Restless Legs Syndrome	
Medications category	**Examples**
Antidepressants	Selective-serotonin reuptake inhibitors (SSRIs), tricyclic antidepressants (TCAs), monoamine oxidase inhibitors (MAOIs)
Antipsychotics	Clozapine, olanzapine, quetiapine
Antiemetics	Metoclopramide, chlorpromazine
Antihypertensives	β-Blockers, α-2 agonists, calcium channel blockers
Anticonvulsants	Phenytoin, zonisamide

Treatment of Restless Legs Syndrome

In patients with RLS who are not iron deficient, treatment involves avoiding alcohol and stimulants (eg, caffeine, nicotine); maintaining regular sleep patterns; participating in regular physical activity, a warm bath, and leg stretching before bed; and reducing stress. For patients with infrequent symptoms who do not require daily treatment, immediate-release carbidopa-levodopa can be used on an as-needed basis. In patients with symptoms two or more nights per week who do not respond to the nonpharmacologic interventions listed earlier, medications may be considered (Table 29.7).

First-line treatment is with pregabalin or gabapentin. If these agents are not tolerated due to their sedating effects, a dopamine agonist (eg, pramipexole, ropinirole, or rotigotine patch) may be considered, though these agents carry a risk of impulse control disorders (such as pathologic gambling) and a progressive worsening of restless legs symptoms called augmentation (see later) and should be avoided when possible. In patients refractory to or intolerant of gabapentinoid or dopamine agonist treatment, low-dose opioids such as oxycodone or methadone may be considered, though these medications carry the risk of addiction.

Augmentation refers to a worsening of restless legs symptoms with prolonged use of dopamine agonists. Patients may report earlier onset of symptoms, increased intensity of symptoms, and spread to the upper extremities. In such patients, dopamine agonists should be tapered to the lowest effective dose or switched to a gabapentinoid medication.

CIRCADIAN RHYTHM DISORDERS

Circadian rhythm disorders are a group of sleep disorders that occur due to disruptions or abnormalities in an individual's internal body clock, known as the circadian rhythm. The circadian rhythm is a natural, approximately 24-hour cycle that regulates various physiologic processes, including sleep-wake patterns, alertness levels, hormone release, and body temperature. When there is a significant misalignment between the internal rhythm and the required timing of a patient's school and/or work, circadian rhythm disorders can have a significant impact on an individual's overall daily functioning. The most common circadian rhythm disorders include:

- **Delayed sleep phase disorder (DSPD)**: Individuals with DSPD develop a delayed sleep phase, leading to difficulty falling asleep at a typical bedtime and waking up at a desired morning time. As a result, they often experience excessive daytime sleepiness and have difficulty meeting morning obligations. DSPD is most common among adolescents and young adults.
- **Advanced sleep phase disorder (ASPD)**: In contrast to DSPD, individuals with ASPD have an advanced sleep phase, meaning they tend to fall asleep much earlier than usual and wake up early in the morning, feeling fully alert during the early hours but tired later in the day. In contrast to DSPD, advanced age appears to be the most important risk factor.
- **Shift work sleep disorder (SWSD)**: SWSD affects individuals who work nontraditional hours, such as night shifts or rotating shifts. The constant change in work schedules can disrupt the body's natural circadian rhythm, leading to difficulty sleeping during designated rest periods.

TABLE 29.7	Treatment of Restless Legs Syndrome	
Medication	**Most common side effects**	**Special considerations**
Gabapentin	Dizziness, drowsiness, nausea	It can be scheduled in divided doses in proximity to bedtime
Pregabalin	Dizziness, drowsiness, nausea	
Pramipexole	Dry mouth, headache, nausea, dizziness, impulse control disorders, risk of augmentation	
Ropinirole	Nausea, dizziness, drowsiness, headache, impulse control disorders	
Rotigotine	Skin irritation, nausea, headache, dizziness, impulse control disorders	Metabolized by the liver, to be used with caution in patients with liver disease

Diagnosis of Circadian Rhythm Disorders

Diagnosing circadian rhythm disorders involves a comprehensive evaluation of a patient's sleep-wake patterns, daily routines, and lifestyle habits. A patient's chronotype, which determines their natural preference for being a "morning person" or a "night owl," can play a significant role in understanding circadian rhythm variations. Objective assessments, such as actigraphy or sleep diaries, need to be used to monitor sleep patterns and determine the diagnosis.[3] Once a diagnosis is established, individualized management strategies can be implemented to help realign the circadian rhythm.

Treatment of Circadian Rhythm Disorders

Management of circadian rhythm disorders typically involves a combination of behavioral and lifestyle modifications along with the use of light therapy and/or medications when necessary. Establishing a consistent sleep schedule with regular bedtime and wake-up times is a fundamental step in entraining the circadian rhythm. For example, in individuals with DSPD, exposure to bright natural light during the morning and avoiding bright light exposure in the evening can help advance the sleep phase. For certain cases, timed evening melatonin supplementation may be recommended to facilitate circadian rhythm alignment. For individuals with more severe circadian rhythm disruptions, such as shift workers, other pharmacologic interventions may be necessary. To mitigate the effects of irregular work hours on their circadian rhythm, shift workers can benefit from strategic shift scheduling and taking short naps during breaks. In cases where circadian rhythm disorders significantly impact functioning, strategically timed waking-promoting agents may be used.

SUMMARY

Sleep is a vital biological function that impacts every aspect of our lives, from physical health to emotional well-being. Sleep disorders are common. It is important to recognize the common symptoms and signs of sleep disorders in order to effectively counsel patients on sleep hygiene, provide appropriate diagnosis and treatment, and refer patients for a sleep study or evaluation by a sleep specialist when necessary.

EDITORS' KEY POINTS

- Sleep disorders have a significant impact on an individual's quality of life.
- Sleep disorders can be classified as those causing excess sleepiness (hypersomnias, such as sleep apnea and narcolepsy), inability to sleep (insomnia), sleep-related events (parasomnias such as REM sleep behavior disorder and sleep-related movement disorders such as RLS), and disruptions to the sleep-wake cycle (circadian rhythm disorders).
- The sleep cycle is made up of three NREM stages (stage 1 through stage 3, from lightest to deepest) and one REM stage. During REM sleep, dreaming occurs and muscle tone is normally absent (referred to as REM atonia) to prevent acting out of dreams.
- The circadian cycle is a 24-hour rhythm that is influenced by environmental cues, particularly light exposure, and regulates physiologic processes, including sleep-wake patterns, hormone release, body temperature, and metabolism.
- Sleep apnea is a common cause of hypersomnia. It is diagnosed by polysomnography, and treatment options include lifestyle changes, CPAP, oral appliances, and surgery.
- Narcolepsy is a central disorder of hypersomnolence categorized as narcolepsy type 1 (previously known as narcolepsy with cataplexy [the sudden, temporary loss of muscle tone triggered by strong emotions]) and narcolepsy type 2 (previously known as narcolepsy without cataplexy). Narcolepsy is associated with hypnogogic hallucinations and sleep paralysis. Treatment includes wakefulness-promoting agents, agents for cataplexy if needed, and encouraging good sleep hygiene.
- Insomnia may be due to difficulty falling asleep (sleep initiation) or difficulty staying asleep (sleep maintenance) and can be caused by a variety of medical and psychiatric conditions, medications, and primary sleep disorders. Chronic insomnia is treated with a combination of cognitive behavioral therapy, patient education, herbal/nutraceutical remedies, and medications.

▶ REM sleep behavior disorder is a parasomnia characterized by the lack of normal muscle atonia during REM sleep, leading to dream-enactment behavior that may injure the patient or bed partner. REM sleep behavior disorder is associated with an increased risk of later development of neurodegenerative diseases associated with α-synuclein accumulation, such as Parkinson disease. Treatment of REM sleep behavior disorder includes melatonin or clonazepam.

▶ Patients with RLS describe an uncomfortable feeling in the legs when trying to fall asleep that improves with walking. This condition may be idiopathic, due to underlying neuropathy, or caused by iron deficiency. Therefore, patients with RLS should be evaluated with serum iron studies. Treatment includes oral iron in iron-deficient patients, avoidance of alcohol or stimulants, and treatment with gabapentin, pregabalin, or dopamine agonists (although dopamine agonists carry a risk of impulse control disorders and augmentation and have largely fallen out of favor unless patients do not respond to safer/better tolerated agents).

▶ Circadian rhythm disorders (such as DSPD, ASPD, and SWSD) occur due to disruptions in an individual's approximately 24-hour internal body clock and are managed with a combination of behavioral and lifestyle modifications along with the use of light therapy and medications when necessary.

REFERENCES

1. Schneider L. Neurobiology and neuroprotective benefits of sleep. *Continuum (Minneap Minn)*. 2020;26(4):848-870. doi:10.1212/CON.0000000000000878

2. Kapur VK, Auckley DH, Chowdhuri S, et al. Clinical practice guideline for diagnostic testing for adult obstructive sleep apnea: an American Academy of Sleep Medicine clinical practice guideline. *J Clin Sleep Med*. 2017;13(3):479-504. doi:10.5664/jcsm.6506

3. American Academy of Sleep Medicine, ed. *International Classification of Sleep Disorders*. 3rd ed. American Academy of Sleep Medicine; 2014.

4. Maski K, Trotti LM, Kotagal S, et al. Treatment of central disorders of hypersomnolence: an American Academy of Sleep Medicine clinical practice guideline. *J Clin Sleep Med*. 2021;17(9):1881-1893. doi:10.5664/jcsm.9328

5. Edinger JD, Arnedt JT, Bertisch SM, et al. Behavioral and psychological treatments for chronic insomnia disorder in adults: an American Academy of Sleep Medicine clinical practice guideline. *J Clin Sleep Med*. 2021;17(2):255-262. doi:10.5664/jcsm.8986

6. Howell M, Avidan AY, Foldvary-Schaefer N, et al. Management of REM sleep behavior disorder: an American Academy of Sleep Medicine clinical practice guideline. *J Clin Sleep Med*. 2023;19(4):759-768. doi:10.5664/jcsm.10424

Head Trauma

Erika J. Sigman and Catherine S. W. Albin

INTRODUCTION

Traumatic brain injury (TBI) occurs when an external force on the head results in temporary or permanent brain dysfunction. Mechanisms of TBI include collision of the head with an object, penetrating injury to the brain, acceleration/deceleration impacts, and exposure to blast forces.

TBI can result in a variety of cranial injuries, including:

- Skull fracture
- Intracranial hemorrhage: epidural hematoma (EDH), subdural hematoma (SDH), intraparenchymal hematoma, and traumatic subarachnoid hemorrhage
- Cerebral contusion
- Diffuse axonal injury
- Cerebrovascular injury (eg, cervical artery dissection)

Head trauma can also cause symptoms in the absence of obvious structural injury seen on neuroimaging.

DEFINITIONS

TBI severity is classified as mild, moderate, or severe based on the Glasgow Coma Scale (GCS) at the time of evaluation after initial injury (Table 30.1). Mild TBI is defined as initial GCS 13 to 15 and may be accompanied by a brief loss of consciousness, though loss of consciousness does not always occur. Mild TBI typically results in temporary brain dysfunction (less than 24 hours), manifesting as a decreased level of alertness and/or amnesia. *Concussion* refers to the constellation of symptoms (eg, dizziness, fatigue, headache, vomiting) that may accompany mild TBI. Moderate TBI is defined as initial GCS of 9 to 12. Moderate TBI causes loss of consciousness for minutes, alteration of consciousness for greater than 24 hours, and amnesia for up to a week. Severe TBI is defined as initial GCS of 3 to 8. Severe TBI leads to prolonged alteration of consciousness for greater than 24 hours and amnesia that may last more than a week.

EPIDEMIOLOGY

The annual global incidence of TBI is estimated at 30 to 60 million cases.[1] In the United States, annual TBI-related hospitalizations are estimated at over 200 thousand and annual TBI-related deaths at about 64,000.[2] Since many patients with mild TBI and sports-related concussion may not seek medical evaluation, the true burden of TBI is likely underestimated. The annual economic costs of TBI related to acute care, long-term disability, and caregiver expenses are estimated at $400 billion globally and $40 billion in the United States.[3,4]

TABLE 30.1	The Glasgow Coma Scale (GCS)	
Eye-opening response	Eyes open spontaneously	4 pts
	Eyes open to verbal command, speech, or shouting	3 pts
	Eyes open to pain (not applied to face)	2 pts
	No eye opening	1 pt
Verbal response	Oriented	5 pts
	Confused conversation, but able to answer questions	4 pts
	Inappropriate response, words discernible	3 pts
	Incomprehensible sounds or speech	2 pts
	No verbal response	1 pt
Motor response	Obeys commands for movement	6 pts
	Localizes to painful stimulus	5 pts
	Withdraws from pain	4 pts
	Abnormal (spastic) flexion, decorticate posture	3 pts
	Extensor (rigid) response, decerebrate posture	2 pts
	No motor response	1 pt

Traumatic brain injury (TBI) severity is classified as mild, moderate, or severe based on the scoring of eye-opening response, verbal response, and motor response.

The most common causes of TBI are falls, road traffic accidents, firearm-related suicide attempts, and assaults. The highest TBI incidence is in younger and older populations, resulting from increased risk of motor vehicle collisions and falls, respectively. Sports-related TBI is increasingly reported, particularly in collision sports (eg, American football, hockey, and lacrosse). The majority of TBIs are mild.

DIAGNOSTIC EVALUATION OF PATIENTS WITH TRAUMATIC BRAIN INJURY

Patients with TBI may have extracranial trauma, which should be evaluated and stabilized. As in all emergencies, the initial focus should be on the "ABCs." Once these are addressed, clinicians may focus on assessing disability and classifying the TBI as mild, moderate, or severe based on the GCS. Patients with moderate and severe TBI should be immediately transferred to the nearest emergency department for urgent evaluation and head imaging with a computed tomography (CT) scan.

Approach to the Patient With Mild Traumatic Brain Injury/Concussion

Not all patients with mild TBI/concussion require hospital evaluation, although all patients with head injury should be evaluated by a health care provider to assess for disorientation, determine the GCS, and screen for focal neurologic deficits. Evaluation rubrics (eg, Standardized Assessment of Concussion and the Military Acute Concussion Evaluation [MACE], which has been validated in civilian populations[5]), can be used to evaluate a patient's mental status and document symptoms.

A helpful framework for deciding which patients require immediate emergency department evaluation is to refer all patients who require head CT. The Canadian Rule for head CT imaging in patients with minor head trauma[6] recommends head CT for all patients aged 60 years or above and patients of any age with a dangerous injury mechanism (eg, pedestrian struck by motor vehicle, ejection from motor vehicle, fall from >3 ft or fall of more than 5 stairs), or if the GCS has not returned to 15 after 2 hours, there is a suspected skull fracture or any sign of basal skull fracture (eg, concern for cerebrospinal fluid [CSF] leak), two or more episodes of vomiting, or amnesia for events greater than 30 minutes before the impact. The Centers for Disease Control and Prevention (CDC)[7] also recommends emergent evaluation in patients exhibiting any "Concussion Danger Signs": seizures, new focal neurologic deficits (such as weakness, anisocoria, Horner syndrome, or visual changes), vomiting, or restlessness and agitation (ie, mental status disturbances that may not be captured by the GCS). In addition, emergent evaluation and head CT should be strongly considered in any patient on antithrombotic agents, given the increased risk of intracranial hemorrhage after even minor head injury. All patients requiring head imaging should be referred to the emergency department for immediate evaluation.

Head CT may reveal one or more of the findings demonstrated in Table 30.2, the management

TABLE 30.2	Pathophysiology and Imaging Characteristic of Blunt Traumatic Brain Injuries		
	Pathophysiology	**Imaging characteristics**	**Example**
Epidural hematoma	Most often due to injury of the temporal bone and resultant laceration of the middle meningeal artery May also result from injury to the middle meningeal vein, diploic vein, or venous sinuses	A lens-shaped (convex) collection of blood Does not cross suture lines	 Noncontrast CT of the head with convex shaped hyperdensity consistent with epidural hematoma (red circle) abutting the left temporal lobe.
Subdural hematoma	Rupture of the bridging veins Often associated with brain atrophy Chronic accumulation occurs due to neovascularization and associated hemorrhage of the membranes that form within the subdural hemorrhage	Crescent shaped Crosses suture lines	 Noncontrast CT of the head with crescent shaped hyperdensity consistent with subdural hematoma (red circle) with mass effect on right frontal and temporal lobes.

TABLE 30.2   Pathophysiology and Imaging Characteristic of Blunt Traumatic Brain Injuries (*continued*)

	Pathophysiology	Imaging characteristics	Example
Contusion	Hemorrhagic necrosis due to acceleration/ deceleration injury	Brain hemorrhage in close proximity to skull May have a "coup" and "contra-coup" pattern: injury at the site of impact and contralateral to the site of impact	 Noncontrast CT of the head showing small hyperdensitiy with surrounding hypodensity consistent with left frontal contusion (red arrow).
Traumatic subarachnoid hemorrhage (SAH)	Tearing of small pial vessels	Blood is located over the cerebral convexities within the sulci and fissures.	 Noncontrast CT of the head with diffuse hyperdense material within the sulci of the left hemisphere consistent with traumatic SAH (red arrow).

(*continued*)

TABLE 30.2	Pathophysiology and Imaging Characteristic of Blunt Traumatic Brain Injuries (*continued*)		
	Pathophysiology	**Imaging characteristics**	**Example**
Diffuse axonal injury (DAI)	Shearing of axons due to rotational force	Punctate hemorrhages may be present in the white matter on CT. MRI has a much higher sensitivity and may show GRE/SWI signal within the white matter at sites of injury.	MRI of the brain, susceptibility-weighted imaging (SWI) sequence, with small areas of parasagittal susceptibility artifact (red arrows) consistent with diffuse axonal injury.
Diffuse cerebral edema	Interrelated cellular and cytotoxic mechanism, breakdown of the blood-brain barrier, and vasogenic edema	Compression and obliteration of the basal cisterns, effacement of sulci	Noncontrast CT of the head demonstrating diffuse cerebral edema with compression of basal cisterns (red circle) and effacement of sulci (red arrow).

CT, computed tomography; GRE, gradient recalled echo; MRI, magnetic resonance imaging.

of which is discussed in the next section. Even if the patient has a normal GCS, patients with evidence of intracranial hemorrhage, contusion, or diffuse edema should be transferred to a hospital with neurosurgeons available for 24 hours of observation and a repeat head CT to document the stability of the imaging findings.

Patients with mild TBI and no indication for neuroimaging (ie, returned to neurologic baseline within 2 hours) should still be closely monitored for 24 hours. For patients with a reliable family member or person able to provide 24-hour care, this observation can occur at home. Patients should be counseled to return to the hospital if any of the following are present: recurrent vomiting, seizure, decline in arousal, or development of any focal neurologic deficits. Patients who live alone or without a reliable observer may either be observed for a 24-hour hospitalization or undergo a head CT. If the head CT is normal, these patients can usually be safely discharged. There is no indication for prophylactic antiseizure medication in patients with mild TBI and a normal head CT or mild TBI and no indication for neuroimaging.

Approach to Sports-Related Concussion

Sports-related concussion should be considered in an athlete with disorientation and memory deficits after a head impact with or without loss of consciousness. All patients suspected of concussion should be evaluated by an experienced licensed health care professional. The Standardized Assessment of Concussion is a screening tool assessing orientation, cognition, and motor function that can be administered by any personnel at the time of injury.

All players suspected of concussion should be immediately removed from play and should not be permitted to return until they have been assessed by an experienced health care professional. Athletes should be restricted from returning to play until they are symptom free without the use of medications. Neurocognitive testing may be useful in determining concussion resolution.

The American Academy of Neurology's Evaluation and Management of Sports-Related Concussion Guideline[8] notes that ongoing neurologic symptoms (eg, headache, fatigue/fogginess, amnesia, disorientation) within the first 2 weeks after injury are associated with persistent neurocognitive impairment by objective testing.

Approach to the Patient With a Moderate-to-Severe Traumatic Brain Injury

Patients with moderate or severe TBI should be urgently triaged to a Level 1 Trauma Center whenever feasible. When this is not possible, patients should be triaged to the nearest emergency department for initial stabilization and then transferred to a higher level of care if needed. Initial stabilization should focus on the "ABCs." Once stabilized, disability should be assessed with the GCS, and the patient should be emergently evaluated for signs of elevated intracranial pressure (ICP): pupillary asymmetry (in size or sluggishness in response to light), bradycardia, hypertension, and irregular respiration. Patients with signs of elevated ICP

should be urgently managed by elevation of the head of the bed, hyperventilation, and/or administration of hypertonic fluids (mannitol or hypertonic saline).

Hypotension (systolic blood pressure [SBP] <90 mm Hg) and hypoxia (PaO_2 <60 mm Hg) should be prevented. Patients with severe TBI (GCS ≤8) should be intubated for airway protection and to prevent hypoxia. Cervical spine precautions must be maintained during intubation unless it has been definitively established that there is no cervical spine injury.

Head CT should be rapidly obtained in all patients with moderate and severe TBI. CT angiogram of the head and neck to evaluate for cervical artery dissection should be considered in patients with a GCS <6, evidence of basilar skull fractures, whiplash injury, and/or cervical spine injury.

Findings on head CT guide subsequent management. Surgical intervention in patients with SDH or EDH is based on imaging characteristics and clinical features. Surgical evacuation is indicated in all patients with SDH >10 mm or midline shift >5 mm or EDH that is >30 cm³. In patients with smaller hematomas, surgery is considered in patients in coma, patients with signs of herniation (eg, asymmetric pupil size or reactivity), and patients who deteriorate clinically.[9,10]

Patients with cerebral contusions, cerebral edema, and/or diffuse axonal injury are at risk of developing elevated ICP. Per the Brain Trauma Foundation Guidelines,[11] invasive ICP monitoring is indicated in any patient with head trauma with a GCS ≤8 and an abnormal head CT or GCS ≤8 and age >40, SBP <90 mm Hg, or motor posturing. Whether ICP is being followed invasively or noninvasively (ie, with serial CT scans, pupillometry, or optic nerve sheath diameter on ultrasound), patients with moderate or severe TBI should be followed closely for evidence of elevated ICP that may require treatment with hyperosmolar therapy. Refractory elevated ICP may require sedation, paralysis, induced hypothermia and, decompressive hemicraniectomy.

Seizures occur in up to a quarter of patients after TBI, with an increased incidence in patients with moderate and severe TBI. Up to half of all seizures occur within the first 24 hours after TBI.[12] Risk factors include intracranial hemorrhage, injury severity, and alcohol use.[12] Generalized tonic-clonic seizures are the most frequent seizure type after TBI, but focal seizures become increasingly common after 24 hours. Seizures at the moment of head trauma are sometimes referred to as "convulsive concussions," and it is unclear whether these are true epileptic seizures; when associated with mild TBI or concussion, these are unlikely to lead to future seizures or development of epilepsy.[13]

Given the incidence of seizures after TBI, continuous video electroencephalogram (EEG) monitoring should be considered in patients with moderate or severe TBI if there are fluctuations in mental status, neurologic deficits not explained by imaging, or sedation or paralysis that confound the neurologic examination.

In patients with head trauma who have not had seizures, 7 days of prophylactic antiseizure medication should be considered in patients with moderate or severe TBI, intracranial pathology on CT (eg, hemorrhage), depressed skull fractures, or penetrating head injury. Although the initial studies establishing this practice used phenytoin, levetiracetam is generally the preferred antiseizure medication due to its better safety and side-effect profile.[14-16] While helpful in preventing early seizures, prophylactic antiseizure medication unfortunately has not been shown to decrease the incidence of post-traumatic epilepsy or improve mortality. For patients who develop early post-traumatic seizures within the first 7 days, antiseizure medication should be maintained at least until the initial outpatient follow-up, after which a joint decision can be made about continuing treatment based on initial injury severity, seizure burden, and patient preference.

MANAGEMENT OF LONG-TERM SEQUELAE OF TRAUMATIC BRAIN INJURY

TBI of any severity can result in long-term neurologic sequelae, including epilepsy, headache, cognitive symptoms, and post-concussion syndrome. In addition, traumatic SDH may reaccumulate after evacuation, so patients with traumatic SDH who develop new or worsening neurologic deficits should be evaluated with repeat head CT. In patients with recurrent SDH, embolization of the middle meningeal artery may be considered.

Post-traumatic epilepsy is defined as one or more seizures occurring more than 1 week after head trauma and occurs in about 10% of patients following TBI. The risk of developing post-traumatic epilepsy is increased in patients with intracranial hemorrhage, severe head injury, alcohol use, and seizure within the first 7 days after head trauma. For patients with moderate or severe TBI who have seizures beyond the first 7 days after injury, sustained use of antiseizure medication is indicated, although the ideal duration needed is not well established.

Post-traumatic cognitive deficits include changes in memory, learning, attention, language, sleep-wake cycles, and mood. In patients with mild TBI and normal head CT, if cognitive symptoms occur, they usually resolve within 3 months. In patients with moderate or severe TBI, cognitive symptoms may last longer: up to one third of patients have cognitive symptoms that last beyond 1 year.[17] Depression and anxiety may be underreported in patients with TBI and should be screened for and treated.

Patients with TBI should also be screened for sleep-wake cycle disturbances, including insomnia, excessive daytime sleepiness, early awakening, and decreased sleep efficiency.[18] Diagnosis and treatment of sleep disorders are discussed in Chapter 29.

Post-traumatic headache is defined as the onset of a headache within 7 days of trauma with no alternative diagnosis to explain the headache. Post-traumatic headache is reported in the majority of patients after TBI and may have features of migraine, tension headache, or, more rarely, trigeminal autonomic cephalalgia (eg, cluster headache). If headaches worsen or new neurologic symptoms develop, neuroimaging should be obtained to evaluate for secondary causes, such as SDH, cervical artery dissection, or intracranial hypotension due to CSF leak. Post-traumatic headache usually resolves within 3 months but may be persistent in some cases, lasting beyond 24 months. Symptomatic treatment of post-traumatic headache is determined based on the primary headache disorder that the patient's headaches most closely resemble (see Chapter 15).

Post-traumatic vertigo is common after TBI.[19] Etiologies include benign paroxysmal positional vertigo (BPPV), vestibular migraine, convergence insufficiency of the eyes or other visual disturbances, medullary infarct due to vertebral artery dissection, and injury to cochlear and/or vestibular structures. For discussion of diagnosis and treatment of these conditions, see Chapters 9 and 22. Convergence insufficiency can present with dizziness and impaired near-point convergence on bedside examination; this requires ophthalmology referral. Injury to cochlear and vestibular structures can cause hearing loss, tinnitus, aural fullness, or episodic vertigo and/or hearing loss exacerbated by Valsalva maneuvers; such symptoms require otology referral.

Post-concussion syndrome or post-TBI syndrome is a complex array of symptoms such as dizziness, headaches, and neurocognitive symptoms lasting for approximately 3 months. There does not seem to be a correlation between injury severity and development of post-TBI syndrome, but female sex, increasing age, and concussive symptoms in the acute period are risk factors. Treatment is symptomatic and should also include counseling and education regarding the limited duration of symptoms, which usually resolve within 3 months.

SUMMARY

TBI is common and causes a significant impact on individuals, their families, and society due to disability and cost of acute and chronic care. Acute management requires medical stabilization, assessing the type and extent of cranial injury with CT to determine whether urgent neurosurgical intervention is needed, and management of complications such as seizures and elevated ICP. Although most patients with mild TBI will recover completely within weeks to months, post-TBI sequelae are common after moderate and severe TBI requiring screening for and treatment of seizures, headache, cognitive symptoms, and mood disorders.

EDITORS' KEY POINTS

▶ Patients with moderate or severe TBI (defined as GCS 9 to 12 for moderate and GCS 3 to 8 for severe) should be referred to the emergency department for urgent CT scan of the head.

▶ Patients with mild TBI (GCS 13 to 15) should undergo CT of the head if they are over 60 years old, on antithrombotic agents, intoxicated, have a dangerous mechanism of injury (eg, motor vehicle collision, fall from more than 3 ft or more than 5 stairs), have two or more episodes of vomiting, have amnesia for more than 30 minutes, do not return to normal consciousness after 2 hours, have seizures or new focal deficits, or have suspected skull fracture.

▶ Patients with moderate and severe TBI should be referred to a Level 1 Trauma Center for management of TBI including monitoring for and treatment of elevated ICP and seizures as well as for potential neurosurgical intervention.

▶ Patients with moderate and severe TBI, traumatic intracranial hemorrhage, skull fracture, and penetrating head injuries should be given 7 days of antiseizure medication prophylaxis to prevent early seizures. There is no indication for longer-term antiseizure medications unless the patient develops seizures.

▶ Concussion refers to symptoms such as dizziness, fatigue, headache, and amnesia caused by mild TBI. Patients with sports-related concussion should be removed from play and evaluated by a healthcare professional. Concussion symptoms are treated symptomatically and generally resolve over months.

REFERENCES

1. GBD 2016 Traumatic Brain Injury and Spinal Cord Injury Collaborators. Global, regional, and national burden of traumatic brain injury and spinal cord injury, 1990-2016: a systematic analysis for the Global Burden of Disease study 2016. *Lancet Neurol.* 2019;18:56-87.
2. Centers for Disease Control and Prevention. *National Center for Health Statistics: Mortality data on CDC WONDER.* 2022. https://wonder.cdc.gov/mcd.html
3. Miller GF, DePadilla L, Xu L. Costs of nonfatal traumatic brain injury in the United States, 2016. *Med Care.* 2021;59:451-455.
4. Howe EI, Andelic N, Fure SCR, et al. Cost-effectiveness analysis of combined cognitive and vocational rehabilitation in patients with mild-to-moderate TBI: results from a randomized controlled trial. *BMC Health Serv Res.* 2022;22:185.
5. Stone ME Jr, Safadjou S, Farber B, et al. Utility of the military acute concussion evaluation as a screening tool for

mild traumatic brain injury in a civilian trauma population. *J Trauma Acute Care Surg.* 2015;79:147-151.

6. Steill IG, Wells GA, Vandemheen K, et al. The Canadian CT head rule for patients with minor head injury. *Lancet.* 2001;357:1391-1396.

7. Center for Disease Control and Prevention. *Concussion danger signs.* Accessed April 23, 2023. https://www.cdc.gov/heads-up/

8. Giza CC, Kutcher JS, Ashwal S, et al. Summary of evidence-based guideline update: evaluation and management of concussion in sports: report of the guideline development subcommittee of the American Academy of Neurology. *Neurology.* 2013;80:2250-2257.

9. Bullock MR, Chesnut R, Ghajar J, et al. Surgical management of acute epidural hematomas. *Neurosurgery.* 2006;58:S7-S15; discussion Si-iv.

10. Bullock MR, Chesnut R, Ghajar J, et al. Surgical management of acute subdural hematomas. *Neurosurgery.* 2006;58:S16-S24; discussion Si-iv.

11. Carney N, Totten AM, O'Reilly C, et al. Guidelines for the management of severe traumatic brain injury, fourth edition. *Neurosurgery.* 2017;80:6-15.

12. Laing J, Gabbe B, Chen Z, Perucca P, Kwan P, O'Brien TJ. Risk factors and prognosis of early posttraumatic seizures in moderate to severe traumatic brain injury. *JAMA Neurol.* 2022;79:334-341.

13. Majidi S, Makke Y, Ewida A, Sianati B, Qureshi AI, Koubeissi MZ. Prevalence and risk factors for early seizure in patients with traumatic brain injury: analysis from National Trauma Data Bank. *Neurocrit Care.* 2017;27:90-95.

14. Temkin NR, Dikmen SS, Wilensky AJ, Keihm J, Chabal S, Winn HR. A randomized, double-blind study of phenytoin for the prevention of post-traumatic seizures. *N Engl J Med.* 1990;323:497-502.

15. Lee ST, Lui TN. Early seizures after mild closed head injury. *J Neurosurg.* 1992;76:435-439.

16. Szaflarski JP, Sangha KS, Lindsell CJ, Shutter LA. Prospective, randomized, single-blinded comparative trial of intravenous levetiracetam versus phenytoin for seizure prophylaxis. *Neurocrit Care.* 2010;12:165-172.

17. Pavlovic D, Pekic S, Stojanovic M, Popovic V. Traumatic brain injury: neuropathological, neurocognitive and neurobehavioral sequelae. *Pituitary.* 2019;22:270-282.

18. Mathias JL, Alvaro PK. Prevalence of sleep disturbances, disorders, and problems following traumatic brain injury: a meta-analysis. *Sleep Med.* 2012;13:898-905.

19. Fife TD, Giza C. Posttraumatic vertigo and dizziness. *Semin Neurol.* 2013;33:238-243.

INDEX

Note: Page numbers followed by *f* indicate figures; those followed by *t* indicate tabular material